PHARMACY CLERKSHIP MANUAL

A Survival Manual for Students

RUTH E. NEMIRE, PHARMD
Director of Clinical Education
Assistant Professor of Pharmacy Practice
Nova Southeastern University College of Pharmacy
Fort Lauderdale, Florida

KAREN L. KIER, PHD, MSC, RPH
Professor of Clinical Pharmacy
Director of Drug Information
Director, Nontraditional Doctor of Pharmacy
Ohio Northern University College of Pharmacy
Ada, Ohio

D1452292

McGraw-Hill
Medical Publishing Division

New York   Chicago   San Francisco   Lisbon   London   Madrid
Mexico City   Milan   New Delhi   San Juan   Seoul
Singapore   Sydney   Toronto

McGraw-Hill

A Division of The McGraw-Hill Companies

Pharmacy Clerkship Manual: A Survival Manual for Students

1 2 3 4 5 6 7 8 9 0   DOC/DOC   0 9 8 7 6 5 4 3 2

ISBN 0-07-136195-2

This book was set in Times Roman by Matrix Publishing Services.
The editors were Steve Zollo, Julie Scardiglia, Kitty McCullough, and Barbara Holton.
The production supervisor was Lisa Mendez
The cover designer was Mary McKeon
The index was prepared by Katherine Pitcoff

R. R. Donnelly and Sons was printer and binder.

This book is printed on acid-free paper.

Library of Congress Cataloging-in-Publication Data is on file for this title at the Library of Congress.

DEDICATION

This book is dedicated to the life and spirit of Dr. Bruce Parks. I hope that you are soaring with the eagles, playing ball with St. Peter, and finding out to whom the ring really belongs! We loved you in life. Your memory lives with all who know your kind and gentle spirit.

CONTRIBUTORS

Dean L. Arneson, PharmD, PhD
Assistant Dean for Student Academic
  Affairs
Associate Professor of Pharmacy
  Administration
Nova Southeastern University College
  of Pharmacy
Fort Lauderdale, Florida

Michelle Assa, PhD
Assistant Professor of Pharmacy
  Administration
Nova Southeastern University College
  of Pharmacy
Fort Lauderdale, Florida

Jacci Bainbridge, PharmD
Assistant Professor
School of Pharmacy and
Department of Neurology
University of Colorado Health Sciences
  Center
Denver, Colorado

Cristina E. Bello, PharmD
Assistant Professor of Pharmacy
  Practice
Nova Southeastern University College
  of Pharmacy
Fort Lauderdale, Florida

Karen Daniel, PharmD
Assistant Professor of Pharmacy Practice
Nova Southeastern University College
  of Pharmacy
Fort Lauderdale, Florida

Sandra B. Earle, PharmD, BCPS
Assistant Professor of Pharmacy Practice
Oregon State University
Oregon Health Sciences University
Portland, Oregon

A. Timothy Eley, PhD
Assistant Professor of Pharmaceutical
  Sciences
Nova Southeastern University College
  of Pharmacy
Fort Lauderdale, Florida

**Elizabeth Frenzel-Shepherd,
BS Pharm, MBA**
Assistant Professor of Pharmacy
  Practice
Director Experiential Education
Nova Southeastern University College
  of Pharmacy
Fort Lauderdale, Florida

Stephenie D. Garrett, PharmD
Assistant Professor
Department of Pharmacy Practice
Nova Southeastern University College
  of Pharmacy
Fort Lauderdale, Florida

Tracy S. Hunter, RPh, PhD
Assistant Dean and Chair
Department of Pharmacy Administration
Nova Southeastern University College
  of Pharmacy
Fort Lauderdale, Florida

Janina Z.P. Janes, PharmD, MBA
Neurology Specialty Resident
Clinical Instructor
University of Colorado Health Sciences
  Center
Denver, Colorado

Karen L. Kier, PhD, MSc, RPh
Professor of Clinical Pharmacy
Director of Drug Information
Director, Nontraditional Doctor of
  Pharmacy
Ohio Northern University College of
  Pharmacy
Ada, Ohio

Daniel Krinsky, MS, RPh
Director, Pharmacotherapy Sales and
  Marketing
Lexi-Comp, Inc.
Hudson, Ohio

**Darlene M. Mednick, RPh, MBA,
PAHM, NPDP**
Vice President, Pharmacy Relations
Merck-Medco Managed Care, L.L.C.
Franklin Lakes, New Jersey

Cathy Meier, PharmD
Clinical Pharmacist
Detroit Medical Center
Ann Arbor, Michigan

Ruth E. Nemire, PharmD
Director of Clinical Education
Assistant Professor of Pharmacy
  Practice
Nova Southeastern University College
  of Pharmacy
Fort Lauderdale, Florida

Bruce Parks, PhD, FCCP
Chair and Professor, Department of
  Pharmacy Practice
Associate Professor, Neurology and
  Pediatrics
Schools of Pharmacy and Medicine
University of Mississippi
Jackson, Mississippi

Pat Partaleno, PharmD
Assistant Professor of Pharmacy
Assistant Director of Drug Information
Ohio Northern University College of
  Pharmacy
Ada, Ohio

Joel R. Pittman, PharmD
Assistant Professor, Pharmacy Practice
School of Pharmacy
University of Mississippi
Jackson, Mississippi

Kelly Rogers, PharmD
Assistant Professor, Pharmacy Practice
School of Pharmacy
University of Mississippi
Jackson, Mississippi

Nancy W. Spencer, MD
Assistant Professor of Neurology and
  Internal Medicine
Indiana University
University Hospital
Indianapolis, Indiana

Ruth C. Taggart, MSN, ANP-C
University of Colorado Multiple
  Sclerosis Center
Denver, Colorado

Ming Wang, PharmD
Instructor-Ambulatory Care Resident
Nova Southeastern University
Fort Lauderdale, Florida

CONTENTS

3   The Basics of Communication: An Overview 35

Michelle Assa

4   Legal Requirements for Filling a Prescription 65

Dean L. Arneson

5   Interpretation of Clinical Laboratory Data 81

Karen Daniel

10   **Monitoring Drug Therapy** **251**
        Bruce Parks, Joel R. Pittman and Kelly Rodgers

11   **Practical Pharmacokinetics** **275**
        Sandra B. Earle

12   **Meeting Preceptor's Expectations: Rounding,**
     SOAP Notes, Patient Education **317**
        Jacci Bainbridge, Ruth C. Taggart, and Janina Z.P. Janes

13   **Charting New Pathways: An Introduction to Managed-**
     Care Pharmacy Experiential Learning Rotation **331**
        Darlene M. Mednick, Tracy S. Hunter, and Cristina E. Bello

PREFACE

Pharmacy faculty and students need a textbook to use for learning about etiquette, ethics, law, and other topics. It should be a pocket-sized book that can be used for referencing information when on early and advanced rotations. We feel this text will fulfill that need for both students and preceptors.

This text should be used both in the classroom to introduce ideas and practice communication skills and on rotation to help guide students in learning terminology, organizing case information, improving problem-solving skills, and rounding. In the first four chapters, the authors discuss expectations for early experience, etiquette and communication skills, ethical issues, and facts of federal law that students need to know before entering the realm of pharmacy practice as an intern. Communication skills are some of the most important tools a pharmacist uses in every day practice. The oral, nonverbal, and written communication nuances reviewed in the communications chapter help the student develop an awareness of his or her own style. Appropriate use and practice of these skills is encouraged. This chapter includes pharmacy-related scenarios set in the hospital, community, and others areas of practice as exercises. In these settings, students may take on the role of a pharmacist, patient, family member, nurse, or physician.

The chapter on pharmacokinetics may be used in a beginning pharmacokinetics class when students need to understand concepts; it will supplement the regular textbook. The information in the chapter will be helpful to the advanced practice student, who will easily be able to look up the formulas used for calculating doses, integrate the case information, and then provide good information to the medical team or pharmacist.

Instructive chapters dealing with the technical and interpretive aspects of the practice of pharmacy, such as calculations, medical terminology, physical assessment, and laboratory testing are included in this handbook. These supply the facts that the student needs as he or she works through everyday problems of the early or advanced rotations. Students will be able to use this book early in their pharmacy school days, keep note of their learning, and indicate "pearls" that they will use later during advanced rotations.

The chapter on drug monitoring is unique. This chapter encourages students to choose the investigative route to monitoring patient and drug therapy. This chapter could be used to augment a text or in the therapeutics class to help students practice a process for critical evaluation of a patient. During the practical experience rotations, students can refer to this chapter to understand the processes they need to develop to become good problem solvers. Included are examples and definitions of information required to evaluate a patient and his or her drug therapy. The critical steps to the evaluation process are identified, and examples are provided for the student; model cases are included for discussion and practice. There are tables included in this chapter that the student can use to review the drug indices that need monitoring.

The pharmaceutical care chapter of this book should help tie all the information from previous chapters together so that the student can work effectively and efficiently at learning the skills needed to become an excellent practitioner. This inspiring chapter encourages students to work with patients and all members of the healthcare team in a professional manner and to provide pharmaceutical care. It encourages the student to go beyond the tasks of daily rounding and chart review and to learn everything possible while on rotations. Students are expected to take the information gained from previous chapters and integrate their knowledge to prioritize problems, create notes, and present cases in a formal, organized manner.

Community pharmacy rotations that incorporate the concept of pharmaceutical care are becoming common around the country. Many pharmacists, organizations, and patients are demanding a higher quality of care in the community. This call is being answered by a "pharmacy practice" model in the community setting that incorporates patient counseling on specific disease states, providing screening programs, and pharmacists working with patients to improve compliance. This chapter is the first to address how this sort of rotation can be implemented in the community and what goals and objectives should be achieved by students both early and later in their school years. The chapter addresses how faculty can participate in the program either full time or part time and what expectations there should be on the student.

Finally, the last two chapters of the book are real patient cases, with chart information that can be assigned to the student before sending her or him off to look at patient charts. Students may need to ask questions in a role-playing mode to get all the information they need to present the case in an organized manner. This patient information is presented in a "chart" format so that students can begin to understand what it is they need to look for.

This "pocket brain" is written for the student to use from start to finish in a college of pharmacy curriculum.

TO THE STUDENT

There are times when it is prudent to invest in books that will aid you in preparing for your life as a pharmacist. Getting ready for your rotations is one of those times when it is difficult to keep all the information in your head. This handbook is one of a few books that you will use through your entire pharmacy school years. So take a pencil or pen and start scribbling notes in the margins.

This handbook is divided into chapters. Some chapters in this book you can read once, dedicate the information to memory, and move on. There are many reference chapters in this book. These are the chapters that you will return to time and time again as you prepare for classes or participation in activities at your site. Several places within the text, you and your preceptor will find activities that can be used for practicing and improving your skills in certain areas. The communications and pharmacokinetics chapters are two examples. There are case chapters at the end of the book that contains six inpatient and six outpatient flowsheets. These data can be used to work up a patient, write a SOAP note, and present to your faculty member or preceptor as practice before looking through charts. This book should become your peripheral brain, where information is stored that you can readily retrieve when needed.

The chapters are organized with goals at the beginning and questions at the end. The goals should be contemplated before you read the chapter so that by the end you can easily answer the questions. I have been known as an instructor to take questions directly from the back of books like these, knowing that most students do not take the time to read them. Your faculty members or preceptors can help you with the correct answers.

The appendices of this book are included to enhance your peripheral brain power. They contain facts that did not directly fit within a certain chapter, enhance information given in the chapter, or supply tools necessary for you to use on your rotation.

There is no one right way to use this handbook. The important thing is that it not sit on your shelf as a required text, never to be opened. You bought the book; take the time to see what information is contained within. Think how good it will be not to have to carry your calculations, kinetics, drug information, and lab book all in your pocket at the same time. Your experiential education is never over. Once you leave the hallowed halls of your alma mater, you will still find use for the information contained within this book.

TO THE FACULTY/PRECEPTOR

It is difficult to choose a text for students that is useful to both of you. Our efforts in writing this book are to provide you with the most useful peripheral brain for students who have no experience in pharmacy but are expected to start interacting as professionals on matriculation into pharmacy school. It is also written for the advanced student who is just getting ready to round with physicians and needs to function at the higher level. We hope that this book will grow with the students as they progress through pharmacy school.

This handbook is written so that it can be used in the classroom to supplement the activities and learning that occur during the experiential education portion of your curriculum. Some of the chapters are mostly text format and can be assigned for reading. Other chapters are included for reference purposes but can be combined with casework in a therapeutics course as well as being used on advanced rotations.

There are two chapters we feel are unique to pharmacy literature. They are the community rotation chapter and the drug-monitoring chapter. Many schools are moving toward providing early and advanced community pharmacy experiences for students. The author of the community chapter provided an advanced clinical community rotation. He includes goals and objectives for setting up such a rotation, includes many intricate details of the operation, and identifies the areas of the community pharmacy for students who have never worked behind the counter. He discusses the decline of the independent pharmacist and the differences in operation between large chain stores and grocery store pharmacies. The chapter highlights for students how they can become involved in the community and make a difference.

In the textbook marketplace you will find many chapters on drug monitoring that include only the indices that need to be monitored. We included a different kind of drug-monitoring chapter because our experience is that many students do not start on advanced rotations ready to problem solve. This chapter guides students through a process for working up a patient and solving his or her therapeutic problems. The student may not choose to continue in this exact manner, as it is an individual process. But, the chapter provides a place for students to refer to when in doubt about what they should be doing. As a faculty member, when you see students struggling with the concepts of drug monitoring, having them review this chapter may help them advance. Having the student do the practice cases in Chapters 15 and 16 along with the information from this chapter should give them the confidence they need to proceed to monitoring "real" patients.

There are several ways this text can be used. It can be used in the classroom to supplement an early experience course, or it can be used by students beginning rotations in their first years of pharmacy school. There are exercises in the chapters that you as faculty can use as in-class activities or student assignments. The communication chapter scenarios were developed as part of an early experience classroom exercise. Students divided into small groups and took turns being the patient or the health care professional. The questions at the end of the communications scenarios can be answered by the audience and/or the participants in the exercise. The section of the physical assessment chapter can be used in the classroom session to teach blood pressure monitoring and pulse. Other information within the chapter will be more valuable as students start their advanced practice rotations.

This book can be a peripheral brain for students on early or advanced experiential education courses. Information in many chapters is provided in table and figure format for quick reference. The laboratory chapter not only contains the normal values expected but has information for the student on why a lab value might be abnormal. This should help the student in determining a differential diagnosis and potential therapeutic problems.

The appendices should not be overlooked in this particular handbook. They supplement the information in the chapters. They include goals and objectives for the community rotation, blank forms for the patient cases that students can copy and use when they go to monitor patients, and medical terminology and a glossary required for students who have not yet been exposed to some of the terms they will encounter while on rotations.

We hope that you find this book useful to your coursework and for your preceptors.

ACKNOWLEDGMENTS

This book comes to fruition due to the efforts of many friends and colleagues. To the Editors, Steve Zollo, Julie Scardiglia, and Barbara Holton, thank you for your ideas, and hard work to put this book together. Julie, your faith and patience make you queen among editors in my book. To my friends who read, and wrote chapters at the last minute and to others who listened to my concerns over the value of this book, I can only say thank you. Thanks, Marijke, for your extra eyes. Tim and Cristina, thank you is not enough.

C H A P T E R 1

TACKLING YOUR FIRST ROTATIONS IN PHARMACY SCHOOL

Elizabeth Frenzel Shepherd

Goals: After reviewing the information in this chapter, you should be able to:

1. Explain what a professional appearance and attitude is.
2. Describe what will happen on the first day of rotation.
3. Compose an appropriate cover letter.
4. Develop a student curriculum vitae.
5. Describe the goals and objectives of early practical experience.

INTRODUCTION

This chapter introduces you to the practice of pharmacy so that you are prepared to start rotations, whether you are a first-year student or advanced standing student. Dress and attitude are primary goals in developing your professionalism. Many colleges of pharmacy start early to help you train for your role. There are goals and objectives in this chapter that will support the structure of the experiential education at your college of pharmacy. In this chapter the goals are limited to what you should strive to attain on your early experience rotations. Later chapters of this book provide you with advanced goals and objectives for specific rotations.

Never underestimate the value of the first impression!

A checklist for preparing for your first day of rotation is given in Table 1.1.

ATTRIBUTES

Appearance

Let's begin with appearance. "Dress for success" is a very common cliché, but there is a lot of punch in that statement. Now that you are in professional school, appearance counts. Professional attire is important. Neatness and cleanliness are priorities. An ironed lab jacket should be worn over your clothes. The lab jacket

---

TABLE 1.1. PREPARATION CHECKLIST

- Mail preceptor curriculum vitae and cover letter.
- Phone preceptor one week before beginning the rotation.
  (Remember to ask about parking, directions to site, readings before beginning rotation.)
- If preceptor is unavailable, speak to her designee.
- Review goals and objectives in COP Early Professional Experience Manual.
- Confirm transportation to the site and/or drive by site before beginning the rotation.
- Prepare list of student goals for the rotation.
- Make copies of immunization records and have them available.
- Complete additional site-required paperwork.
- Review wardrobe for enough professional attire and comfortable shoes.
- Put a smile on my face and get a good night's sleep.

---

should have your college of pharmacy school insignia in the chest area or upper arm area or elsewhere as required by your school. Always have your pharmacy intern identification badge attached to your lab coat. For men, a shirt and tie are appropriate with dress or casual pants. Shoes should be comfortable but not look like sneakers or be sneakers. Remember to wear socks. For women, slacks, skirts, and dresses are all appropriate. Skirts and dresses should be no more than two inches above the knee. Shoes should be flat and comfortable for wearing all day long. Hosiery is a must. Jewelry should not be excessive. Earrings should not hang down to your shoulders. Do not wear more than two bracelets on one wrist. You do not want to look like a Gypsy pharmacist. Long hair should be tied back or put up. Wouldn't you be embarrassed if a patient returned a prescription because hair was in the vial with the medicine? Early experience rotations allow you to meet people every day and help you to begin making your professional contacts in your first year of pharmacy school. A professional appearance will help you create a professional image about yourself, and you will make an appropriate first impression.

Attitude

The next step in creating a professional image is having a professional attitude. You worked very hard completing your prerequisites and maintaining your high GPA. Be positive. Let everyone know you are glad to be in pharmacy school. Have a smile on your face. Be energetic and eager. Your preceptors will notice your positive attitude. Be honest. Pharmacists are regularly considered by the public to be highly ethical and trusted professionals.[1,2] Your preceptor and patients will notice your positive attitude and may even change theirs.

Let's talk about how to handle yourself when small problems arise outside or even inside the pharmacy. Consider your attitude on a day you don't feel well or have a test in the afternoon or received a speeding ticket on the way to your rotation site because you overslept. Keep the sharing of your personal problems to a minimum. Always call the preceptor as soon as you know you will unable to reach your rotation site on time. You may explain that you will be late because you received a speeding ticket. You are not the first person to receive a speeding ticket that caused him or her to be late for school or work. Don't overexaggerate. Leave your personal issues at the door of the pharmacy. Remember that your preceptor was a pharmacy student once and had to juggle tests, work, school, and home life all at the same time too. All pharmacists have gone to work when they were not feeling well. A cold and an exam are not excuses for a less than positive attitude or lack of attendance. Clients who come to the pharmacy are patients. They need your help and attention. Poor attitude and personal problems cannot be allowed to affect your rotations.

Timeliness

Before your first day, you should map out your route to the rotation site. If you're going to be driving to your rotation, you should do a practice drive by the site to see how long the commute is from your home. If you do this on the weekend, when traffic is light, remember to add additional travel time. If you're commuting by train or bus, make sure you have a schedule and know when and where you may have to transfer. Five minutes before you are scheduled to start at your site is sufficient time to arrive. Do not arrive too early, no more than 15 minutes before you are scheduled. Even though you are eager and want to put your best foot forward, your very early arrival will be distracting to your preceptor.

Your preceptor should be notified as soon as possible if you will be tardy or absent from rotation. Time off for holidays should be discussed with your preceptor at the beginning of the rotation. Not all pharmacies will close for holidays, and you may be expected to be at your rotation site on a holiday, especially if your preceptor is working on the holiday.

CURRICULUM VITAE AND COVER LETTER

To allow your preceptor to prepare for your arrival, you should be sure he or she has your cover letter (Fig. 1.1) and CV about 5 to 10 days before you are scheduled to begin the rotation. In the cover letter introduce yourself and include the

Your Address

Date

Preceptor Name

Preceptor Title

Name of Institution

Address of Institution

Dear Dr. Smith:

This letter is to introduce myself. My name is Student Pharmacist. I am a student at Smart College of Pharmacy. I will be at your site from 00/00/00 through 00/00/00 for an early experience rotation. My phone number is 123-4567. I will be calling you Monday morning of next week to receive directions to your facility, where and what time I should meet you, and which readings or other preparatory work I can do before I begin the rotation. I am looking forward to meeting you and learning from your experience.

Sincerely,

Smart Pharmacy Student

Figure 1.1. Cover Letter.

start and stop dates of the rotation, your address, e-mail address, telephone number, and when you will be verbally contacting him or her. Make sure you know the appropriate title for your preceptors and if they should be addressed as Doctor, Mister, or Ms. Include in the cover letter that you are looking forward to meeting them and learning with them. Figure 1.1 illustrates a sample cover letter.

You may include in the letter specific comments about the facility if you know them to be true. Examples of such comments include how you look forward to working with a specific team in the pharmacy or at the busiest outpatient pharmacy in the country.

Your curriculum vitae should include your name, address, phone number, e-mail address, previous college attendance, current college attendance, professional experience, work experience, and any awards and honors you have received during your college years. If you read, write, or speak any languages other than English, include this in your CV. High school honors and awards should not be included. The term "references on request" should also be omitted because the college of pharmacy is your reference. Your professional experience should include any positions you have held in the field of pharmacy. Describe what you have done in pharmacy using action verbs. Examples of action terms are filled prescriptions, communicated with health care professionals, managed inventory. You may have counted capsules and tablets, spoken to nurses on the phone, and put away the stock, but on your CV you should use professional terms to describe your activities. Also include your specific job title for all jobs (technician, data entry clerk). If you worked as a professional other than a pharmacist, for example, a teacher or an engineer, you may include this as other professional experience. Be sure to include the dates of attendance at all colleges, any degrees you have earned, and the dates on which they were conferred. As you progress through rotations, include them on your CV. Put your most recent experience first, the rest in reverse chronological order. Remember that professional experience is gained while you are a pharmacy intern. Even though rotations are part of your academic requirements, they still are part of your professional experience. Figure 1.2 illustrates a sample curriculum vitae.

There are numerous primary and secondary sources on resumes and writing a curriculum vitae. Your college library should have these, both in hard copy and online. *Drug Topics,* a pharmacy professional publication, gives graduating students tips on resume writing and interviewing skills in their March/April publication every year.

Make sure that you know the paperwork procedure for your sites, and send all required information with your cover letter, or earlier if required. Some early experience sites may require special applications. The Veterans Administration Medical Centers require that student have background checks and require students to submit their social security numbers as well as two different application forms. Some early experience sites, especially schools and school programs, may require fingerprinting and photo identification badges.

Smart P. Student
123 Birch Street
College Town, US 12345
123-4567
smarts@abc.efg

Education

0/00–present   Smart College of Pharmacy, University of City
                  City, State

0/00–0/00   ABC Community College
                  City, State. AA in Pharmacy 0/00

Professional Experience

Green's Pharmacy • Pharmacy Technician • Responsibilities included answering the telephone, managing inventory, assisting clients, and assisting in prescription filling.

Work Experience

Greenwood Elementary School • Teacher's Aid • Responsibilities included helping third grade students with their homework in the after-school care program and assisting the kindergarten teacher with all art projects.

Honors and Awards

Dean's List • 0/00,0/00,0/00
Rho Chi Honor Society President • 0/00–0/00
Language • Speak and write Portuguese

Figure 1.2. Student Curriculum Vitae.

AT THE SITE

Expectations

On your first day you arrive at the pharmacy. What can you expect? It really depends on what type of practice setting you are scheduled to attend. Most likely, you're at a hospital or a community pharmacy, or you may find yourself at a nursing home pharmacy, a prison, a methadone facility, or a home healthcare agency. All of these facilities require the services of a pharmacist. Wherever you are assigned for your first experience, you should expect to be busy. There will be phones ringing and people talking. The staff in the pharmacy or facility will be in constant motion, and you will not. By your third week, you will be in motion too. Don't become upset after your first day. You will feel that you are in the way, and in some respects you will be. But you won't be in the way for very long. Everyone who starts a new job feels that way on the first day.

Orientation

The best first day you can have in a pharmacy is to be early and for the preceptor to give you a tour of the facility and pharmacy and a full-day orientation. This orientation will cover preceptor expectations, objectives for the rotation, assignments, and outcomes expected for the student. You will be introduced to all staff members. Preceptors should inform the student of the role of each staff member. It is essential that you understand the role of each staff member. You should share with the preceptor what you expect to get out of the rotation, your concerns, and your desired goals. The objectives of the rotation will be discussed at length. You should develop a plan with the preceptor to meet the discussed objectives. Most preceptors will provide you with grading forms and a calendar of assignment due dates and meetings. What I just described is the ideal situation and truly the best way to begin a rotation. It may not always happen this way, and you must remember that you are in an experiential learning situation and that flexibility is the next most important attribute after attitude.

Pharmacy Technicians

Pharmacy technicians will be working in the pharmacy along with the pharmacists. Most states will allow the pharmacist to work with two technicians at a time. Technicians do not have the same responsibilities as pharmacy interns. Pharmacy interns must follow pharmacist laws, whereas technicians do not. Pharmacy interns may be disciplined by their State Board of Pharmacy. In most states, the technicians are not yet required to have a license and will be disciplined by the supervisor. Some pharmacy technicians are certified, but others are not. Technicians are in the pharmacy to assist the pharmacist.

The civil responsibilities are different between an intern and a technician. You may find, however, that the job responsibilities are very much the same. You will find yourself doing what you think is "technician work" or work that you feel is "beneath" you. Because this is the job that you will be doing as a pharmacist if you do not have the help of a technician, it is never "beneath" you. You must know how to do every job in a pharmacy. You can't supervise or run a pharmacy if you don't know how the jobs are done. You will be a better supervisor if you have done "technician" work.

You must develop a positive working relationship with the technicians. Good technicians keep the workflow smooth and steady. A good technician can make your day much easier and the learning better. Respect these people, as many have more experience than the pharmacist, and they are good resources for learning about pharmacy that may not be directly related to information about medication. As a student and pharmacist, you will come to depend on good technician support.

Confidentiality and Success

You discuss with your preceptor your goals for the rotation, and you get started. How do you have a successful rotation? There are a few things to keep in mind at all times. Remember your professional behavior and conduct while on rotations. You will have access to patients' medical records, charts, and data. Keep all information you know and have access to in the strictest confidence. Do not discuss patient information outside the pharmacy. If you must use patient information for a presentation or a school project, remember to use initials and not full names. Also keep confidential all fee systems and professional policies that you may encounter. Always be courteous and respectful of your preceptor. If you witness your preceptor giving out incorrect information or practicing in the gray area of the law, do not confront him or her in front of others. Wait until you can discuss the matter in private. You may not be correct in your interpretation of the circumstance and might embarrass yourself or your preceptor needlessly. If you believe your preceptor is violating any pharmacy laws and cannot discuss the issue with him or her, seek advice of a faculty member at your college. The experiential director is probably the best person to share this information with because she is in a position to take action.

Never dispense prescriptions before being checked by your preceptor or another pharmacist. You do have liability as a pharmacy intern if you make a mistake in filling a prescription. Do not make professional decisions without first discussing them with your preceptor. Your answer may be incorrect or may violate policies of the institution. Always let your preceptor know of any information you will be giving to patients or healthcare professionals.

Do not let the above cautionary statements keep you from initiating communication with other health care professionals. As a pharmacy intern you will be expected to call physicians and nurses on the phone. Always identify yourself as a student and be courteous and professional on the telephone. Use common sense when interacting with patients and other healthcare professionals. Always state why you are calling and remember to include the patient's name. Most of the time a nurse will be clarifying prescriptions written incorrectly by physicians. Make sure the nurse understands what you need. If the strength of a medication is missing from a prescription, inform the nurse of the available strengths. Remember that it is possible that the physician does not know. When the nurse clarifies the prescription with the physician, she will give him the strength options. If you do not supply the information, it is possible the physician will indicate a strength he believes is available when it is not, and you will be starting the telephone process of seeking the medication strength all over again.

You should be aware of the laws governing the practice of pharmacy. You should have a copy of all the state and federal laws that apply to the practice of pharmacy. Read the laws. If you are unsure of something being done in the pharmacy, look up the law first before going to your preceptor. Then your preceptor will be able to clarify any points that are unclear to you and explain the gray areas of the law. Some laws apply only to hospital pharmacies and not to community pharmacies. The opposite is also true. Your preceptor is the best person to clarify any questions you may have.

Stick with the schedule that you and your preceptor agree to, or if your schedule is determined by your college, adhere to the predetermined hours. Remember it will be necessary to devote more time at home and in the library to meet the goals of your practical experience rotations than are scheduled at the site. Most likely you will also have to spend additional time at your site to take advantage of unique experiences.

GOALS OF PRACTICAL EXPERIENCE

What are the goals of early experience rotations? The main goal of the early experience rotations is to apply concepts learned in the classroom to practical experience immediately. Early experience rotations are also designed to aid you in developing the practical aspects of the profession. You will also begin to develop communication skills with patients and with other health care professionals while on the early experience rotations.

Advanced professional practice rotations allow you to apply all didactic knowledge learned to clinical practice. On advanced practice rotations you become part of the healthcare team, assuming the position of the pharmacist. On advance practice rotations you will learn to manage patients' disease states and endpoints of therapy. Students on advanced practice rotations are supervised in learning practical applications while advancing their clinical judgment skills.

Most colleges of pharmacy provide students with objectives and outcomes for the early experience rotations. Faculty at colleges and universities want students to be exposed to hospital and community practices as early experience rotations. Some college curricula may require that students be assigned to public health activities, community service activities, nursing homes, and home health care agencies as early experience rotations. Others emphasize continuity of patient care, and students are assigned to monitor one patient's disease states for an entire year or years. The goals for service learning, community, and hospital are discussed in further detail below.

Service-Learning Experience

What can you expect if you are assigned to a community service rotation? Most likely you will serve similar functions as those who volunteer for the agency.

You will have your own personal goals that you expect to achieve on a service-learning rotation as well as time that you will spend reflecting on your rotation experiences. Barbara Jacoby defines service learning as "a form of experiential education in which students engage in activities that address human and community needs together with structured opportunities intentionally designed to promote student learning and development." Reflection and reciprocity are key concepts of service-learning.[3] Most likely you will work on a project that will contribute in some way to the community. Examples of projects that you will be conducting include food and clothing drives, after-school care programs, and holiday community programs. A community service rotation will help you develop a sense of community involvement. You will learn to be a team player. Service-learning rotations help students improve their listening and observation skills. Service-learning rotations are designed to help you grow as a professional and develop your professional demeanor. Learning through service will help you to meet community needs while developing your critical thinking skills and group problem-solving skills.

As a student doing an early experience service-learning rotation, you will attend to the needs of the community that are not being met, see aspects of illness or dying that cannot be learned through the classroom and readings, and learn the importance of developing and nuturing a moral and ethical conduct individually and among peers. Awareness of community needs and social problems helps pharmacy students discover empathy and feelings of compassion. Service rotations also aid pharmacy students in developing ethical and moral values. Early experience service rotations will also help you to appreciate why community service should be a significant and ongoing part of life. The service rotation will enhance your awareness of the need and role of volunteers in the community. Ideally, your service rotation will help you develop a volunteer niche for the rest of your life (Table 1.2).

Hospital Experience

What can you expect if you are assigned to an early experience hospital rotation? As a pharmacy student you will be assigned to all areas of a hospital pharmacy. You will be working with pharmacy technicians, clinical pharmacists, staff pharmacists, administrative pharmacists, IV pharmacists, and delivery technicians. Most likely you will spend your intern hours learning about a different aspect of hospital pharmacy each time you are at your site. Learning how to fill a prescription in a hospital pharmacy and interacting with other healthcare professionals are the two major goals of an early experience hospital rotation.

As a student doing an early experience hospital rotation you will participate in various aspects of hospital pharmacy practice, including dispensing, and management. Early experience rotations in a hospital promote early exposure to hospital pharmacy drug distribution and enhance a pharmacy student's awareness of

TABLE 1.2. SERVICE LEARNING GOALS AND OBJECTIVES

Upon completion of a service-learning rotation a pharmacy student will be able to:

- Display attitudes, habits, and values appropriate to a pharmacist.
- Promote awareness of health and prevention of disease.
- Articulate personal values and ethical principles.
- Display an understanding of unmet community needs and be able to provide examples in the community.
- Explain how social attitudes cause or cure unmet community needs.
- Discuss issues of diversity.
- Choose appropriate levels of communication.
- Adapt and pursue solving or correcting any given challenge.
- Understand a health care professional's role in the community.
- Work as a group leader and a team member.

the many aspects of pharmacy practice in a hospital. These experiences will include the role and responsibilities of a professionally oriented hospital pharmacist; the importance of effective communication between pharmacists and other health care providers; the importance of monitoring drug utilization; the organizational requirements necessary to achieve efficient operations; and the application of local, state, and federal regulations governing the prescription process. Early practical experience in a hospital setting also enhances a student's awareness of the role and responsibilities of the pharmacist in the healthcare delivery system. Students doing an early experience rotation in a hospital will immediately be able to apply information learned in pharmacodynamics, pharmacy law, and basic sciences at their rotation site. As a pharmacy student on an early experience hospital rotation, you can expect to be introduced to pharmacy operations, use reference materials common to hospital pharmacy practice, understand and use a unit dose system, be exposed to computerized order entry, and perform prescription preparation.

A pharmacy student on an early experience hospital rotation will be expected to develop skills and knowledge in all areas of hospital pharmacy practice (Table 1.3).

Community Experience

What can you expect if you are assigned to an early experience community rotation? As a pharmacy student assigned to an early experience community rotation, you will learn all aspects of managing a community pharmacy. Every detail of filling a prescription will be reviewed including the ordering of prescription

---

TABLE 1.3. HOSPITAL GOALS AND OBJECTIVES

Upon completion of an early experience hospital rotation, a pharmacy student will be able to:

- Explain the process of receiving, interpreting, clarifying, and verifying medication orders for accuracy and completeness.
- Select the appropriate drug product to be used in filling medication orders.
- Package and label medication in compliance with hospital pharmacy policy and local and federal pharmacy laws.
- Describe the process for drug control, storage, and security functions in drug distribution.
- Describe the process for recording the medication order following established pharmacy policies and procedures.
- Participate in the drug distribution process for timely delivery of ordered medications, including STAT orders, to the appropriate location.
- Communicate effectively with other members of the health care team including nurses, technicians, and other staff members.
- Observe aseptic technique in the IV room and recognize its importance.
- Demonstrate knowledge of reference material.
- Discuss hospital pharmacy management issues as they pertain to inventory, formularies, budgets, regulation of narcotics, and quality assurance.

---

medications. Some of the activities you will be exposed to include inventory management, patient counseling, third-party plans, and state and federal pharmacy laws.

An early experience rotation in a community pharmacy will promote competency in drug distribution and enhance student awareness of many aspects of community pharmacy practice. Students will be exposed to the role and responsibilities of the professionally oriented community pharmacist; the importance of effective communication among pharmacists, patients, and other healthcare providers; and the application of local, state, and federal regulations governing the prescription-filling process. The student is expected to enhance patient care and contribute to the practice of pharmacy. The goal of an early experience community clerkship is to facilitate the application of skills, concepts, and knowledge acquired in the classroom. Activities completed while on a community clerkship will be selection of drug products; prescription dispensing; interactions with patients; and interactions with nurses, physicians, and other healthcare professionals (Table 1.4).

TABLE 1.4. COMMUNITY GOALS AND OBJECTIVES

Upon completion of an early experience community rotation, a pharmacy student will be able to:

- Receive, interpret, check, and verify prescriptions for accuracy and completeness.
- Select the most appropriate drug product to be used in filling a prescription, taking into account factors that will enhance patient care.
- Interact with health insurance companies to provide the patient with the most effective and lowest-cost medication.
- Describe the legal constraints governing the dispensing process.
- Package and label the prescription in compliance with local, state, and federal laws.
- Dispense the prescription to the patient in a professional manner that complies with all legal requirements including OBRA '90.
- Maintain the confidentiality of patient information, especially during data collection, patient interviews, prescription clarification, and patient counseling.
- Participate in interactions with patients to obtain information relevant to filling the prescription.
- Participate in interactions with patients to create and/or expand the patient profile.
- Participate in interactions with other health care providers with regard to the provision of pharmaceutical care.

CONCLUSION

After reading this chapter you should have a better understanding of the professional role you play as a pharmacy student. There are certain important attributes that you must strive to master early in your career, such as appearance, attitude, and timeliness. It is important to write an appropriate cover letter and curriculum vitae as directed by college faculty and send them to your site. Setting goals for yourself before beginning your rotation and letting your preceptor know what they are is how you can make the most of your rotation. Practice learning every day. Being comfortable in your environment is important. The definitions, goals, expectations, and ideals discussed here may help you achieve your desired level of learning and comfort.

The information in this chapter is meant to support goals and objectives set forth by your own college of pharmacy. In all cases, follow the directions of your own faculty, and where this book disagrees, it is because the practice of pharmacy is not perfect, and many ways of doing things may be correct. That is why they call it practice.

QUESTIONS

1. What is considered professional dress for male and female pharmacists?
2. What is a professional attitude?
3. What can a student expect on the first rotation day in a pharmacy?
4. What goals will a pharmacy student have completed at the end of his or her early experience rotations?
5. How do hospital and community rotations differ in the experience offered?

REFERENCES

1. Facts about Pharmacists and Pharmacies. http://www.pharmacyandyou.org/about/pharmacyfacts. html.
2. Carlsen DK. Nurses remain at top of honesty and ethics poll. http://www.gallup.com/poll/releases/ pr001127.asp, 2000.
3. Jacoby B, et al. *Service Learning in Higher Education.* San Francisco: Jossey-Bass, 1996.

ETHICS IN PHARMACY PRACTICE

Nancy W. Spencer

Goals: After reviewing the information in this chapter, you should be able to:

1. Understand why the core of clinical ethics is the doctor/clinician–patient relationship, what responsibilities and potential abuses are inherent in that relationship, and why there need to be guidelines for clinicians so the clinicians can recognize what behavior is ethically their duty to provide to the patient and what is ethically unacceptable behavior.
2. Use the Siegler "four box" system of (1) Medical Indications, (2) Patient Preferences, (3) Quality of Life, and (4) Contextual Features when approaching cases of ethical decision making.
3. Know the four Georgetown bioethics principles of autonomy, beneficence, nonmaleficence, and justice.
4. Understand and follow codified ethical practices such as those published by the American College of Physicians.
5. Understand that your ethical duties also extend to the family, your profession, to society, and to patient research.

INTRODUCTION

This chapter is addressed to clinicians; a clinician is a professional involved in clinical care of patients. This includes physicians, nurses, pharmacists, Pharm. D.'s, physical therapists, occupational therapists, and others. Ethical decision making is involved in every case of clinical decision making.

The chapter is set up in five sections:

1. The Hippocratic Oath is the foundation of the doctor–patient relationship and of the code of clinical ethics in medicine.
2. Two philosophical theories are often referred to in biomedical ethics: utilitarianism and deontology.
3. History of (a) how biomedical ethics evolved and the fundamental principles of biomedical ethics, (b) how clinical ethics evolved, and (c) clinical applications of those principles (clinical ethics) with case examples.

4. Codes of conduct in the professions and, specifically, clinical ethics.
5. Conclusion. The doctor/clinician–patient relationship is the core of clinical ethics.

HIPPOCRATIC OATH IS THE FOUNDATION OF THE DOCTOR/CLINICIAN–PATIENT RELATIONSHIP AND OF THE CODE OF PROFESSIONAL ETHICS IN MEDICINE

When we choose a career in a health profession, there comes with it the power to restore health or, at the very least, lessen the suffering of the patient. In this very special relationship, the patient must assume the patient role, that of asking for help from the clinician, and the clinician must assume the clinician role, that of trying to restore health or at least lessen the suffering of the patient. These roles will always put the patient in the less powerful position and the clinician in the more powerful one. It is important that the clinician understand and accept the responsibilities and potential abuses of the power in that relationship. Through the centuries it was recognized that because of this power differential, there needed to be guidelines for clinicians so that once a patient entrusted his or her health to the clinician's care, the clinician could recognize what behavior was ethically his or her duty to provide to the patient and what was ethically unacceptable behavior.

It has been recognized since the days of Hippocrates that physicians needed a shared understanding of the goals of medicine, their role in the practice of medicine, and what behavior was appropriate and what behavior was not appropriate toward patients. Written documentation of "professing" the ethical principles involved in patient care date back to the Hippocratic Oath taken by physicians. Therefore, the doctor–patient relationship is used in this chapter as the classic model of the clinician–patient relationship. The principles are the same for all clinicians.

The Hippocratic Oath is a physician's obligation to safeguard the life and welfare of the patient. The moral centerpiece of the Hippocratic Oath is that "the physician will use judgment to help the sick according to his ability and judgment, but never with the view to injury and wrongdoing." In book I on "Epidemics" attributed to Hippocrates, it is also said that "Physicians must take a habit of two things—to help or at least to do no harm. The art of medicine has three factors, the disease, the patient, and the physician. The physician is the servant of the Art. The patient must cooperate with the physician in combating the disease."[1] Once the patient seeks the physician's help, the patient must ultimately trust that the Hippocratic physician will provide the best available treatment for the medical condition and end treatment if it turns out to be harmful.

Figure 2.1 is an interpretation of the Hippocratic Oath by Dr. Steven Miles.

I swear by Apollo the Physician and by Asclepius, Hygia, and Panacea, and by all the deities, making this testimony before them that I will keep this oath to the best of my power and judgement. I will regard those who taught me this art and science as equal to my patients. I will share with my teachers according to their necessities. I will impart the art, science, lectures, and all the rest of learning to those students who have sworn to live up to this profession. I will use treatments for the benefit of the ill according to my ability and judgement and from what is to their harm or injustice I will keep them. I will not give a poison to anyone if asked for it, nor will I suggest such a course. Likewise I will not give a woman a destructive pessary. In a pure and holy way, I will guard my life, my art, and my science. Into the households I enter, I will go to benefit the ill, while being far from all voluntary and destructive injustice, especially from sexual acts upon women's or men's bodies whether they be free or enslaved. Of whatever I see or hear in my personal or professional life that should not be aired, I will remain silent, holding such things to be unspeakable. If I observe this oath, and do not blur and evade it, may I enjoy the benefits of life and of this work and be held in good repute by all persons for all time. However, if I transgress and perjure myself, may the opposite befall me.

Figure 2.1. Hippocratic Oath as interpreted by Steven Miles.[2]

TWO PHILOSOPHICAL THEORIES ARE OFTEN REFERRED TO IN BIOMEDICAL AND CLINICAL ETHICS: UTILITARIANISM AND DEONTOLOGY

When you look through textbooks on ethics, you will see thousands of pages devoted to many philosophic theories. However, when these theories are applied to clinical practice, two are highly regarded as sound ethical principles.

Utilitarianism philosophy is based on the belief that the morality of an act is based solely on the basis of its consequences. In the words of the most famous of the utilitarian philosophers, John Mill, "Actions are right in proportion as they tend to promote happiness, wrong as they tend to produce the reverse of happiness." The degree of moral rightness of an act is directly proportional to its net utility, defined as the difference between its overall utility and disutility[3] or, in medical terminology, its benefits and burdens.

Deontological philosophy is based on the belief that the morality of an act is based solely on the basis of the moral rightness of intentions, termed the "categorical imperitive." In this paradigm, the intentions and sense of duty behind a given act determine the degree of moral rightness of an act. Immanuel Kant is the most famous of the philosophers of deontologism.

HISTORY OF (a) HOW BIOMEDICAL ETHICS EVOLVED AND THE FUNDAMENTAL PRINCIPLES OF BIOMEDICAL ETHICS, (b) HOW CLINICAL ETHICS EVOLVED, AND (c) CLINICAL APPLICATIONS OF THOSE PRINCIPLES (CLINICAL ETHICS) WITH CASE EXAMPLES

(a) History of How Biomedical Ethics Evolved and the Fundamental Principles of Biomedical Ethics

Nuremberg Code

After the Second World War, the Nuremberg trials revealed the terrible abuses, called "medical experimentation," perpetuated by Nazi doctors on concentration camp prisoners. The Nuremberg Code, 10 rules set down to protect human subjects in medical research in perpetuity, was formulated in August 1947 in Nuremberg Germany by American judges sitting in judgment of 23 physicians and scientists accused of murder and torture in the conduct of medical experiments in the concentration camps. These rules were a merger of the physician-centered duties set down in the Hippocratic oath and the patient/subject-centered assertion of patient/subject protections. Within the text of the Nuremberg Code was the assertion of the unequivocable, absolute protection of the rights of patients/subjects and of their autonomy. Those protections affirmed two important rights—that of informed consent and the right to withdraw from research.

Since that time, the informed consent requirement of the Code is now seen as an ethical necessity not only in research but also in treatment.

Famous Historical Examples of Ethical Dilemmas and Scandals in the 1960s: Recognition of Medical and Nonmedical Selection Bias while Attempting to Ethically Ration Hemodialysis; Exposure of the Flagrant but Unrecognized Racial Bias in the Tuskegee Syphilis Study; Beginnings of Debate over Definition of Death in Organ Transplantation and in Brain Death

After the Nuremberg Code, more ethical dilemmas were recognized in the United States. In the early 1960s, with the advent of hemodialysis, there were many more candidates than hemodialysis machines. Determination of selection of patients for hemodialysis was ultimately recognized as an ethical dilemma—what medical and nonmedical criteria should be used to select suitable candidates?

Later, the research carried out over several decades (1932–1972) by the US Public Health Service in Tuskegee, Alabama, on hundreds of black men with known syphilis who were never offered penicillin in order that the progression of the disease could be studied was made known. This led to acknowledgment of physician bias, racial arrogance, and unethical treatment of racial minorities in the United States.[4]

In 1967, Dr. Christiaan Barnard transplanted a human heart from a dead (or dying) person into a patient with a terminal cardiac disease. This led to some wondering about the organ donor's state—was the source truly dead, and what were the wishes of the donor about donating his heart while living?

In the early 1960s ventilators had been invented, and patients with polio were being saved from certain death. However, other patients, including those in irreversible coma, were placed on ventilators as well. This led to a large number of cases where physicians were faced with the ethical dilemma of withdrawing ventilator support from patients who had functioning cardiorespiratory systems but who had had cessation of total brain functions. The standard definition of death was when a doctor determined that the heart and/or lungs ceased to function. However, these patients on ventilator support had functioning hearts and lungs, but brain function had ceased. Adding to this concern was the growing recognition that these patients' organs were of great value in transplantation. Therefore, in 1968, the Harvard ad hoc Committee on Brain Death was established and published their definition and recommendations for the diagnosis of brain death. Under these criteria, patients who met the brain death criteria were considered medically unequivocally dead, and ventilator withdrawal was deemed medically and ethically appropriate. Also, organ removal for transplantation from these patients was deemed ethically appropriate (assuming consent from the family) because these patients were medically unequivocally dead.

Famous Historical Examples of Ethical Dilemmas in the 1970s and 1980s: Ethical Dilemmas Arising from Famous Cases of Patients in Persistent Vegetative State (Recognition and Definition of Persistent Vegetative State; Who Can Make Decisions Regarding Administering and Withdrawing Hydration and Nutrition in These No Longer Autonomous Patients); Belmont Report's Critical Role in Codifying Protection of Human Subjects in Research and Stating the Three General Principles of Biomedical Ethics[5] (Respect for Persons, Beneficence, Justice) and Their Applications (Informed Consent, Assessment of Risks and Benefits, and Fair Selection of Subjects); the Four Principles of Biomedical Ethics[6]

By the 1970s and 1980s, several court cases arose concerning patients (Quinlan, Cruzan, Brophy) in persistent vegetative state (a state in which the brain stem, which controls various "vegetative" functions such as wake/sleep cycles, breathing, and pupillary responses, is still functioning but the higher levels of cortical functioning such as meaningful interaction with the environment permanently cease to function), raising questions of the ethics surrounding the withdrawal of ventilator, hydration, and nutrition in *nonautonomous* patients (see Appendix O for the consensus statements and practice parameters published by the professional organizations American Academy of Neurology and the American Neurological Society).

By 1974, the Congress established the National Commission for the Protection of Human Subjects of Biomedical and Behavioral Research to recommend policies that would guide researchers in the design of ethical research. That commission, which sat from 1974 to 1978, engaged the help of a wide variety of scholars from many disciplines and solicited public opinion on many issues. Out of this Commission developed *The Belmont Report; Ethical Principles and Guidelines for the Protection of Human Subjects of Research* (April 18, 1979) published by the Department of Health, Education and Welfare. The Belmont Report asserted three "general principles" of "biomedical ethics"[5]:

1. *Respect for persons,* which includes two moral requirements, (a) the requirement to acknowledge *autonomy* and (b) the requirement to protect those with diminished autonomy).
2. *Beneficence,* which is the obligation to secure the patient's well-being. Two general rules apply: (a) do no harm and (b) maximize possible benefits and minimize possible harms.
3. *Justice,* fairness in distribution; the importance of explaining in what respects people should be treated equally.[5]

Applications of the three general principles include[5] (1) informed consent, which includes three elements: (a) information, (b) comprehension, and (c) voluntariness; (2) assessment of risks and benefits, which include (a) the nature and scope of risk and benefits and (b) the systematic assessment of risks and benefits; and (3) selection of subjects, with fair procedures and outcomes in the selection of research subjects.[5]

The publishing of The Belmont Report then led to the publishing of the landmark work of Beauchamp and Childress, *The Principles of Biomedical Ethics.*[6] This system is taught at the Kennedy Institute of Ethics at Georgetown University and is labeled the "Principles of Biomedical Ethics." In this system there are four essential ethical principles[6]:

1. *Respect for Autonomy: Autonomy* is the moral right to choose and follow one's own plan of life and action. Respect for autonomy is the moral attitude that disposes one to refrain from interference with others' autonomous beliefs and actions in the pursuit of their goals.
2. *Nonmaleficence: Nonmaleficence* is the moral duty to do no harm.
3. *Beneficence: Beneficence* is the moral duty to assist persons in need.
4. *Justice: Justice* is the ethics of fair and equitable distribution of burdens and benefits within a community.[6]

These ethical principles of *beneficence, nonmaleficence, autonomy*, and *justice* as set forth by Beauchamp and Childress remain well established in the bioethics field. However, at the bedside or clinic, it was often difficult to see how these principles can be applied to medical decision making in individual cases. This led to the development of clinical medical ethics decision making as described in the next section.

(b) History of How Clinical Ethics Evolved

The term "clinical ethics" was coined by Siegler in the 1970s.[7] Clinical ethics is an approach to assisting clinicians in identifying, analyzing, and resolving ethical issues in clinical medicine. Albert Jonsen, Mark Siegler, and William Winslade published their first of four classic editions of "Clinical Ethics" in 1982. In it they wrote,

> The practice of good clinical medicine requires some working knowledge about ethical issues such as informed consent, truth telling, confidentiality, end of life care, pain relief, and patient rights. Medicine, even at its most technical and scientific, is an encounter between human beings, and the physician's work of diagnosing disease, offering advice, and providing treatment is embedded in a moral context. Usually values such as mutual respect, honesty, trustworthiness, compassion, and a commitment to pursue shared goals make a clinical encounter between physician and patient morally unproblematic. Occasionally physicians and patients may disagree about values or face choices that challenge their values. It is then that ethical problems arise. Clinical ethics is both about the ethical features that are present in every clinical encounter and about the ethical problems that occasionally arise in those encounters.[8]

(c) Clinical Applications of Biomedical Ethics Using the Siegler Method of "Four Boxes"

When you are seeing patients in the outpatient or inpatient setting and a dilemma arises as to how to best resolve an ethical question, I suggest you use the following "four box" system developed by Siegler, Winslade, and Jonsen[8] (Fig. 2.2). It was developed because clinicians have long found it difficult to see how ethical principles of autonomy, beneficence, nonmaleficence, and justice, as valued as they are, can be brought back down to practical application at the bedside or clinic setting. In their book, *Clinical Ethics,* Siegler, Winslade, and Jonsen pooled their extensive experiences and incorporated all the important bioethical principles into a "hands on" practical approach to solving ethical dilemmas in clinical practice. In the Siegler, Winslade, Jonsen approach, each clinical case, when seen as an ethical problem, should be analyzed by means of four topics[8] (Fig. 2.2).

1. Medical Indications: Medical indications refers to the relation between the pathophysiology presented by the patient and the diagnostic and therapeutic interventions that are "indicated," that is, appropriate to evaluate and treat

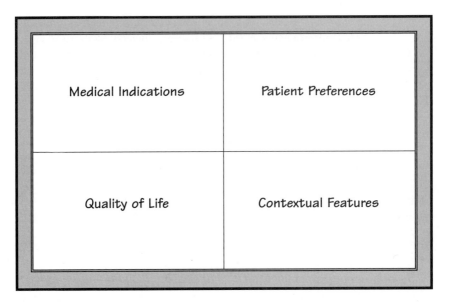

Figure 2.2. The "four box" method for ethical decision making. *(From Jonsen A, Siegler M, Winslade W. Clinical Ethics: A Practical Approach to Ethical Decisions in Clinical Medicine, 4th ed. New York: McGraw-Hill, 1998.)*

   the problem. The ethical discussion will not only review the medical acts but also focus on the purposes and goals of any indicated interventions.

2. Patient Preferences: The preferences of the patient, based on the patient's own values and personal assessment of benefits and burdens. This is the clinical application of autonomy. The systematic review of this topic requires further questions including decision-making capacity, informed consent, who has the authority to decide on behalf of the patient (surrogate decision maker), the legal and ethical limits of that authority, etc.

3. Quality of Life: This is less worked out in the literature of medical ethics but is important in all medical situations. Any injury or illness threatens patients with actual or potential reduced quality of life. The clinician has a duty to duty to restore, maintain, or improve quality of life. However, it is usually a third party such as the clinician or family members rather than the patient who is involved in quality-of-life decisions. Because the patients themselves may not be able to assert their own preferences, and it is third parties rather than the patient who are trying to judge the patient's quality of life, these decisions are perilous and must be recognized as such because these decisions open the door for bias and prejudice. Nevertheless, quality-of-life issues must be confronted in the context of analysis of clinical ethical problems.

4. Contextual Features: The doctor–patient relationship, defined by the patient's asking for help and the the physician's fiduciary duty to help, is at the core of clinical ethics. But every medical case is embedded in a larger context of persons, religious beliefs, institutions, and financial, legal, and social arrangements. These contextual features are important in understanding and resolving clinical problems.[8]

Each topic organizes the varying facts of the case and identifies the moral principles appropriate to the case. These topics help clinicians understand where the moral principles meet the circumstances of the clinical case.[8]

Notice in the "four box" system above, there is a double line separating *Medical Indications* and *Patient Preferences* from *Quality of Life* and *Contextual Features.* This is intentional. Although in any clinical situation all four aspects should always be thoroughly explored, the top two, Medical Indications and Patient Preferences, "trump" the bottom two, Quality of Life and Contextual Features.

To illustrate the "clinical ethics" approach, here are two cases that involve some ethical dilemmas.

Case 1: Quality of Life

A 26-year-old Gold Medal Olympic bicyclist was struck by a car, flung 30 feet into the air, and fell into an embankment. He was training for his second Olympic trial and was well known in the community as being devoted to his sport. He was unconscious at the scene. After stabilization in the hospital, it was determined that his spinal cord was completely severed below T10. He sustained a serious head injury, but it was anticipated that he would probably be able to talk and communicate his wishes over time. However, a long rehabilitation period was anticipated for the head injury with uncertain degree of return to full preaccident mental abilities, and the paraplegia was permanent. During his recovery period he needed proxies to make his decisions for him because of his temporary lack of decision-making capacity. The patient had several medical complications including pneumonia and urosepsis. After several weeks, several family members, including his wife, who was the main proxy decision maker, voiced their concern that the patient, given his athletic prowess, would "never want to be a cripple" and suggested that, because of the patient's poor quality of life, antibiotics be withheld and the patient be allowed to "die with dignity." Both the patient and his wife were avid athletes, and the subject of paraplegia had never been discussed. But because of his love of the sport and their life style of athleticism, she was sure he would not want to be a "cripple." You, as the pharmacist, are approached by the family to cease administration of antibiotics.

Case 1 Recommendation

It is difficult to know what a patient's preferences are when he can not speak for himself. Quality-of-life assessment is often made by a third party making pronouncements about someone else's quality of life. It is important to note that there is significant bias introduced here.

Studies consistently show that physicians (not to mention family members) consistently rate the quality of life of their patients lower than the patients do themselves. Rehabilitation literature abounds that documents that although the initial grief and shock of disability are profound, paraplegics, even quadriplegic patients, gradually learn to find life worthwhile and cope with the disabilities and find pleasures in life.

Case 1 Outcome

In this patient's case, he is temporarily in need of proxy decision makers but will ultimately be able to state his own patient preferences. It is appropriate to continue antibiotics until the patient is able to communicate his own preferences. Because the patient had not communicated his wishes beforehand (and because you know that people, once disabled, often accept their disability), you are able to convince the family to wait until his speech therapy is successful and he is able to communicate his wishes.

CASE 2: FAILURE TO COOPERATE WITH MEDICAL RECOMMENDATIONS AND CONTEXTUAL FEATURES OF RESOURCE ALLOCATION AND THE RISK OF CLINICIAN BIAS/DISCRIMINATION

A 45-year-old man with insulin-dependent diabetes experienced frequent episodes of ketoacidosis and hypoglycemia and traumatic and poorly healing foot ulcers. He has been noncompliant with a diabetic diet and has begun abusing alcohol after a stormy divorce. He has been hospitalized several times for diabetic and alcohol-related complications. On several admissions he was found to be eating excessively in the hospital cafeteria. His physician and pharmacist wonder if they should withdraw from the therapeutic relationship because it appeared "futile"—the patient continued to engage in behavior that posed serious risk to health and even life despite many hours of cumulative time given by clinicians regarding recommendations and consequences of his noncompliant and risky behavior. There were some who began to wonder if the patient should continue to be admitted, especially if his situation wasn't critical because his risky behavior was self-imposed and he was "wasting resources" taking up bed space that other patients who did not engage in these behaviors might be able to use that bed (case based largely on one reported by Seigler et al.[8]).

Case 2 Recommendation

In this patient's case, and in similar cases of patients who continue to engage in behaviors that result in worsening health (such as patients with emphysema who are repeatedly admitted for respiratory failure or obese patients who overeat with consequent medical complications), the situation is frustrating to healthcare providers and puts great strain on the clinician–patient relationship. It is important to determine whether and to what extent the patient is acting voluntarily or involuntarily. Some noncompliance may be secondary to emotional disturbance. If the clinician judges the noncompliance to be voluntary, efforts should be made at rational persuasion. If these fail, it is ethical for the clinician to adjust therapeutic goals and to do his or her best in the circumstance. In rare cases, it is ethically permissible to withdraw from the case after advising the patient how to obtain care from other sources. However, keep in mind that clinicians swear in their Hippocratic oath to undertake difficult tasks and even risks in the care of persons in need of medical attention. Inconvenience, frustration, provocation, and dislike are not sufficient reasons to exempt you from that duty. If contextual features such as inability to pay for medicines, inadequate housing, etc. are a source of noncooperation, help should be provided in these circumstances. If noncooperation arises from psychological pathology, the clinician has a strong ethical obligation to remain with the patient, adjusting treatment plans to the undesirable situation. Professional assistance in treating the pathology should be sought.[8] You may feel frustrated, but the frustration is not, in itself, sufficient to justify leaving the patient.

Regarding the issue of distributive justice and resource allocation (also called rationing) that was raised by the bed space argument for nonadmission, this is not a rare complaint voiced by frustrated health professionals. However, in the context of the current American medical system (which is not socialized), it is very important to avoid making rationing decisions at the bedside. The criteria for deciding good from poor uses of societal resources is impossible and inappropriate to do at the bedside. It is the kind of decision that must be made at the policy level. The overall view of social need and the contribution of particular decisions to that need are not known to clinicians. For example, there is no guarantee that whatever is "saved" by refusing this patient will be used in any better manner. Blame for "wasting resources" is better laid on the system than the patient[8].

Also, be very careful of clinician bias as far as deciding who "deserves" to be admitted. One of the important ethical tenets is that those in need should be cared for regardless of race, religion, or nationality. However, clinicians may have beliefs and values (maybe even unrecognized) against certain persons or classes of persons, and these attitudes may affect clinical decisions. The Tuskegee Syphilis Study is one example of clinicians in the US Public Health Service who thought they were doing something valuable and good for humanity in general by withholding penicillin treatment to hundreds of black men with syphilis so that they could study the evolution of syphilis despite the ready availability and known efficacy of penicillin.

The study wasn't secret. It took 40 years before the health professionals realized it was unethical, and the study was halted.

Studies have revealed that clinicians are also biased against elderly patients, termed "agism," and may chose to undertreat. Other studies have confirmed bias against gay patients, women, and those of low "social worth" (such as criminals). Singling out socially disapproved behaviors (such as overeating in patients who are obese, or repeatedly drinking alcohol in patients who may be criminals, for example) as less deserving of treatment reflects social prejudices rather than logic (for example, engaging in dangerous sports is socially tolerated, even praised, and is associated with high risk and consequences).[8]

Case Two Outcome

In this patient's case, it was determined that he was severely depressed. Psychiatric consultation was obtained. Medications and psychotherapy were begun. Over time, the patient's compliance with medical management improved significantly.

CODES OF CONDUCT IN THE PROFESSIONS AND, SPECIFICALLY, CLINICAL ETHICS

A profession is one in which one "professes" or takes an oath. The essence of professionalism is the primary concern for the welfare of those whom the professional serves over his own proprietary interests.[3]

Bernat's *Ethics in Neurology*[3] lists 10 defining characteristics of a learned profession[3]:

1. The profession possesses a circumscribed and socially valuable body of knowledge.
2. The members of the profession determine the profession's standards of knowledge and expertise.
3. The profession attracts high quality students who undergo an extensive socialization process as they are absorbed into the profession.
4. The profession is given authority to license practitioners by the state, with licensing and admission boards made up largely of members of the profession.
5. There is an ostensible sense of community and mutuality of interests among members of a profession.
6. Social policy and legislation that relate to the profession are heavily influenced by members of the profession through such mechanisms as lobbying and expert testimony.
7. The profession has a code of ethics that governs practice, the tenets of which are more stringent than legal controls.

8. A service orientation supersedes the proprietary interests of the professionals.
9. A profession is a terminal occupation; that is, it is the practitioner's singular and lifelong occupational choice.
10. A profession is largely free of lay control, with its practitioners exercising a high degree of occupational autonomy.[3]

The focus of clinical ethics is set on the duties physicians/clinicians owe to their patients. Physicians also have ethical duties toward families of patients, other physicians, and to the medical profession, to society, and in patient research.

The physician's duty to his or her patients is the cornerstone of clinical medical ethics. Application of moral rules and ethical theories is codified into practice by professional societies. The following are excerpts from the American College of Physicians *Ethics Manual.*[9] It incorporates principles of *beneficence*— duty to promote good and prevent harm to patients; *nonmaleficence*—the duty to do no harm to patients; respect for a patient's *autonomy*—the duty to protect and foster an individual's free and uncoerced choices as well as rules for *truth telling, disclosure,* and *informed consent*. It includes the basic tenets of the doctor–patient relationship. The codes of conduct would be the same for you in the pharmacy profession:

- The patient's welfare and best interests must be the physician's main concern. The physician should treat and cure when possible and help patients cope with illness, disability, and death. In all instances, the physician must help maintain the dignity of the person and respect the uniqueness of each person.
- Confidentiality is a fundamental tenant of medical care. It respects the privacy of patients, encourages them to seek medical care and to discuss their problems candidly, and prevents discrimination based on their medical condition. The physician must not release information without the patient's consent. Confidentiality, like other ethical duties is not absolute. It may have to be overridden to protect others or the public—for example to warn sexual partners that a patient has syphilis or AIDS. Before breaching confidentiality the physician should make every effort to discuss the issues with the patient and minimize harm to the patient.
- The physician is obligated to ensure that the patient is informed about the nature of the patient's medical condition, the objectives of the proposed treatment, treatment alternatives, possible outcomes, and the risks involved. This doctrine of informed consent must not be coerced.
- Lack of *decision-making capacity* can usually be determined by the physician when it has been carefully determined that the patient is incapable of understanding the nature of the proposed treatment, the alternatives, the risks and benefits, and the consequences. When a patient lacks *decision-making capacity,* an appropriate surrogate should make decisions with the physician. Ideally the surrogate decision makers should know the patient's choices and values and

act in the best interests of the patient. If the patient has designated a proxy, as through a durable power of attorney for health care, that choice should be respected. When patients have not selected surrogates, the standard clinical practice is for family members to serve as surrogates. Some states designate the order in which family members will serve as surrogates, and physicians should be aware of legal requirements in their state for surrogate appointment and decision making. Physicians should take reasonable care to assure that the surrogate's decisions are consistent with the patient's preferences. Physicians should emphasize that decisions be based on what the patient would want and not on what surrogates would choose for themselves. In order of priority, decisions should be based on advance directives (competent patients state what treatments they would accept or decline if they lost decision-making capacity) substituted judgments (the surrogate attempts to make the judgment that the patient, if competent, would have made), and best interests of the patient.

- It is unethical for a physician to refuse to care for a patient solely because of medical risk, or perceived risk, to the physician.
- Requests by patients for treatment outside the recognized methods of medical care pit the physician's judgment on optimal medical therapy against the patient's right to choose what care to receive and from whom. The physician should be sure that the patient understands the condition, traditional medical treatment, and expected outcomes. The physician should not abandon the patient who elects to try an unorthodox treatment and should regard the patient's decision with grace and compassion. In general, the physician should not participate in such treatment. When the treatment is clearly harmful to patients, the physician should seek the best means by which to protect the patient and, where possible, have dangerous therapy challenged.
- Physicians should be discouraged from treating close friends or family members. Potential problems include feelings of constraints on time or resources, incomplete disclosure of patient information, or limited physical examination.
- It is unethical for a physician to become sexually involved with a current patient even if the patient initiates or consents to the contact. Issues of dependency, trust, transference, and inequalities of power lead to increased vulnerability of the patient and require that a physician not cross the boundary.
- Financial arrangements should be clarified, and means of payment or inability to pay should be established. Fees for physician services should accurately reflect services provided. As professionals dedicated to serving the sick, physicians should contribute services to the uninsured and underinsured and do their fair share to ensure that all people receive adequate medical care.
- When conflicts of interest arise, the moral principle is clear. The welfare of the patient must at all times be paramount, and the physician must insist that the medically appropriate level of care take primacy over fiscal considerations imposed by the physician's own practice, investments, or financial arrangements. Trust in the profession is undermined when there is even the appearance of impropriety.

- Physicians should distinguish among withdrawing life-sustaining treatment, allowing the natural process of death to occur, and taking deliberate actions to shorten a patient's life. Physician involvement in deliberately hastening a patient's death has long been prohibited in professional codes. Uncontrolled pain may lead patients to request assisted suicide. Physicians should make relief of suffering in the terminally ill patient their highest priority as long as this accords to the patient's wishes. In most cases the patient will withdraw the request for assisted suicide when pain management, depression, and other concerns have been addressed.
- Physicians should obtain consultation when they feel a need for assistance in caring for the patient.
- Patient care must never be compromised because a physician's judgment or skill is impaired. Every physician is responsible for protecting patients from an impaired physician and for assisting a colleague whose professional capability is impaired.
- It is unethical for a physician to disparage the professional competence, knowledge, qualifications, or services of another physician to a patient or a third party or to state or imply that a patient has been poorly managed or mistreated by a colleague without substantial evidence, especially when such behavior is used to recruit patients. Of equal importance, it is unethical for a physician not to report fraud, professional misconduct, incompetence, or abandonment of a patient by another physician. All physicians have a duty to participate in peer review.
- Society has conferred professional prerogatives on physicians in the belief that they will use such power for the benefit of patients. In turn, physicians are responsible and accountable to society for their professional actions.
- All physicians must fulfill the profession's collective responsibility to be advocates for the health of the public.
- Decisions on resource allocations must not be made in the context of an individual patient–physician encounter but must be part of a broader social process.
- The physician should help develop health policy at the local, state, and national levels by expressing views as an individual and as a professional.
- The interests of the patient have primacy in all aspects of the patient–physician relationship. All health professionals share a commitment to work together to serve the patient's interests. The best patient care is often a team effort, and mutual respect, cooperation, and communication should govern this effort.
- Ethics committees and consultants contribute to achieving patient care goals primarily by developing educational programs in the institution coordinating institutional resources, providing a forum for discussion among medical and hospital professionals, and assisting institutions to develop sound policies and practices. Although it is generally agreed that neither ethics committees nor consultants should have decision-making authority, they can advise physicians on ethical matters.

- Physicians should remember that all citizens are equal under the law, and being ill does not diminish the right or expectation to be treated equally.
- Although physicians cannot be compelled to participate as expert witnesses, the profession as a whole has the ethical duty to assist patients and society in resolving disputes.
- It is unethical for physicians to withhold medical services through strikes when patients will be harmed or when the strike is for the physician's benefit.
- Advances in the diagnosis and treatment of disease are based on well-designed, carefully controlled, and ethically conducted clinical studies. Subjects must be equitably selected and instructed concerning the nature of the research; consent from the subject or an authorized representative must be truly informed and given freely; research must be planned thoughtfully, so that it has a high probability of yielding significant results; risks to patients must be minimized; and the benefit/risk ratio must be sufficiently high to justify the research effort.
- When there is no precedent for innovative therapy, consultation with peers, an institutional review board, or other expert group is necessary to assess whether the innovation is in the patient's best interest, the risks of the innovation, and probable outcomes of not using a standard therapy.[9]

Notice within the codes of conduct, the physician also has some ethical duties beyond the patient, including to the patient's family, to the medical profession, to society, and in patient research. The patient's family is often a partner in patient care. Duties to other physicians and to the medical profession include teaching other clinicians as well as the patients and participation in peer-reviewed activities to protect patients from impaired and incompetent physicians. Duties to society include protecting the safety of the general public. This may even override the very important oath of confidentiality. The President's Commission for the Study of Ethical Problems in Medicine and Biomedical and Behavioral Research stipulated five conditions for which a physician may override his ordinary ethical duty to maintain the confidentiality of a patient's clinical information[3]:

1. Reasonable efforts to elicit voluntary consent to disclosure have failed.
2. There is a high probability that harm would occur if the information is withheld.
3. There is a high probability that the disclosed information would avert that harm.
4. There is a high probability that the harm inflicted on the third party would be serious.
5. Appropriate precautions would be taken to ensure that the only information conveyed is that necessary to avert the harm.

Duties to society require physicians to promote measures to improve the public health of all citizens. The physician who conducts clinical research should have the research be critiqued and approved by institutional review boards to safeguard patient/subject safety.[3]

CONCLUSION: THE DOCTOR/CLINICIAN–PATIENT RELATIONSHIP IS THE CORE OF CLINICAL ETHICS

The doctor/clinician–patient relationship is at the core of clinical ethics. Dr. Mark Siegler published an article entitled "Falling off the Pedestal: What is Happening to the Traditional Doctor–Patient Relationship?" in *Mayo Clinic Proceedings* in 1993[10] in which he described the Doctor–Patient Accommodation Model that respected the autonomy of both patients and physicians. This model is a shared decision-making model in which both physicians and patients make active and essential contributions. Physicians bring their medical training, knowledge, and expertise, including an understanding of the available treatment alternatives, to the diagnosis and management of the patient's conditions. Patients bring their own subjective aims and values through which the risks and benefits of various treatment options can be evaluated. The Doctor–Patient Accommodation Model relies heavily on communication, discussion, and negotiation. It incorporates Plato's description of "medicine befitting free men" (in Plato's "The Laws"). Plato wrote that the citizen physician "treats a disease by going into things thoroughly from the beginning in a scientific way and takes the patient and his family into confidence. Thus, he learns something from the sufferers. . . . He does not give prescriptions until he has won the patient's support, and when he has done so, he steadily aims at producing complete restoration to health by persuading the sufferer into compliance."[10]

You, as a practicing pharmacist in the outpatient or inpatient setting, make clinical decisions every day. After reading this chapter it is hoped that you now recognize that ethical decision making is involved in every clinical interaction you have with patients. As clinicians with the best intentions of "doing the right thing," you can refer to your professional society, which has codes of conduct, and the legal system, which has statutes and laws, but the core of how to decide what is ethically acceptable and not acceptable is found within yourself, vigilantly keeping in mind the duties and biases you bring to the clinician/doctor–patient relationship. If in the course of clinical decision making you encounter situations in which you find yourself trying to sort out which course of action would have acceptable ethical grounding, this chapter was incorporated into this book to help you think these situations through as thoroughly as possible. Use the information from this chapter. Remember the history of events that led to the development of the field of clinical ethics. Remember the four biomedical principles (*autonomy, beneficence, nonmaleficence,* and *justice*). Then apply the "four boxes" clinical ethics analysis method of Siegler et al. (*medical indications, patient preferences, quality of life, and contextual features*) to assist yourself in identifying, analyzing, and resolving ethical issues in your clinical case.

QUESTIONS

1. In Siegler's four boxes of clinical medical ethics decision making, the four are not weighted equally. Which two "trump" the other two?
2. If conflicts of interest arise, what is the overriding moral principal?
3. What are the four bioethics principles?
4. What are Siegler's four boxes in clinical medical ethics decision making?
5. What is the core of clinical medical ethics?

Answers

1. Medical indications and patient preferences.
2. When conflicts of interest arise, the moral principle is clear. The welfare of the patient must at all times be paramount, and the clinician must insist that the medically appropriate level of care take primacy over fiscal considerations imposed by the clinician's own practice, investments, or financial arrangements. Trust in the profession is undermined when there is even the appearance of impropriety.
3. Autonomy, beneficence, nonmaleficence, justice.
4. Medical indications, patient preferences, quality of life, contextual features.
5. The doctor/clinician–patient relationship is the core of clinical ethics.

REFERENCES

1. Shuster E. The Nuremberg Code; Hippocratic ethics and human rights. Lancet 1998;1351:974–977.
2. Miles S. Translations of the oath. Presentation at University of Chicago McLean Center for Clinical Medical Ethics Conference. November 2001.
3. Bernat JL. Ethical Issues in Neurology. Boston: Butterworth-Heinemann, 1994.
4. Wolinsky H. Steps still being taken to undo damage of "America's Nuremberg." Ann Intern Med 1997;127(4):I43–I44.
5. The National Commission for the Protection of Human Subjects of Biomedical and Behavioral Research. The Belmont Report: Ethical principles and guidelines for the protection of human subjects of research. OPRR Reports. Washington: US Government Printing Office, 1978;1–8.
6. Beauchamp TL, Childress JF. Principles of Biomedical Ethics, 3rd ed. New York: Oxford University Press, 1989.

7. Siegler M. Communication during his address to the University of Chicago McLean Center for Clinical Medical Ethics Conference. November 2001.
8. Jonsen A., Siegler M, Winslade W. Clinical Ethics: A Practical Approach to Ethical Decisions in Clinical Medicine, 4th ed. New York: McGraw-Hill, 1998.
9. American College of Physicians. Ethics Manual, 3rd ed. Ann Intern Med 1992;117:947–960.
10. Siegler M. Falling off the pedestal: what is happening to the traditional doctor–patient relationship? Mayo Clin Proc 1993;68:461–467.

C H A P T E R 3

THE BASICS OF COMMUNICATION: AN OVERVIEW

Michelle Assa

Goals: After reviewing the information in this chapter, you should be able to:

1. Articulate the importance of communication skills.
2. Explain the process of communication including the types of messages (verbal or nonverbal), barriers, and the participants' backgrounds.
3. Discuss types of listening behaviors and appropriate responses.
4. Describe how to conduct an efficient, effective patient interview.
5. Use assertiveness to deal with difficult situations.
6. Explain the dimensions of nonverbal communication.
7. Structure written communication effectively.

INTRODUCTION

Contrary to many peoples' understanding, communicating with someone is far from "just talking" to him. In fact, people may hold several false assumptions regarding communication. For one, many people assume that when children learn to talk, they also learn to communicate well. Another is that communication competence is something inherent in one's personality, that one can naturally communicate well or not well at all. Both of these are generally misconceptions.

At some point, communication skills become very important to a person's success in his or her chosen profession. For you, that is happening now. As you learn how to be a pharmacist, you must also learn to evaluate your communication skills and to improve them where necessary. Personality is a factor in communication style, but people can learn to be better communicators. And, although there are requisite skills to master, you should definitely be yourself when you are talking with others, especially in a professional setting. People can pick up on whether or not you are sincere. Trying to fake an interest in someone else's life is usually transparent. When patients recognize this lack of interest, they are unlikely to cooperate with you or provide you with the information that you need. As a pharmacist you will be interacting will people from many different backgrounds, all in the same day. You may have to talk to physicians and nurses more than patients or vice versa, depending on your chosen practice site. This chapter reviews techniques you can use to work with health care providers, patients, or your employers/employees. The chapter maintains a focus on interactions with patients and patient-interviewing skills because patient interaction is one of the most significant types of communication for pharmacists. After a discussion of the importance of communication skills and a review of a model of communication, sections in this chapter are devoted to oral communication, barriers to communication, nonverbal communication, patient interviewing, education, and, finally, written communication. You, too, can be an effective communicator even if you do not feel confident in your abilities right now. Some of you may feel you already know everything you need to know. Because applying communication techniques in a pharmacy is different than in social settings, it is likely that you will pick up a few good ideas in this chapter to help you develop professionally. As you read, try to leave your assumptions aside and envision how you can incorporate these skills into your daily communication, whether professionally or socially.

IMPORTANCE OF COMMUNICATION SKILLS

Communication skills are crucial to helping you develop your practice. Your position as a pharmacist will require you to communicate well verbally with healthcare professionals and with patients. Writing skills are equally important as presenting a professional image with your oral communication. This section discusses the significance of fostering your good communication skills for yourself, your patients, and the healthcare professionals with whom you work.

Early communication research[1] has shown that communication skills play an important role in career advancement. The skills that were identified as crucial included speaking, listening, and working well with groups. You may benefit in your career by improving your communication skills; however, your patients will also benefit. As Ley[2] describes, improving healthcare provider communication has been shown to have several positive outcomes for patients. Specifically, better communication with healthcare providers leads to a higher level of patient recall of information. This improvement in recall can help patients better manage their medications and their disease state. Further, enhanced communication has been found to be associated with patient satisfaction. Although this may seem trivial, patient satisfaction plays a large role in a patient's decision to return to a healthcare provider and in the trust they place in that provider. Improved communication with providers can also have a moderate effect on patients' compliance with their medication regimens. Finally, communication has been shown to reduce the length of hospital stays for some patients. Clearly, there are advantages for patients when their providers have become skillful in the art of communication.

Other healthcare providers may benefit from your improved communication because they will be better able to learn from you. Having a pharmacist as part of the healthcare team can prove to be extremely valuable for all of the professionals involved. Yet, a pharmacist who is unable to make her points heard and understood will not be an effective member of the team. Conversely, a pharmacist with good communication skills can make valuable contributions to the team. More importantly, these contributions can be made without creating tension among other professionals who may not fully understand the pharmacist's newly expanded role.

Whether the improvement in your skills makes an impact on patients or other professionals, the benefits of a well-communicating pharmacist are immeasurable. In order to understand the factors that make up an interaction and the skills necessary to make sure those interactions go smoothly, we now turn to an exploration of a model of communication. By investigating these factors, you become better able to recognize the important points of communication that will help you develop your own approach.

MODEL OF COMMUNICATION

Many researchers have investigated the nature of human communication. Since the inception of the field of study, people have tried to explain and label the components associated with communication. Thus, there are many models of communication. A model attempts to explain a phenomenon and lend a structure to an otherwise amorphous concept. Models help us better understand such concepts by allowing us to test the premises of the models and build on them. Even the earliest communication researchers developed models to guide their study.

Many factors can influence the process of communication. Think about the last time you had a conversation with a close friend. You probably paid close attention to the way he or she responded to you, both verbally and nonverbally. But what you may not have considered are all the background factors that go in to your interpretation of other people's behavior and their interpretation of yours. Your experience with them, your experiences with communicating with other people, your personality, your beliefs in general, your beliefs about the interaction you are having, and your desired outcome all affect the way you interact with a friend. Although each of these factors is important, not all models of communication include them. Early models took a more simplistic view of the process. Let's briefly review the history of these models and their contributions to a more inclusive one.

Several models such as the SMCR model,[3] the Shannon-Weaver model,[4] and the transaction model[5] offer good insight into the communication process. As Northouse and Northouse[6] explain, the Shannon-Weaver model[4] illustrates the flow of a message from its source to its receiver. According to this model, a message is transmitted as a signal from an information source through a receiver in order to reach its destination. Central to this model is that the signal being transmitted is subject to interference, or "noise," as it is labeled in the model. Noise may represent any type of barrier including background noise or a personal barrier one of the participants may have. On the other hand, one of the disadvantages of this model is the fact that it is linear; messages flow in only one direction, from the source to the destination.

In contrast to the Shannon-Weaver model, the SMCR model does not attempt to illustrate the flow of messages. Rather, it suggests that a *source,* based on his or her knowledge, communication skills, attitudes, social system, and culture, formulates a *message.* This message has unique components and dimensions and is conveyed via one or more *channels.* Potential channels include any of the five senses: seeing, hearing, touching, smelling, or tasting. Finally, the message, traveling through the channels, reaches the *receiver.* Just as the source formulates the message based on a number of personal factors, so does the receiver interpret the message according to those personal factors. This model exemplifies the complexity of each of the components of communication, yet it does not illustrate the flow of messages.

The important contribution of the transaction model[5] is the premise that messages flow both ways. Although the model is a simple one, it was this model that originally suggested a more dynamic explanation of the stream of messages. A more complete description of these models in addition to diagrams can be found in the references provided. In our discussion of a model, let us consider the model illustrated in Fig. 3.1. This model, adapted from those listed above, incorporates many of the positive aspects of each of the previous models. Communication models often label one person the "sender" and one the "receiver" of messages

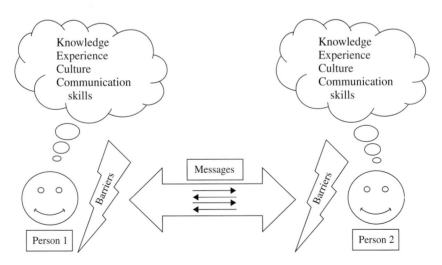

Figure 3.1. Integrated model of communication.

for simplicity. In truth, based on the transactional perspective described by Wilmot,[5] both parties simultaneously send and receive messages, whether verbal or nonverbal. Throughout the course of a conversation, the parties may take turns sending verbal messages but are likely to be communicating even without an oral message during the entire exchange. Thus, in our model, the two participants are labeled "person 1" and "person 2."

From the SMCR model, we know that both people bring to the interaction their past experiences with each other and with other people. It is impossible to separate a person's background from the way he or she will perceive a message. Thus, two people's cultures, including the rules of interaction that they share, will shape their interactions. For example, in some cultures it is considered rude to interrupt when another person is talking. Yet, in other cultures, the person who talks the loudest over the other is the one who is given the floor. You can see how this may impact the way one talks to another person. For further reading on cultural differences in communication, see the additional reading list in Appendix B. Other examples of factors that may influence how a person interacts include his knowledge in the area being discussed as well as his communication skills. You can imagine a situation in which a pharmacist is sharing information with a physician regarding a new prescription medication. Because the pharmacist has a great deal of knowledge about the topic, she is going to be doing more of the talking. The interaction between pharmacist and physician is also going to be affected by the pharmacist's communication skills. Perhaps the physician is not interested in learning about the new dosing regimen. However, with sufficient skill, the pharmacist may be able to underscore the importance of appropriate prescribing and teach the physician what he needs to know.

Notice that, in the integrated model depicted in Fig 3.1, messages are flowing back and forth between the two people at the same time. These may be verbal or nonverbal messages. For example, nonverbal messages may be sent via facial expressions while the other person is speaking. Further, although the model appears linear, communication is in fact a dynamic process. Each interaction helps frame the next. Each interaction provides the participants with experience from which to base expectations regarding future interactions. Finally, notice that messages are subject to barriers that may inhibit their transmission. Barriers may include preconceived ideas about the message, physical barriers such as a high counter, or noise in the area preventing the message from being heard. A further discussion of potential barriers to communication is presented in the next section.

POTENTIAL BARRIERS TO PHARMACIST'S COMMUNICATION

Much research has been conducted on the barriers to pharmacists' communication with patients, especially in the retail setting.[7-9] Pharmacy environment, as well as barriers that were pharmacist-related, patient-related, informational/philosophical, and miscellaneous have been addressed.

Herrier and Boyce[9] offer the most comprehensive evidence with results from workshops with nearly 30,000 pharmacists. Participating pharmacists were asked to identify barriers to patient counseling at their practice sites. Common themes emerged in the discussions. Barriers in the pharmacy environment may include the store layout, lack of privacy, workload issues, and a lack of reimbursement for the counseling services. Pharmacists' personal barriers to provision of counseling services in the community setting may include their feelings of competence and their willingness to communicate. Pharmacist-related barriers included lack of formal education in patient counseling or lack of knowledge about the prescribed drug or poor counseling skills.

Patient-related barriers were most frequently identified as the patient being in a hurry or uninterested in receiving information about the medication. Philosophical or information barriers were related to pharmacists' questioning of their abilities to affect patient outcomes through counseling activities. Finally, miscellaneous barriers include concerns over liability and lack of reimbursement as barriers to providing counseling services.

In practice, as in the model of communication, these barriers prove to be a challenge for pharmacists who hope to establish and maintain good communication with their patients in the retail setting. Other practice settings may share similar barriers, or other issues may create problems. Overcoming these barriers is essential to ensuring that your messages are received and understood by the receiver. Now, let's further explore the types of messages that can be sent from one person to another including both verbal and nonverbal messages.

ORAL COMMUNICATION SKILLS

As we can see from the model of communication, there are many components to an interaction with another person. In order to have an interaction, we must be able to act as senders and receivers of messages. In this section, skills necessary to accomplish that end are reviewed. They include listening, responding, phrasing questions, and assertiveness. There are many equally valuable skills that are also necessary in communicating verbally. We focus here on the crucial skills for pharmacist-related interactions.

Listening

The best way to show your commitment to developing and maintaining relationships with those you work with, whether patients or colleagues, is to listen to them. Listening, like communication in general, does not come naturally to some people. The first step in listening is to stop talking. However, being quiet is not sufficient to qualify you as listening. In order to listen to someone, you must have an environment that is conducive to the interaction. Both nonverbal and oral communication can give someone the impression that you are in fact listening to them. Central to this idea is that you should not be distracted when you are listening to someone. In a busy pharmacy, it can be difficult to stop all tasks in order to listen to a patient, but unless the patient has your undivided attention, you will have a difficult time understanding them. It is imperative that you find a quiet place with some degree of privacy in order to consult with patients. Even in the busiest of pharmacies, there is likely to be a corner of the store that has less traffic and can be used for consultation. Having a private area enables you to listen better and also provides the patient with the sense that he/she is not opening themselves up to the general public when discussing a concern with you.

When listening to another person, one must attempt to truly understand her point of view and then convey that understanding to her. Several methods exist for demonstrating that understanding. By responding to the person in a manner that demonstrates that understanding, you are communicating that you have in fact heard what she has to say. At times, health care professionals do not respond to patients in the most appropriate ways. It is common to want to solve problems or to want to tell people how to handle their situations.

For example, consider Mr. Nodough, a patient who is picking up a prescription at the pharmacy. During the exchange, he says, "these prescription prices are so high. The pharmacist must be making a mint." As Tindall et al.[10] describe, many types of potential responses are possible, yet few will have the desired effect. We briefly review less effective response strategies and then discuss better ways to demonstrate that you have heard and understood Mr. Nodough.

Types of Responses

Judging

A judging response is made when one tells someone that he should not have the feelings he does about a particular situation. Alternatively, a judging response may also tell someone that he should feel a certain way. A judging response to Mr. Nodough might be "you shouldn't complain. These medications are helping to keep you healthy." Judging responses are not effective because they invalidate a person's feelings. This may in turn discourage him from sharing his feelings with you in the future.

Reassuring

Another type of response that is less desirable is a reassuring response. "Don't worry about it; I'm sure you'll manage to figure out something" is an example of a reassuring response. Like the judging response, it tends to invalidate the feelings a person is having. Although given with the best intentions of making someone feel better; a reassuring response is not usually helpful. It is unlikely that you are truly able to know how things will work out. Therefore, by suggesting that everything will be all right, you are offering false reassurance. This type of response is often given when one is unsure how to respond. In that situation, it is usually better to respond empathically, which will be discussed shortly.

Probing

A third type of common response is the probing response. Probing responses are usually in the form of a question designed to elicit additional information. Although probing questions do have their place in a patient interview, a probing response to a situation where a patient may be upset is not the best option. In keeping with the example above, a probing response to the patient may be "how much money do you spend on prescriptions each month?" This response does not address the patient's main concerns about the cost of his medication. Rather, it redirects the interaction. Healthcare professionals often use this response in an attempt to help the patient solve the problem at hand. Although well intentioned, this type of response does not give the patient the satisfaction of feeling understood. In gathering information, a probing question is helpful, but when you are trying to convey that you are listening to someone, it falls short.

Generalizing

A generalizing response is one that, as the name suggests, generalizes what the patient may be feeling. Examples may include global statements such as "everyone feels that way sometimes" to more specific examples such as "I feel the same way when I get a prescription filled." This type of response takes the focus away from the patient. Although many people think this is helpful because it lets the patient know that she is not alone, the problem with this type of response is that you cannot know exactly what the patient's situation is or how the patient is feeling. In addition to shifting the focus from the patient to you in the case of the latter response, some may feel that this type of response trivializes their feelings.

Distracting

A distracting response is a response that does not acknowledge what the patient has said. It may be as drastic as a complete change of subject. In response to Mr. Nodough, a pharmacist who says, "Well, your prescription is ready now," is distracting the patient from his initial feelings and comments. Like the other responses discussed here, this type does little to convey that you care about the patient and his feelings. Often this type of response is used when one has difficulty dealing with the subject matter at hand or does not feel comfortable exploring the issue at hand. Again, an empathic response is most likely to make the patient feel at ease and understood.

Advising

This type of response suggests what a person should do. For example, the pharmacist may say, "You should find a better health insurance company; one that covers prescriptions." As healthcare professionals, many times pharmacists cannot help but offer advice. After all, that is part of their job. However, unless there is something you can do to directly solve the problem, you should refrain from advising responses. You may find that offering alternatives is a way of helping the patient identify his own solution. Often there is little, if anything, you can do to solve the patient's problem, but conveying that you have heard and understood it can go a long way in helping him or her feel better.

Understanding

As the name implies, this type of response allows a person to convey his understanding of a message. This can also be considered a response in which paraphrasing is used. An understanding response to Mr. Nodough may be, "I understand you feel the prescription prices are too high." The pharmacist is paraphrasing what the patient has already said in order to demonstrate understanding of the patient's statement. This can be a helpful tool. In fact, it is essential that you understand the message you are attempting to receive. Therefore, if clarification is necessary, you will be sure to get it. This type of response can help minimize misunderstandings.

In practice, this type of response should be used with caution. You may not completely understand the patient's concern or situation, and implying that you do may make the patient feel uncomfortable. Like the generalizing response, although you may have had similar experiences, you will never be able to fully appreciate the patient's experience. To say you understand or to suggest that you do may offend some people.

Empathy

An empathic response goes beyond an understanding response to address the feelings that underlie a statement. This type of response demonstrates not only that you heard and understood what the person said but also that you recognize the emotions that led her to say what she did. To Mr. Nodough, a pharmacist may say, "It must be very frustrating trying to pay for all your prescriptions and other costs of living." This pharmacist acknowledges that she has heard Mr. Nodough's concern and also that she understands how this makes Mr. Nodough feel.

Empathy is a useful tool. It can be most helpful when you may feel that you do not know what to say or that you cannot do anything to help the person. By recognizing and responding to the feelings the person has, you are demonstrating true listening and also caring. It is important to note that empathy is difficult if not impossible to fake. People can easily see through a false attempt at empathy and are likely to respond negatively to it. Unless you are genuine in your willingness to understand and relate to another person, empathy will be difficult to master.

In most cases, an empathic response is a beginning to a dialogue. It is not the only thing you will say to the patient. However, as you first recognize their feelings and demonstrate your understanding, the patient will be reassured of your sincere caring about his or her concern. This will help you foster a helping relationship with the patient and will encourage him to begin a further discussion of the issue. At that point, you may be able to offer additional assistance. For Mr. Nodough, you may be able to suggest financial assistance programs or equivalent medications at a lower cost. If nothing else, you will have made Mr. Nodough feel that you have heard his concern.

Listening to patients and responding empathically to their concerns are both important skills to master. In order to elicit information from them, however, you will need to initiate a dialogue. To do this, appropriate phrasing of questions is essential. The next section focuses on this skill.

Phrasing Questions

The way a question is phrased impacts the amount and type of information one receives in response. A closed-ended question, for example, is a question that is phrased to elicit a "yes" or "no" response. One example of a closed-ended question is "Are you taking your medication as prescribed?" The patient responding to this question may either say "yes" or "no" but is unlikely to provide any additional information. Closed-ended questions are useful in a patient interview when you are following up on information you already have. There are times when a closed-ended question is appropriate, such as when probing for additional information or when you need to have something confirmed. An example of this may be when you check your understanding of information a patient has provided. You might say, "Is it correct that you experience headaches 1 hour after taking your blood pressure medication?" This will tell you if you are right; however, if you are looking for additional information about the type of headache the patient has, you are likely to learn more from an answer to a question that encourages the respondent to elaborate. Contrast this style of question with an open-ended one.

An open-ended question is a question that allows the person responding to elaborate on the topic. This is particularly useful when you are beginning an interview and would like to get as much information as possible. One way to phrase an open-ended question is to begin with the word "how." For example, "How are you taking your medication?" provides a patient with the opportunity to talk about his response to a medication. When asking patients open-ended questions, one should avoid beginning with the word "why." For example, asking a patient "Why isn't your medication working for you?" may put her on the defensive. The patient may feel that you are accusing her of improper use of the medication or suggesting that she is in some way at fault for the ineffectiveness of the medication. There are times when it is appropriate to use the word "why"; however, it should be used cautiously. It can be used in combination with other key phrases such as in the case of the question, "Why do you think you are forgetting to take your medication?" In this example, the pharmacist is eliciting the patient's opinion rather than challenging her.

To follow open-ended questions, probing questions can be used. A probing question helps you gather detailed information along the lines of the open-ended question. Often, these are closed-ended questions, yet they can also be open-ended. Consider a situation in which a patient shares with his pharmacist that he has been having difficulty adhering to a medication regimen. He further offers that when he does take his medication properly, he suffers from stomach discomfort. The pharmacist agrees that the stomach problems may be caused by the medication but knows they may also be related to the patient's ulcer. The pharmacist also knows that if the patient takes the medication with food, the stomach discomfort will likely dissipate if it is caused by the medication. In this case, a closed-ended probing question may be "Are you taking the medication with food?" An example of an open-ended probing question may be "Would you describe the discomfort you've experienced?" Both of these questions are probing questions because they both search for additional information based on what the patient has already said. Both will enable the pharmacist to gather the additional information that is needed to make a recommendation for this patient.

One type of question that is common among healthcare professionals but is best to avoid is the leading question. A leading question is phrased such that it prompts a patient to answer a certain way. Healthcare professionals use these questions, often inadvertently, because they have an idea in mind about what the patient is experiencing. For example, when a pharmacist says, "You're having a hard time sticking with the medication because of the side effects, aren't you?" to a patient who is late for a refill, she is using a leading question. Although there are many other reasons the patient may be late picking up the refill from the pharmacy, the pharmacist has made an assumption about the patient's situation.

In another example, when a pharmacy technician says to a patient, "You don't have any questions for the pharmacist, do you?" he implies that the patient should say that she does not in fact have any questions for the pharmacist. Contrast this with the following way of phrasing the same question. If the pharmacy technician were to say, "Would you like to ask the pharmacist any questions?" the patient is likely to perceive that he or she does have the option of speaking with the pharmacist. It is of particular significance to avoid leading questions when discussing sensitive subjects such as noncompliance. Consider the following example.

Pharmacist Dexter is speaking with Mrs. Green about her untimely refill of an antihypertensive prescription. In the course of the conversation, Pharmacist Dexter says, "Well, it's not that you can't afford these medications, is it?" Mrs. Green, obviously flustered, responds by saying "No, no, of course not. . . . I guess I'm just forgetful." Although the pharmacist may feel he was asking Mrs. Green if she had financial concerns about her medication, Mrs. Green perceived the question as judgmental and was unable to respond truthfully. Had the pharmacist phrased the question differently, such as "Is it sometimes difficult to pay for the medications all at once?" perhaps Mrs. Green would have felt more comfortable discussing her financial situation with him. This would have allowed the pharmacist to potentially solve the problem of noncompliance by working out a payment schedule for Mrs. Green or by recommending another less expensive therapeutic option to the physician.

In summary, it is generally best to begin by asking open-ended questions. This will enable the person to elaborate on the issue at hand and will give you insight into her perspective. Following up on the answers with closed-ended questions can help you pinpoint specific information you need or help you better understand the other person's view. Finally, it is better not to phrase questions in a leading manner to ensure that you truly understand their perspective.

Dealing with Difficult Situations: Assertiveness

Often you will be faced with situations in which people are being difficult. Examples may include a situation in which a patient is upset with something that has happened at the pharmacy, an employee is unhappy with an administrative decision, or a physician chooses to debate a suggestion you have made regarding medication therapy. In each of these cases, in order to keep the situation from escalating into an argument, depending on your personality, you may want to concede your point and allow the other person to have his or her way. In the extreme, this would be considered passive behavior. Although passive behavior is effective in avoiding conflict, it can create other problems by leaving situations unresolved or poorly resolved. Some people may choose to handle the situation by fueling it and allowing it to escalate. This type of behavior would be considered aggressive. A mature, professional approach would be to handle these situations and others like them with assertiveness. Assertiveness allows you to maintain your position without responding aggressively to a situation. The following techniques can help you develop ways to respond assertively. Tindall et al.[10] offer a strong explanation of the following techniques. Here, we briefly summarize each.

Fogging

Fogging is a technique with which you acknowledge the truth about a statement yet ignore the implicit value judgment contained within it. For example, a physician who is unfamiliar with the clinical role pharmacists can play on the health-care team says, "In attempting to manage a patient's medications, you pharmacists are crossing the line!" Your response to him may be "Yes, clinical pharmacists are expanding the boundaries of their practices." With this response, you are acknowledging the truth of the physician's comments in that pharmacy has a newly expanded role. What you are not acknowledging, however, is the underlying suggestion that pharmacists are impinging on the physician's role and that they should not participate in the management of a patient's medication therapy.

Acknowledging the Truth

Another technique is acknowledging the truth in a criticism. When someone confronts you with a criticism or a complaint, the natural tendency is to try to explain why you did what you did. This can sound defensive and may escalate the situation. For example, if a patient complains about the long wait for her prescription, you could respond by explaining that each prescription is processed in the order it was received and that there are several steps involved in filling a prescription. However, it is unlikely that the patient is interested in learning about the processing of a prescription. Rather, she is frustrated by the length of time it will take her to complete her task of picking up the prescription. By acknowledging that the wait is long, you are demonstrating that you understand her concern, but you are neither apologizing for it nor making excuses. In apologizing for the wait, you are behaving less assertively in your attempt to avoid a conflict with this patient. If you begin to explain to the patient the entire process for accurately and safely filling a prescription in an attempt to justify your position, it will appear that you are becoming defensive about the situation. This would illustrate a more aggressive response to the patient.

The truth of the matter is that the patient may have to wait a long time for her prescription. In responding to her, acknowledging the truth of the situation will be beneficial. The patient will notice that you are not attempting to disagree with her or change her mind about her perception of the situation. She will also notice that you are not going to be able to do anything to change the situation.

Disagreeing with Criticism

In contrast to those times when a criticism is valid, when you are confronted with criticism that is unfounded, it is equally important to disagree with it. For example, your employer observes an interaction with a patient in which perhaps you did not provide the patient with all the information he needed and mentions to you that you "never give patients enough time." The implication that you are not practicing pharmacy at the level required by your employer is implicit in her comment to you. If this criticism is untrue or unfounded, it is best to address it immediately. Using an aggressive response is not recommended. However, when you do acknowledge that you did not spend sufficient time with a particular patient, it is appropriate to identify it as an isolated incident rather than a general pattern of behavior. For example, you may say, "You're right. I didn't spend enough time with Mr. Quinn today. I usually take much more time with my patients." In making it clear to your employer that you disagree with her general characterization, you are responding assertively.

Broken Record Technique

A technique that has many applications is the broken record technique in which your response does not change as long as the person with whom you are speaking repeats the same request. Consider a situation in which a physician wishes to prescribe a medication for a hospitalized patient that is not on that hospital's formulary. It may be the pharmacist's responsibility to review the physician's request and make a decision regarding that prescription. If, in the pharmacist's best professional judgment, that nonformulary medication is not necessary, she may experience resistance from the physician in accepting that decision. In this situation, the pharmacist might respond to the physician by saying, "In my professional judgment, this situation does not call for a nonformulary medication; there are sufficient therapeutic choices on the formulary." For each argument made by the physician, the pharmacist using the broken record technique will respond again that the nonformulary medication is not called for in her professional judgment.

This type of response can be difficult to employ when the other party responds aggressively. With this response, you are merely stating your position; not attempting to escalate the interaction into an argument. Neither are you conceding your point and allowing the physician, in this case, to declare victory. It may be frustrating for the physician to continue to discuss the issue with the pharmacist because it will become clear that she has no intention of changing her mind.

Getting Useful Feedback

When you find that a criticism is vague, it is best to get useful feedback in order to understand the nature of the criticism. For example, if your preceptor tells you that you "don't know how to practice pharmacy," it would be easy to become upset and disregard the comment entirely. However, the preceptor probably has something in mind that he would like you to master. By asking the preceptor, "What specifically do I need to work on?" you will get the precise information you need. You may discover that you made an error on a prescription and that you will need to be more careful with your work. You can then utilize one of the other assertive response techniques to deal with the situation. However, without an understanding of the true concerns the preceptor has, you would be unable to respond to the situation in an assertive way. Another situation where this technique would be helpful may occur if a patient accuses a pharmacist of not responding to his concerns. The pharmacist would be better able to respond if she knew what had happened to make the patient feel that way.

Delaying a Response

On occasion, you may find that someone pressures you for a response. In general, the assertive response to this situation is to delay a reply until you have had sufficient time to ponder your answer. For example, consider a situation in which a physician demands to know why you recommended a particular medication for a patient. If you do not have that patient's chart readily available or do not recall the specific situation to which the physician is referring, how can you respond? You could agree to change your recommendation to the physician's choice, yet that would be seen as passive. On the other hand, an assertive response may be to tell him that you will review your notes and meet with him at a later time to discuss the patient's medication therapy. In contrast to passive behavior, which may include bowing to the physician's authority and making the therapeutic change he requests, this assertive technique helps avoid an escalating conflict with the physician as well as giving you the time you need to prepare to have the discussion with him.

In summary, assertive responses, such as the types reviewed in this section are useful in many situations. With practice, they will come naturally to you and not feel so awkward. Being assertive allows you to avoid conflict and at the same time hold your position. This section of the chapter has reviewed basic verbal communication skills including listening, responding, phrasing of questions, and assertiveness. These skills can be used to overcome many barriers to communication, both personal and environmental. We move now to a discussion of nonverbal communication skills. As we have seen from the model of communication, these too can play a dramatic role in the way messages are sent and perceived.

NONVERBAL COMMUNICATION SKILLS

In addition to specific oral questioning techniques, nonverbal cues help people interpret the meaning behind your words. Whether you are aware of it or not, people routinely consider the words they hear within the context of the accompanying nonverbal communication. Nonverbal communication can be defined as a message or messages that are conveyed without using language. It includes everything from the way you stand to the maintenance of eye contact as you are talking to someone. Sometimes nonverbal communication can give someone an impression about the message you are trying to send that is incongruent with your intentions. For example, consider a pharmacist in a busy community pharmacy asking a patient if he has any questions while she is simultaneously typing something in the computer and speaking on the telephone. That pharmacist is likely to convey the message that she is too busy to talk to the patient rather than the message that she is sincerely interested in talking to the patient and answering his questions. A similar situation exists when a pharmacist enters a hospital room to conduct discharge counseling, stands near the doorway, and rushes through the information being presented. This pharmacist is likely to give the patient the impression that she is too busy to review the medications the patient will be taking home with him. Consider the same scenario when the pharmacist comes into the room, sits by the bed, and reviews each medication thoroughly with the patient. The nonverbal act of sitting down gives the patient the impression that the pharmacist is there as long as she needs to be. An important point to remember is that if there is incongruence between verbal and nonverbal messages, it is the nonverbal cues that are taken as a true reflection of the person's feelings, so pay attention to keeping your nonverbal and verbal signals congruent!

The best way to convey, nonverbally, that you are interested in a patient, or anyone else, and what he is trying to tell you is to face him. Whether you are sitting or standing, unless you are facing the patient and making eye contact, he is likely to perceive you as uninterested in what he is saying. Next, be aware of your arms. Keeping your arms crossed in front of you, folded across your chest, suggests a closed posture. This does not invite patients to share with you; rather, it is telling them that you are either upset or preoccupied and are uninterested in their information. It is also helpful to lean slightly in toward the patient while maintaining relaxed, steady eye contact. When the person is speaking, you may nod your head to indicate that you are paying attention and hearing what is being said. This can also encourage him to continue speaking. This subtly conveys that you are listening and that you care. This technique, when used properly with appropriate verbal techniques, will help you establish a good relationship with patients. It will help patients feel more at ease with you and will ultimately make your job easier by allowing you to find out the crucial information you need. Specific nonverbal cues may be based on kinesics, proxemics, chronemis, or haptics. Each of these is discussed briefly.

Kinesics

Kinesics is the method by which messages are conveyed through one's posture. The way one holds one's body sends a message to others with whom we are interacting. Think about going for a job interview. During that interview, you sit straight in the chair and keep you hands folded in your lap. This will generally present a professional, mature image to your prospective employer. Contrast this with a person who slouches down in the chair and is tapping her foot throughout the interview. It is possible that the sloucher is nervous about the interview, but the message that she is sending is that she is not interested in obtaining the position. Another example is the position of your arms. Keeping your arms crossed in front of your body suggests that you are not open to hearing another person's ideas. This is definitely a position to avoid when trying to engage in a dialogue. In your interactions with patients, giving them the impression that your attention is elsewhere can be easy with kinesics. By maintaining eye contact, ceasing other tasks, and maintaining a relaxed but professional posture, you will be sending the desired message of interest and concern for the patient.

Proxemics

Proxemics refers to the messages that are conveyed by the use of space and distance. Usually, different types of communication occur at different distances. A message that is sent to another person from very far away is likely to be a public one because it is one that the sender will have to shout. One example of such a message may be greeting a classmate who is quite a distance down the hall from you.

More private types of communication occur at closer distances. When you are sharing a secret with your best friend, you are probably quite close to him or her, which enables you to quietly convey your message without being overheard. In between these two extremes is the distance that is comfortable in social or professional situations. This distance varies among cultures. In the United States, a comfortable distance is approximately 2 to 4 feet. Of course, individuals have their own preferences as well. There are no clear-cut guidelines about what is too close or too far away. Distance is generally negotiated during an interaction. If someone feels that you are invading his personal space, he will back away from you. Instead of moving closer to him, allow him to define the distance between you. Finding the comfortable distance from which to talk with patients or other healthcare professionals will make productive interactions easier.

Chronemics

Chronemics refers to the messages that are sent by the use of time. This may sound confusing, but the best example of chronemics generally occurs in physicians' offices. Patients are kept waiting until the physician is free to see them. This is often a source of frustration for patients because as anecdotal evidence suggests, appointments are rarely kept on schedule. Thus, patients are left waiting and given the feeling that the physician does not respect their time. Likewise, in the pharmacy, chronemics can play an important role in your relationship with patients. The amount of time patients spend waiting to speak with someone about a prescription as well as the time they wait for the prescription to be filled can send a strong message to them about the value you place on their patronage. Although it is not always possible to fill prescriptions as quickly as a patient would like, addressing patients' concerns about these issues can help mitigate potentially frustrating situations for everyone involved.

Haptics

Haptics refers to the messages that are conveyed through touch. Touch is an integral portion of human communication. It is the first form of communication that babies sense and is used to show caring and support for those around us. Healthcare professionals, for example, on a regular basis offer a handshake as a greeting or a reassuring hand on a patient's shoulder providing comfort during a time of emotional distress. Even a pat on the back or a high five given to a child can help create warmth in a provider–patient relationship. A word of caution is needed, however. Not all patients respond well to touch. Cultural and personal differences will dictate the extent to which you incorporate touch into your practice.

In summary, the use of nonverbal cues can reinforce your verbal messages. Thus, it is essential to be aware of all the messages you are sending to your receiver. Each dimension of nonverbal communication discussed here is important, but the most important seems to be kinesics. That concept will prove to be most true when working with patients. Next, we discuss ways of integrating the skills presented thus far in performing patient consultation.

PATIENT INTERVIEWING

Gathering information from patients is probably one of the most important and most common functions pharmacists perform. It is also one that requires the most awareness of your communication skills. By correctly phrasing questions to the patient within the context of a sincere desire to help, you can get most patients to provide the information you need to know. In this section the phrasing and ordering of questions are explored. It is crucial to prepare and organize when approaching a patient so that you will not inadvertently omit important questions or be surprised at that patient's response to you. It is important to remember that the patient is the only one who has key bits of information you need. It is not sufficient to ask patients how they are doing with their medication. Patients may feel that you are not really interested in how they are doing and will tell you everything is just fine, even when it may not be.

Sometimes it is hard for patients to differentiate between something that is of importance and something that is not. Therefore, it is your job to ask the right questions, to help patients formulate their questions, and to make sure patients understand the information presented. In the real world, pharmacists are often unable to spend as much time with a patient as they would like. In this case, it becomes important to prioritize the information you wish to give. Even more important is developing an ongoing relationship, as some things can wait a month or two until you see the patient again, but others require immediate attention. In the community setting, when a patient is picking up a new prescription, there is a lot of information the patient should receive. For a refill prescription, the type of information you should gather may be different. In this case, perhaps the most important information to assess is how that patient has been taking the medication. Table 3.1 provides a checklist of items to be included in a full initial patient interview. Take a moment to review the components.

Process

We have already discussed the importance and use of open-ended and closed-ended questions. Prudent use of both types of questions will help the interview flow smoothly. We have also reviewed the concept of empathy and the importance of responding empathically to patients. In this section, we focus on the process of patient interviewing and the order in which questions are asked.

First, you must establish the goal for the interaction. A patient interview may consist solely of gathering information from the patient. Alternatively, following the patient interview, a patient education session may be conducted. In this section we focus on the interviewing process as a systematic way of gathering information from patients. The key to this is in the structure or system employed. By developing your own system for asking questions, you will be less likely to inadvertently leave out questions. You will also be able to guide the interview to flow quickly and smoothly. One way to maximize the time you have

TABLE 3.1. CHECKLIST FOR THE EVALUATION OF THE CONTENT AND STRUCTURE OF A PATIENT INTERVIEW[a]

During the patient interview, did the pharmacy student/pharmacist perform the following:

1. Identify the patient (or caregiver)   YES   NO   N/A
2. Introduce self   YES   NO   N/A
3. Explain purpose of the interview   YES   NO   N/A
4. Estimate the length of time necessary for interview   YES   NO   N/A
5. Explain how patient will benefit from interview   YES   NO   N/A
6. Obtain patient consent to proceed   YES   NO   N/A
7. Obtain a complete and accurate history of
      a. present medical problems   YES   NO   N/A
      b. past medical problems   YES   NO   N/A
      c. present prescription drug use   YES   NO   N/A
      d. past prescription drug use   YES   NO   N/A
      e. present OTC use   YES   NO   N/A
      f. past OTC use   YES   NO   N/A
      g. patient compliance with drug regimen(s)   YES   NO   N/A
      h. social-behavioral factors that may influence
         medicine use patterns   YES   NO   N/A
      i. suspected/documented drug allergies or sensitivities YES   NO   N/A
         (i) date of occurrence   YES   NO   N/A
         (ii) type of reaction   YES   NO   N/A
8. Verify accuracy of the information already in the
   chart   YES   NO   N/A
9. Assess, through open-ended questions, the patient's
   understanding:
      a. of medication dosage   YES   NO   N/A
      b. of dosage frequency   YES   NO   N/A
      c. of method of administration   YES   NO   N/A
10. Assess patient's actual use of medication(s)   YES   NO   N/A
11. Obtain from patient information regarding factors
    that may affect compliance:
       a. lifestyle   YES   NO   N/A
       b. compliance history   YES   NO   N/A
       c. attitudes toward disease and medication   YES   NO   N/A
       d. physical and/or mental impairments   YES   NO   N/A
       e. socioeconomic constraints   YES   NO   N/A
       f. patient's perception of the severity of the disease(s) YES   NO   N/A
       g. patient's perception of the importance of the
          prescribed drug(s)   YES   NO   N/A
12. Summarize information gathered from patient to
    assess accuracy and completeness   YES   NO   N/A

(*continued*)

TABLE 3.1. CHECKLIST FOR THE EVALUATION OF THE CONTENT AND STRUCTURE OF A PATIENT INTERVIEW[a] (*Cont.*)

13. Gather complete medication history before providing new information	YES	NO	N/A
14. Determine appropriate dosage regimen based on prescription directions, drug characteristics and patient's compliance factors	YES	NO	N/A
15. Explain new prescription(s) to patient			
a. Provide the indication(s)	YES	NO	N/A
b. Explain dosage regimen(s)	YES	NO	N/A
c. Suggest time(s) of administration	YES	NO	N/A
d. Explain or demonstrate method of administration	YES	NO	N/A
e. Instruct patient in what to do if a dose is missed or an extra dose is ingested	YES	NO	N/A
f. Explain potential side effects	YES	NO	N/A
g. Explain how to recognize the signs and symptoms of a therapeutic response	YES	NO	N/A
h. Explain how to recognize the signs and symptoms of therapeutic failure	YES	NO	N/A
i. Explain what to do if signs and symptoms of therapeutic failure or important side effects occur	YES	NO	N/A
j. Explain methods by which side effects can be minimized	YES	NO	N/A
16. Determine the patient's level of comprehension via open-ended questions such as			
a. How you are going to take this medication?	YES	NO	N/A
b. How will you be able to tell the medication is working?	YES	NO	N/A
c. What will you do if you miss a dose?	YES	NO	N/A
17. Arrange for follow-up with patient	YES	NO	N/A
18. Provide written and/or pictorial information to enhance patient understanding	YES	NO	N/A
19. Make self available to answer questions in the future	YES	NO	N/A
20. Ask patient's permission to contact physician, when needed	YES	NO	N/A
21. Throughout the interview			
a. Communicate at the appropriate level for the patient (caregiver)	YES	NO	N/A
b. Solicit and encourage questions from the patient (caregiver)	YES	NO	N/A
c. Respond empathically to patient's (caregiver's) concerns	YES	NO	N/A

[a]This checklist may be used as an aid in developing your own interview structure. It may also be used as a self-evaluative tool or in a rotation evaluation. The content of this list represents material that may be covered during a complete, initial session. Subsequent sessions with patients may not include each element.

with a patient is to address only those issues of concern to you or the patient. It is not always necessary to address everything about a patient's drug therapy at one time. Neither you nor the patient is likely to have time for that.

In addition to being prepared to meet with the patient, you can also maximize your time with the patient by eliciting what information the patient already has. You do not need to reiterate information that patient already knows. For example, rather than reviewing how to take each medication, you may simply ask the patient how he or she is taking each one. That way, you can assess if the patient already knows how to take the medication and address any issues that may arise as a result of this. Be careful with your questions. Which of the following questions do you think will best help you identify potential problems with patient understanding?

1. Are you taking your medications as prescribed?
2. How are you taking your medication?

If you chose question 1, you may be surprised to learn that all of your patients are in fact taking their medications as prescribed. Question 1 is a closed-ended question. As such, patients are likely to respond with a "yes" or "no." Most people will not want to admit that they are not following their doctor's instructions, so they will respond affirmatively even if they are not taking their medications as prescribed. Question 2, as an open-ended question, allows patients to tell you how they are taking their medication. At that point, you can determine if they are taking them as prescribed or not. You can then follow up and discuss possible solutions to managing their medication regimens.

Introduction

The first thing you will say to the patient is likely to be a greeting of some sort. "Good morning, Mr. Simmons," is a nice way to begin. Let's consider other items to include in your opening. Unless the patient already knows you, he will not know what to expect from talking with you. Therefore, at an initial meeting, after you introduce yourself, you should explain to the patient why you would like to speak with him, how long it will take, and what will be accomplished during the session. For example, one pharmacist might say:

> Good afternoon, Mrs. Hope. I am Stacy Student, the pharmacist here at the clinic. I would like to spend about five minutes discussing your medications with you so that we may prevent any potential problems and resolve any problems you might be having with your medications.

After obtaining the patient's permission to proceed, you may begin asking the patient questions.

Phrasing Key Questions

After the introduction, you may want to proceed by making sure you have a complete list of all the medications a patient is taking. Although you may have a list of medications from the patient profile, the profile may not be current. Also, it may not contain all of the medications the patient is taking. Perhaps he has prescriptions filled at another pharmacy, or perhaps he is taking nonprescription items that may interfere with the prescription medications. In asking, "What prescription medications are you currently taking?" you will be sure to have a complete, updated list from which to work. After gathering that list, you may want to ask the following questions for each of the medications on the list. At this point, it is important not to confuse the patient or yourself by discussing more than one medication at a time. Using a transition such as "let's talk about your blood pressure medication first " will help minimize confusion.

In addition to how patients are taking their medications, important areas to explore include what medications they are taking (both prescription and over the counter), what problems they might be having, if they are experiencing side effects that they attribute to their medications, if they are using any alternative therapies to treat their medical conditions, and if they have other health concerns they would like to discuss. When asking about other health concerns, keep in mind that a patient may be experiencing side effects from a medication that he does not attribute to that medication. It will be up to you to help him determine what issues are medication-related and what issues are not. In either case, if a concern is revealed, resolution may involve a discussion with the patient's physician. Important points to ask about each and every medication include the following:

"How did the doctor tell you to take the medication?"
"How are you taking your medication?"
"Have you noticed any problems with this medication?"
"How effective has the medication been?"
"How can you tell the medication is working?"

Refer again to Table 3.1 for the checklist of items to cover during a patient interview. This may be helpful for you in developing your own interview checklist or for a self-evaluative tool.

Providing Education

After you have gathered your information, you will likely want to make recommendations to the patient. It is wise to wait until after you have collected all the pertinent information before initiating a patient education session. If you respond to each potential problem before getting a clear, complete picture of the patient's medical and pharmacologic state, you may need to modify the information you have given the patient. In addition to taking longer, it is likely to confuse the patient. Therefore, it is best to wait until you have gathered all the information before providing any information.

Much as in the interviewing process, providing patient education should be done in an organized, systematic way. Begin by addressing the most important issue. Prioritization is essential. It is unlikely that you will be able to completely address all the necessary issues with a patient. That is why the development of a strong relationship with patients will be helpful. When you see patients on a regular basis, you can cover one topic at a time and know that you will have other opportunities at a future date to refine the patient's understanding of other issues. Certainly, addressing the most pressing first makes sense. Anything that is potentially life threatening should be addressed immediately. As you work in clinical settings, you will hone your ability to recognize the clinical significance of each patient's issues, and you will be able to determine how quickly you need to address them.

You can maximize your time in patient education by providing only new information for them. It is unnecessary for you to review information that the patient already understands. By asking open-ended questions, you can ascertain what information the patient still needs and provide that information for him or her.

The format of the information you provide is also important. Research has shown that it is not sufficient to merely tell patients about something. It is very helpful for patients to have written information to which they can refer when they are at home.[11,12] Using written information in addition to orally communicating the information reinforces the concepts for patients. This will minimize misunderstandings and will give patients something to refer to if you are not available to answer their questions. Some patients may do research on their own and may come to you with a great understanding of their medical conditions and their medications, yet others may rely on you to provide that information to them. You can be of help to both types of patients and to the majority of patients who will lie somewhere in between those two ends of the spectrum. By making yourself available to answer all levels of questions and being willing to provide information at levels appropriate to each patient, you will be fulfilling their needs. You may need to provide information at a lower level than the computer-generated patient information leaflets or to provide references to scientific journals for patients who want to read the latest clinical trials.

When providing patient education, your ultimate goal is for the patient to retain and utilize the information you have provided. There are certain things you can do to help patients remember the important points. Tindall et. al.[10] offer the following suggestions. First, like students in a classroom who are told that something is important for an exam, patients who are told that something is important will better remember what follows. By telling patients that something is important, you cause them to pay more attention. For example, Pharmacist Noledge may say to her patient, "Mr. Brown, what I'm about to tell you is very important. This medication may cause your eyes to change color." Although the mere mention of such a radical side effect may have been enough for Mr. Brown to remember it, preceding that statement with a declaration that the information to come is important helped the patient focus on the upcoming information. This technique is useful, but only if used sparingly. If every other sentence you utter begins with, "now, this is very important," it will lose its effect, and patients will not demonstrate the desired response to it.

Another way to help patients remember information is to summarize key points after you have given it to them. It is most effective when you have the patient summarize the information for you rather than you summarizing for the patient. By asking the patient to repeat the important points from the education session, you accomplish two things. First, you are able to assess the patient's understanding of the information, and second, you are able to determine if you inadvertently omitted some information. Using probing questions such as "How do you plan to take your medication?" can help you assess patients' understanding of particular portions of the education session. You may also ask the following questions to assess patients' understanding:

"What will you do if you miss a dose?"

"How will you be able to tell if the medication is working?"

"What side effects may you experience from this medication?"

A third way to minimize misunderstandings by providing clear instructions. Telling a patient to take a medication with food, for example, is rather vague. The patient may have questions about how much food would be sufficient or if the medication should be taken only at mealtimes. By being specific about your instructions, you can prevent this confusion. Telling the patient to take the medication with food, such as a small snack or with meals, depending on the dosing regimen, will help the patient take the medication properly in order to gain its full potential benefit.

Finally, explaining to patients just why something is important will help them to understand and remember the point. In the above example, if a patient understands that not taking the medication with food may cause stomach discomfort, he is more likely to follow those instructions. Conversely, if the patient is not aware of the potential consequences of following the instructions, he may not be as motivated to follow the instructions.

To summarize, key ways to help patients understand and remember the information you present to them include the following:

1. Advising patients that important information is to follow.
2. Explaining to patients why the information is important.
3. Giving clear instructions.
4. Providing written information to supplement oral information.
5. Assessing patient understanding.

These five skills will help you optimize the time you have with patients and help you identify areas for exploration and explanation at future encounters with the patient.

The main points in the structure and process of a patient interview include a formal introduction if it is an initial consultation. Following that introduction will be the gathering of information. This may include making sure your patient profile is complete, assessing how patients are taking medications and whether they are having any problems with those medications. After you are sure you have all the information you need, you may proceed to provide information that the patient needs. In order to maximize your time and the patients', only provide information that the patient does not already know. At the conclusion of the exchange, an assessment of patient understanding should take place. Finally, you should arrange for follow-up with the patient, if necessary, and make yourself available in the future should the patient have additional questions or concerns.

WRITTEN COMMUNICATION

Written communication can take many forms in the practice of pharmacy. Perhaps the most common form of written communication for clinical pharmacists in a hospital setting is a note in a patient's chart. This topic is covered elsewhere in this handbook, as are cover letters and the curriculum vitae. In this chapter, we discuss other forms of professional writing. In the course of your practice, you may find occasion to write a letter to a physician or other healthcare professional, to an insurance company, or even to a patient. You may also be called on to submit reports in writing regarding medication protocols, medication errors, or inventory matters. If you are involved in formulary decisions, you may also be responsible for preparing documents for the pharmacy and therapeutics committee. Needless to say, you will want these documents to appear professional and well written. Each document may be slightly different and should be tailored to your specific need. This section reviews some general guidelines for the preparation of such documents.

One of the most important points to remember in preparing any written communication is that if spelling or grammatical errors are present, they severely detract from the effectiveness of the message. It is very tempting to rely on electronic spell checking and grammar checking devices because of their convenience, and these tools are quite useful. Unfortunately, they may not reveal all of the errors in a document. Words such as "know" and "no" are both correctly spelled here but would not appear in an electronic check for spelling. As you know, they have different meanings and cannot be used interchangeably. Many such examples can be found in the English language. As an exercise, you may want to think of as many of these words as you can in order to familiarize yourself with them. Then, when you are typing, it may jog your memory to double-check your work even after the spell check. Grammatical errors may also be reviewed through an electronic screening process. It may seem at times that these are tedious, catching every minor error. Generally speaking, using one is worth the extra time. Few of us recall the detailed grammatical rules we learned in grade school. It is certainly wise to make use of the electronic tools available in this area, but always remember to read the document out loud to yourself, looking for items that may have been missed.

In addition to the importance of an error-free document, a well-organized document is much more powerful than one that does not make its point. As in the structure of a patient interview, organization is the key. Let's take the example of a written letter to a physician in order to explore this concept further.

When you write to a physician, it will likely be on behalf of a patient. Perhaps you have identified a problem that you feel should be brought to the physician's attention. Although there are many communication choices these days, it is difficult to speak to a physician on the telephone for any length of time at your convenience. Therefore, making use of other options seems appropriate. A letter can be faxed to the physician or, if not of great urgency, mailed. A letter to a physician should include the following areas (see example in Fig. 3.2):

1. Statement of the problem.
2. Potential solutions.
3. Specific recommendation for a solution.
4. Support for your recommendation.
5. Description of follow-up.

First, a concise statement of the problem is the way to begin such correspondence. Making reference to the patient and his or her problem in the first sentence will show the physician the importance of your letter and encourage her to keep reading. Going into great detail about the circumstances of the problem is usually unnecessary. The physician does not need to know too much detail regarding the method by which you have uncovered the problem. Further, offering a detailed explanation is also unnecessary. Unless the problem is quite complicated, you should be able to describe it in one or two sentences. Maintaining objectivity is also important in describing the problem. Avoid placing blame on the physician or the patient. The goal of the letter is to help resolve the problem, not to interfere with the physician–patient relationship.

After you have identified and described the problem, you should offer potential solutions. Again, this information should be presented in the most concise fashion possible. The letter should not take longer than a few minutes to read because the physician will be unlikely to have more time than that. In phrasing your options, maintain an objective and neutral tone. This means that you are offering suggestions to the physician rather than telling her what to do. If the tone of the letter suggests that the physician was in error or is lacking sufficient knowledge to practice correctly, it will leave her with a negative opinion about you and your suggestions. In offering your suggestions, explain briefly why each will help address the problem at hand. An explanation of your reasoning will help the physician to understand your train of thought and will reassure her that you have in fact given thought to the problem.

Once you have described one or two options, let the physician know which of the alternatives you would suggest. Make this a clear statement so no confusion exists regarding your choice. The solution should be fully explained in detail, giving, for example, a complete dosing regimen if you are suggesting a

Rx-R-Us Pharmacy
1234 Medicine Lane
Your Town, ST 99999
November 30, 2000

Dr. Jan Jones
5678 Hospital Dr., Suite 200
Your Town, ST 99999

Dear Dr. Jones:

This letter is in reference to our patient, Mrs. Patty Patient. In reviewing Mrs. Patient's profile, I noticed that she is taking the drug Tonsoprobs for cholesterol. She is also taking Lowerthepreser for hypertension. As you may know, recent studies have shown that Tonsoprobs decreases Lowerthepreser's effectiveness. This may pose a problem for Mrs. Patient.

Possible solutions to this problem may include increasing the dose of Lowerthepreser, decreasing the dose of Tonsoprobs or changing thera-peutic agents. A recent study published in the Medical Journal suggests that the best course of action would be to increase the dose of Lowerthepreser. Based on this, I recommend a new regimen of 500mg of Lowerthepreser twice a day for Mrs. Patient.

After this therapeutic change, I will continue to monitor Mrs. Patient's blood pressure and keep you informed of her progress. I have enclosed a copy of the Medical Journal article for your review. I will telephone you next Tuesday to discuss your decision.

Thank you for your attention to this matter.

Sincerely,

Stacy Student

Stacy Student, Pharm.D.
Pharmacy Manager

Figure 3.2. Sample physician letter.

therapeutic change. To give your recommendation more weight, you can supplement it with your rationale. In addition to your clinical judgment, you may have relied on current literature in making your recommendation. If so, include the reference for the article you used or a complete copy of it. This will assure the physician that your recommendations are based on sound clinical evidence.

The final component of such a letter is the explanation of the necessary follow-up. Because you are initiating this correspondence and bringing the problem to the physician's attention, it is your responsibility to follow-up with the physician. This can be accomplished via a phone call several days after the letter is mailed or by additional written correspondence. It should be made clear to the physician that you will in fact follow-up with the patient and make sure that the corrective action taken by the physician is implemented. This will reassure both the patient and the physician that the situation will be adequately resolved.

Inclusion of the five components described above in a concise letter to a physician will help the physician have a clear understanding of the problem and of the solution. A well-written, well-organized letter is a powerful tool in communicating your point of view to another professional. These components of organization and structure apply to other forms of written communication as well. Keep in mind how much easier a reading assignment is when it is short and the important information is clearly presented!

SUMMARY

In this chapter we have reviewed basic communication skills that may be used in various areas of interaction. The careful consideration of nonverbal communication, the phrasing of questions, appropriate use of empathy, and assertiveness are all useful tools when interacting with employers, colleagues, and patients. We reviewed a systematic way to conduct patient medication interviews and patient education sessions. Following a structured format will allow you to make best use of the time that you have with each patient. Last, writing for pharmacists was reviewed in the context of relating to other health care professionals.

As with any new skills, communication skills require practice. As mentioned at the beginning of the chapter, few people are able to instinctively conduct an efficient patient interview. With time and practice you will become both effective and efficient in your role as a patient educator, health care professional educator and pharmacy professional. Refer to Appendix A for several realistic scenarios for practice. Consider how you would handle each of the scenarios and discuss them with your classmates, preceptors, or professors to get a variety of perspectives. Even if you are not sure that you have responded in the best way, having an idea of how you plan to handle difficult situations before they arise will be helpful when they do materialize. Finally, as you practice pharmacy and grow in experience, you will also gain insight into communicating with patients and colleagues. You will develop your own style and gain confidence in your ability to communicate effectively with others.

QUESTIONS

1. What nonverbal cues send a positive message to others?
2. Describe how communication occurs.
3. How would you respond to a patient who says, "This medication isn't working at all. I don't know what else to try"? What techniques would you use?
4. How would you respond to a nurse who says, "It took way too long to get this laxative. We ordered it STAT!" What assertiveness technique would you use?
5. Explain the usage of open-ended and closed-ended questions in a patient interview.
6. When communicating in writing, how will you best structure the information?

REFERENCES

1. Muchmore J, Galvin K. A report of the task force on career competencies in oral communication skills for community college students seeking immediate entry into the work force. *Commun Ed* 1983;32:207–220.
2. Ley P. The benefits of improved communication. In: *Communicating with Patients: Improving Communication, Satisfaction and Compliance*. New York: Croom Helm, 1988.
3. Berlo DK. *The Process of Communication*. New York: Holt, Rinehart and Winston, 1960.
4. Shannon CE, Weaver W. *The Mathematical Theory of Communication*. Champaign: University of Illinois Press, 1949.
5. Wilmot WW. *Dyadic Communication: A Transactional Perspective*. Reading, MA: Addison–Wesley, 1979.
6. Northouse PG, Northouse LL. *Health Communication: Strategies for Health Professionals*. Norwalk, CT: Appleton and Lange, 1992.
7. Nelson AR, Zelnio RN, Beno CE. Clinical pharmaceutical services in retail practice II. Factors influencing the provision of services. *Drug Intell Clin Pharmacy* 1984;18(12):992–996.
8. Raisch DW. Barriers to providing cognitive services. *Am Pharmacy* 1993;33(12):54–58.
9. Herrier R, Boyce R. Why aren't more pharmacists counseling? *Am Pharmacy* 1994;34(11):22–23.
10. Tindall WN, Beardsley RS, Kimberlin CL. *Communication Skills in Pharmacy Practice*. Malvern, PA: Lea & Febiger, 1994.
11. Kimberlin CL, Berardo DH. A comparison of patient education methods used in community pharmacies. *J Pharmaceut Market Manage* 1987;1(4):75–94.
12. Gotsch AR, Liguori S. 1982 "Knowledge, attitude, and compliance dimensions of antibiotic therapy with PPIs." *Med Care* 1982;20(6):581–595.
13. Zelnio RN, Nelson AA, Beno CE. Clinical pharmaceutical services in retail practice I. Pharmacists' willingness and abilities to provide services. *Drug Intell Clin Pharmacy* 1984;18(11):917–922.

LEGAL REQUIREMENTS FOR FILLING A PRESCRIPTION

Dean Arneson

Goals: After reviewing the information in this chapter, you should be able to:

1. Define *drug* according to the FDA.
2. Identify information that is required to be included on a prescription.
3. Identify information that is required to be on the prescription label.
4. Identify the factors that make a prescription legal.
5. Define and distinguish the different controlled substances.
6. List and explain the pharmacist's responsibilities for implementing OBRA '90.
7. List and explain the pharmacist's responsibilities for implementing the Poison Prevention Packaging Act.
8. Define and differentiate between risk assessment and risk management.

INTRODUCTION

To fill a prescription a pharmacist must be aware of all legal requirements. The pharmacist must also keep in mind that his or her actions may be open to civil liability if he or she makes an error in filling a prescription and causes harm to a patient. This chapter discusses the Federal law and briefly touches on some state requirements for filling a prescription. The learning objectives outline the areas to be covered.

This chapter is designed to describe the legal aspects of filling a prescription systematically. One of the first steps is to define what is a drug and then discuss what makes a prescription a legal prescription. The information that must appear on the prescription is also outlined. Information that appears on the label is explained with a discussion of the differences between federal and state requirements. The legal requirements for the container in which the medication is dispensed are also discussed, with the requirements and exemptions presented. Finally, the requirements for the information that the pharmacist must provide to the patient are presented and discussed.

ADMINISTRATIVE AGENCIES

The Food and Drug Administration

The federal government has established an administrative agency, the Food and Drug Administration (FDA), to oversee the area of pharmaceuticals. The FDA oversees all aspects of the pharmaceutical market. One of the most important duties it performs is to approve new medications for use in the United States. In overseeing this function, it has established the procedures manufacturers must follow to perform pharmacologic/toxicologic studies on new chemical entities. These methods determine the potential benefit the entity may have versus the risk of harm it may cause. This is accomplished through the clinical testing of medications on human subjects. The FDA also approves and monitors the manufacturing process established by the drug company. The company must file the exact process they use to manufacture the drug with the FDA, and if the company decides to change the process in any way, they must notify the FDA and obtain approval.

Among the parameters the FDA monitors are the absorption, distribution, metabolism, and elimination of the medication by the body; these comprise its pharmacokinetics. The FDA uses this parameter to approve generic medications. The decision to approve a generic medication is based on the comparison of the bioavailability of the generic medication to the brand-name product. Because the FDA has the authority over the manufacturing process, the federal government has also given them the right to inspect any facility where medication is held.

Other areas that are regulated by the FDA include the approval of all drug advertising to health care professionals, such as in the package insert. They also approve advertising to the public. They regulate the distribution of drug samples. Pharmacists are not allowed to be in possession of sample products except in very structured situations.

The primary goal of the FDA is to protect the safety of the public, and they do this by requiring testing for the safety and efficacy of medicinal products. They monitor the products even after they have been approved and are on the market. The FDA has the authority to require pharmaceutical manufacturers to perform drug recalls to retrieve any product that may pose a danger to the public.

The Drug Enforcement Administration

A second administration agency that is involved with medications is the Drug Enforcement Administration (DEA). It is a branch of the US Justice Department, and its main purpose is to administer the federal Controlled Substance Act. The Controlled Substance Act (CSA) (21 U.S.C. §§ 801-970) regulates a particular set of medications (controlled substances, which are defined later in the chapter) that have a high potential for physical and/or psychological addiction.

The DEA has the authority to perform inspections on pharmacies where controlled substances are held. The inspectors have the authority, through permission of the pharmacist or an administrative warrant, to inspect any pharmacy where they feel illegal activity is taking place. The inspectors have the authority to audit the pharmacy's invoices, inventory, and prescription files to determine if there are any discrepancies between what has been purchased, what is presently in inventory, and what has been dispensed by the pharmacy. If a pharmacist is found in violation of the federal Controlled Substance Act, his or her license may be revoked, and he or she may be incarcerated in a federal prison.

DRUG LAWS

The Food, Drug, and Cosmetic Act of 1938

A major piece of federal legislation that regulates the pharmaceutical industry now is the Food, Drug, and Cosmetic Act (FDCA) of 1938. It was enacted to protect the public's safety and was passed in response to a tragedy involving sulfanilamide (an antibiotic) and diethylene glycol (commonly used in antifreeze). A pharmaceutical company desired to make an elixir of the antibiotic and discovered that sulfanilamide easily dissolved in the diethylene glycol. The product was never tested for toxicity before marketing. One hundred and seven deaths were caused by the drug. Thus, the FDCA of 1938 was passed to set guidelines for the definition of a drug or a cosmetic and to establish methods to determine their safety.

Presently a drug is defined as the following:

1. Articles recognized in the official United States Pharmacopoeia, official Homeopathic Pharmacopoeia of the United States, or official National Formulary.
2. Articles intended for use in the diagnosis, cure, mitigation, treatment, or prevention of disease in man or other animals.
3. Articles (other than food) intended to affect the structure or any function of the body of man or other animal.
4. Articles intended for use as components of any articles specified in Clause (A), (B), or (C), FDCA § 201(g)(1), 21 U.S.C. § 321(g)(1). (Chapter 21 of the Code of Federal Regulation[1] may be accessed through the FDA web site, www.fda.gov).

Certain medications, because of their physical and/or psychological addictive nature, are classified as controlled substances. This means that the prescribing, acquisition, dispensing, and inventorying of these medications is more tightly controlled than other medications. The definition, prescribing, acquisition, dispensing, and inventorying of these medications are outlined in the Controlled Substances Act.

The Controlled Substances Act defines the controlled substances in the following schedules:

Schedule I: High potential for abuse; no currently accepted medical use in treatment in the United States; lack of accepted information on the safety of their use, even under medical supervision (21 C.F.R. § 1300.11). Examples include heroin, marijuana, peyote, mescaline, and dihydromorphine.

Schedule II: High potential for abuse; does have a currently accepted medical use in treatment in the United States or a currently accepted medical use with severe restrictions; abuse of the drug or other substance may lead to severe physical or psychological dependence (21 C.F.R. § 1300.12). Examples include cocaine, morphine, meperidine, codeine, and methadone.

Schedule III: The drug has a potential for abuse less than that of the drugs or other substances in schedules I and II; does have a currently accepted medical use in treatment in the United States; abuse of the drug or other substance may lead to moderate physical or psychological dependence. (21 C.F.R. § 1300.13). Examples include acetaminophen with codeine, anabolic steroids, and paregoric.

Schedule IV: The drug has a low potential for abuse relative to the drugs or other substances in schedules III; does have a currently accepted medical use in treatment in the United States; abuse of the drug or other substance may lead to limited physical or psychological dependence relative to the drugs or other substances in schedule III (21 C.F.R. § 1300.14). Examples include diazepam, chloral hydrate, phenobarbital, and diethylpropion.

Schedule V: The drug has a low potential for abuse relative to the drugs or other substances in schedules IV; does have a currently accepted medical use in treatment in the United States; abuse of the drug or other substance may lead to limited physical or psychological dependence relative to the drugs or other substances in schedules IV (21 C.F.R. § 1300.15). A schedule V drug cannot contain more than 200 mg of codeine per 100 mL or 100 g, 100 mg of dihydrocodeine per 100 mL or 100 g.

Poison Prevention Packaging Act

Another requirement that governs the practice of pharmacy is that a pharmacist must dispense prescriptions according to the Poison Prevention Packaging Act (PPPA) (16 C.F.R. § 1700). This law requires that prescriptions be dispensed in child-resistant closures. A child-resistant container is defined as a container that 80% of children less than 5 years of age cannot open and 90% of adults can. Table 4.1 lists the products that are subject to the Poison Prevention Packaging Act. Because the containers can lose their integrity with use, a new container must be used each time a prescription is filled, whether it is new or a refill.

Patients or their physicians may orally or in writing request that a prescription be dispensed in non-child-resistant containers. To protect themselves from

---

TABLE 4.1. PARTIAL LIST OF PRODUCTS SUBJECT TO THE POISON PREVENTION PACKAGING ACT (16 C.F.R. § 1700.14)

- Oral prescription drugs (exemptions noted in Table 4.2)
- Controlled substances in dosage forms intended for oral human administration
- Liquid preparations containing more than 5% by weight of methyl salicylate
- Oral aspirin preparations containing more than 5% by weight of methyl salicylate
- Oral aspirin preparations (exemptions noted in Table 4.2)
- All drugs and dietary supplements that provide iron for therapeutic or prophylactic purposes and contain a total amount of elemental iron from any source in a single package that is equivalent to 250 mg or more elemental iron in a concentration of 0.025% or more w/v, and 0.05% or more on w/w for non-liquids
- Oral dosage form of acetaminophen in containers holding more than 1 g.
- Ibuprofen in oral dosage forms containing 1 g or more of the drug in a single package
- Diphenhydramine HCl in oral dosage forms containing more that the equivalent of 66 mg of the diphenhydramine base in a single package
- Loperamide in oral dosage forms containing more that 0.045 mg of the drug in a single package
- Mouthwash preparations for human use containing 3 g or more of ethanol in a single package

---

liability, if the request is oral, a pharmacist should document this request in writing with the patient signing a statement to the effect:

I, ___(patient's signature)___, request that my prescription be dispensed in a non-child-resistant container.

This statement should be stamped on the back of each prescription, and the patient should sign each time. Alternatively, a comprehensive blanket statement requesting non-child-resistant containers signed one time by the patient and kept on file is acceptable. If the patient's physician makes the requests, it must be on a per-prescription basis.

Products that are exempt from the Poison Prevention Packaging Act are listed in Table 4.2.

Omnibus Budget Reconciliation Act of 1990

When dispensing the prescription, the pharmacist must follow a law that was part of the Omnibus Budget Reconciliation Act of 1990 (OBRA '90) (P.L. 101-508). The law requires each state that provides Medicaid benefits to establish pharmacy requirements. However, that would create two levels of care for residents

TABLE 4.2. PARTIAL LIST OF PRODUCTS EXEMPT OF THE POISON PREVENTION PACKAGING ACT [16 C.F.R. § 1700.14(a)(10)]

- Sublingual dosage forms of nitroglycerin
- Sublingual and chewable forms of isosorbide dinitrate in strengths of 10 mg or less
- Anhydrous cholestyramine in powder form
- Sodium fluoride products containing not more than 264 mg of sodium fluoride per package
- Methylprednisolone tablets containing not more than 84 mg of the drug per package
- Menbendazole tablets containing not more than 600 mg of the drug per package
- Betamethasone tablets containing not more that 12.6 mg of the drug per package
- Potassium supplements in unit dose forms, including effervescent tablets, unit dose vials of liquid potassium, and powdered potassium in unit dose packets containing not more than 50 mEq per unit dose
- Erythromycin ethylsuccinate granules for oral suspension and oral suspensions in packages containing not more than 8 g of the equivalent erythromycin
- Pancrealipase preparations
- Preparations in aerosol containers intended for inhalation therapy
- Colestipol in powder form up to 5 g in a packet
- Prednisone tablets not containing more than 105 mg per package
- Cyclically administered oral contraceptives, conjugated estrogens and norethindrone acetate tablets in manufacturers's mnemonic dispenser packages
- Medroxyprogesterone acetate tablets

of the state. Because of legal and/or ethical standards, most states will not allow that to happen. Therefore, what applies to the Medicaid patient must apply to all citizens of the state.

One requirement under this act is that the state must perform a retrospective drug utilization review (DUR). To complete this, the state must establish a panel to review medication use to determine that the medication prescribed is therapeutically appropriate and medically necessary and compare the treatment to predetermined standards. They must also look for adverse drug results and monitor for potential abuse. The state must also watch for underutilization and overutilization and be vigilant for any fraud that may be taking place. If it is determined by the panel that there is a problem in any of these areas, an "educational process" for the prescriber or pharmacist is implemented to address and correct the situation.

A second requirement is that pharmacists perform a prospective drug utilization review (DUR) in which he or she is to monitor for:

Drug–drug interactions
Therapeutic duplications
Adverse drug–drug interactions
Incorrect dosages
Incorrect duration
Drug allergy interactions
Clinical abuse/misuse
Drug–food interactions

In order to perform the prospective DUR, the pharmacist must have certain information and is required to make a reasonable effort to obtain a medical history on patients. The minimal information that should be obtained from the history includes name, address, telephone number, date of birth, gender; individual history, including disease state(s), known allergies, and drug reactions; and a comprehensive list of medications and relevant devices.

The pharmacist must also (depending on the state) make an offer to council patients who are having prescriptions filled or answer any questions that the patient may have. Depending on the state, the pharmacist's offer to council may need to be extended on both new and refill prescriptions. The minimal requirements for counseling must include:

• Name and description of the medication.
• Dosage, dosage form, route of administration, and duration of drug therapy.
• Special directions and precautions for preparation, administration, and use by the patient.
• Common severe side effects, or interactions and therapeutic contraindications that may be encountered, including ways to prevent them and the action required if they do occur.
• Techniques for self-monitoring of drug therapy.
• Actions to be taken in case of a missed dose.

Each state is required to establish its own statutes pertaining to OBRA '90, and they vary considerably across the country. A pharmacist must become familiar with his state's requirements before dispensing prescriptions. With the enactment of OBRA '90, the state boards and courts are determining that pharmacists are responsible for patient education and are accountable for counseling.

OBRA '90 implicates the pharmacist in risk management. The pharmacist must help the patient manage the drug therapy that has been prescribed by the practitioner. The practitioner performs a risk assessment in deciding which treatment is the best for the patient. He will compare the risk versus the benefits for the patient and decide on an approved drug therapy. The pharmacist must then assist the patient in managing aspects of the therapy. This includes side effects or indications that the treatment is not working. The courts are increasingly recognizing the pharmacist's responsibility in risk management by upholding OBRA '90 requirements.

THE PRESCRIPTION

The Practitioner

A practitioner is the person who is legally entitled to prescribe medications as determined by each state. It is the state and not the federal government that determines who is entitled to prescribe medication. The states then generally require that the practitioner be licensed and/or registered in that state. This is usually accomplished by having the practitioner pass a competency exam, which evaluates his or her knowledge of the diagnosis and treatment of diseases. Examples of practitioners are allopathic physicians, osteopathic physicians, dentists, veterinarians, and nurse practitioners. Veterinarians are allowed to prescribe only for animals. Nurse practitioners may be allowed to prescribe only under certain protocols or limited to a particular formulary. In the ambulatory setting, the practitioner then writes a prescription for the patient to have filled at a community pharmacy. This does not apply in a hospital or institutional setting, where the patient's chart serves as the medication order record.

Another area that pharmacists must consider when filling a prescription is the scope of practice of each practitioner. Practitioners are generally allowed to prescribe only in their area of expertise. An example of this is a surgeon prescribing analgesic medications and antibiotics. This is within the scope of practice of a surgeon: his patients may need analgesics for any pain they may be suffering, and antibiotics to prevent or treat infection. On the other hand, a dentist prescribing birth control pills will generally be considered beyond the scope of practice. The pharmacist can and should refuse to fill the prescription until he or she has contacted the dentist. In some cases, a pharmacist must use his or her professional judgment when making a decision about the scope of practice. If there is a question, the pharmacist should contact the practitioner to determine if the prescribed medication may be for a new indication.

Presentation of the Prescription to the Pharmacy

Nonscheduled and schedule III, IV, and V prescriptions may be presented in the pharmacy either by the patient or her agent, or it may be telephoned or faxed to the pharmacy by the practitioner or his agent. (21 C.F.R. § 1306.21). Schedule II prescriptions must be physically presented to the pharmacy unless it is an emergency. The DEA defines an emergency as:

Immediate administration of the controlled substance is necessary for the proper treatment of the patient.

No appropriate alternative treatment is available.

It is not reasonably possible for the prescribing physician to provide a written prescription to the pharmacist before dispensing (21 C.F.R. § 290.10).

If the situation is deemed to be an emergency:

The quantity prescribed and dispensed is limited to the amount necessary to treat the patient for the emergency period.

The prescription must be immediately reduced to writing by the pharmacist and shall contain all required information except the signature of the prescriber.

If the prescriber is not known to the pharmacist, the pharmacist must make a reasonable, good faith effort to determine that the oral authorization came from a registered individual practitioner. This reasonable effort could include a call back to the prescriber using the telephone number in the telephone directory rather than the number given by the prescriber over the telephone.

Within 7 days after authorizing an emergency oral prescription, the prescriber must deliver to the dispensing pharmacist a written prescription for the emergency quantity prescribed. The prescription must have written on its face "Authorization for Emergency Dispensing" and the date of the oral order. The written prescription may be delivered to the pharmacist in person or by mail. If delivered by mail, it must be postmarked within the 7-day period. On receipt, the dispensing pharmacist shall attach this prescription to the oral emergency prescription previously reduced to writing. If the prescriber fails to deliver the written prescription within the 7-day period, the pharmacist must notify the nearest office of the DEA. Failure of the pharmacist to do so will void the prescription [21 C.F.R. § 1306.11(d)].

Also, in general schedule II prescriptions cannot be faxed to pharmacies; all schedule II prescriptions must be dispensed pursuant to an original signed prescription. The schedule prescription may be faxed to a pharmacy, but the original must be received before the medication can be dispensed. There are three situations in which a faxed schedule II prescription may be used as the original:

1. If the prescription is faxed by the practitioner or practitioner's agent to a pharmacy and is for a narcotic schedule II substance to be compounded for the direct administration to a patient by parenteral, intravenous, intramuscular, subcutaneous, or intraspinal infusion [21 C.F.R. § 1306.11(e)].
2. If the prescription faxed by the practitioner or practitioner's agent is for a schedule II narcotic substance for a resident of a long-term care facility (LTCF) [21 C.F.R. § 1306.11(f)].
3. If the prescription faxed by the practitioner or practitioner's agent is for a schedule II narcotic substance for a patient residing in a hospice certified by

Medicare under Title XVIII or licensed by the state, the practitioner or agent must note on the prescription that the patient is a hospice patient [21 C.F.R. § 1306.11(g)].

Legitimacy

A prescription is generated for a patient who is in need of medical attention and seeks out a practitioner who determines that the patient needs to have medication, thus creating the patient–practitioner relationship. A prescription must be generated from a valid patient–practitioner relationship. This patient–practitioner relationship must be established so that a prescription is generated for a legitimate medical condition. If it is not a legitimate medical condition, then the prescription is not valid and cannot be filled [21 C.F.R. § 1306.04 (a)]. It is the pharmacist's professional judgment to try to determine if the prescription is valid. The Drug Enforcement Administration has a suggested list of questions for pharmacist to help him or her determine the legitimacy of a prescription.

1. Does the prescriber write significantly larger numbers of prescriptions orders (or in larger quantities) than other practitioners in your area?
2. Does the prescriber write for antagonistic drugs, such as depressants and stimulants, at the same time? Drug abusers often request prescription orders for "ups" and "downs" at the same time.
3. Do patients appear to be returning too frequently? In numerous cases drug abusers have been found to have been receiving prescription orders that ought to have lasted for a month in legitimate use, on a biweekly, weekly, or even a daily basis.
4. Do patients appear presenting prescription orders written in the names of other people?
5. Do a number of people appear simultaneously, or within a short time, all bearing similar prescription orders from the same practitioner?
6. Are numerous "strangers," people who are not regular patrons or residents of community, suddenly showing up with prescription orders from the same physician? Typically, you will find that these individuals are in the 18- to 25-year-old age group, although drug abuse does not necessarily end with the achievement of chronological maturity.
7. Are your purchases of controlled substances rising dramatically? If so, it is time to look at your prescription counter policies. Drug abusers may have found a "vendor" who dispenses prescription orders mechanically, without using professional judgment. (Pharmacist's Manual,[2] pp. 30–31).

These are some of the questions that a pharmacist must ask himself or herself when trying to determine if a prescription is legitimate, and she will have to rely on her professional judgment when presented with a questionable situation.

Information That Must Be Present on the Prescription

The prescription paper must contain certain information, depending on whether it is a controlled substance or a noncontrolled medication. An example of a prescription is depicted in Fig. 4.1. A prescription for a noncontrolled substance must contain the following information; (1) patient's name, (2) date on which the prescription was written, (3) name of the medication, (4) dosage form, (5) strength of the medication, (6) quantity to dispense, (7) directions for use, (8) number of refills, and (9) practitioner's signature in ink or indelible pencil. If the prescription is for a controlled substance (see below), it also requires (10) the patient's address and (11) the practitioner's address and (12) DEA registration number [21 C.F.R. § 1306.05 (a)].

The DEA registration number is a number issued to a practitioner to identify persons authorized by the state and Drug Enforcement Agency to prescribe controlled substances. It consists of nine characters; the first two are letters, and the next seven are numbers. Originally, the first letter was A and the second letter was the first letter of the registrants last name. As an example, Dr. Margaret Brown's number begins with the characters AB. Subsequently, the DEA has used all the available A numbers and has started using the Bs, and it is assumed that they will continue with the Cs when necessary. The second character may be a number if the registrant is registered as a business and the business's name begins with a number. The second group of characters consists of a set of numbers

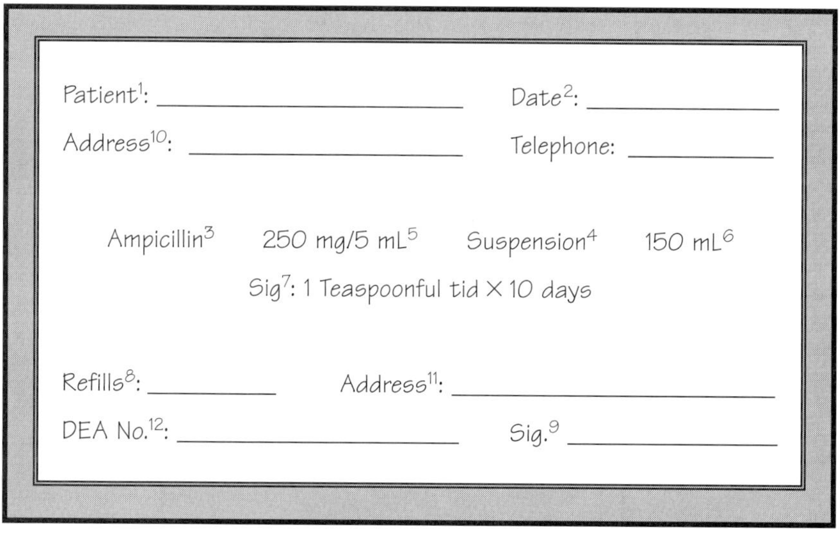

Patient[1]: _____ Date[2]: _____

Address[10]: _____ Telephone: _____

Ampicillin[3]   250 mg/5 mL[5]   Suspension[4]   150 mL[6]

Sig[7]: 1 Teaspoonful tid × 10 days

Refills[8]: _____ Address[11]: _____

DEA No.[12]: _____ Sig.[9] _____

Figure 4.1. Prescription information.

that are unique to each registrant. The last digit is a check number that can be validated by performing three steps:

1. Add the first, third, and fifth digits.
2. Sum the second, fourth, and sixth digits, multiply this sum by 2, and add the results to the first sum.
3. The last digit of the sum should correspond to the ninth character of the DEA number.

As an example, check the DEA number for Dr. Natasha Jones, DEA registration number AJ 1234563:

1. Add the first, third, and fifth digits: $1 + 3 + 5 = 9$.
2. Sum the second, fourth, and sixth digits, then multiplying by two: $(2 + 4 + 6) \times 2 = 24$.
3. Next, sum the two results: $9 + 24 = 33$

Compare the last digit of step 3 with the last digit of the DEA registration number; because they match, it is an indication that the prescription may be from a legitimate practitioner. Individuals who are attempting to obtain controlled substances by forged prescriptions often know this validation check, so it is not an absolute guarantee.

Medications

There are two types of medications to be considered, the type that needs to be prescribed and the type that the person can purchase over the counter (OTC). The 1951 Durham-Humphrey amendment (§ 503:21 U.S.C. §3 53) to the 1938 Food Drug and Cosmetic Act created these two categories of drugs. This amendment created what is referred to as "legend" drugs by requiring the statement "Caution: Federal law prohibits dispensing without a prescription." [Recently changed to "Rx only" U.S.C. 21 § 353 (4) (a)] Legend medications can be dispensed only via a prescription, and the practitioner must authorize refills of the prescription. Over-the-counter medications do not require a prescription to be purchased. These medications are proven able to be used safely by patients without a prescription and are often sold in nonpharmacy settings such as grocery or mass merchandising stores.

Drug Product Selection

State law may allow a pharmacist to select drug products and dispense a generic medication that is bioequivalent to a brand name product. There is no federal law that governs this arena; it is left to the state to determine if pharmacists are allowed to perform this activity. The federal government (FDA) does provide some guidance for the pharmacist in making the decision of what is bioequivalent by publishing the *Approved Drug Products with Therapeutic Equivalence Evaluations.*[3] This book rates the bioequivalence of drugs. Bioequivalence is defined as the rate and extent of absorption of a test drug as compared to the rate and extent of absorption of a reference drug when administered at the same molar dose of the therapeutic ingredient under similar experimental conditions in either a single or multiple dose (*Approved Drug Products with Therapeutic Equivalence Evaluations, 20th ed., p. ix*)[3] of all FDA-approved generic products against the brand name product. Products are given a rating that consists of two letters the first of which can be either A or B. If the rating is an A designation, the product is considered therapeutically equivalent to the brand name product. If the rating is a B designation, the product is considered not to be bioequivalent, or the product has not been tested against the brand name product. The second letter designates the dosage form of the product; examples include the following:

AA: Drugs that are available in conventional dosage forms and have no bioequivalence problems.

AB: Drugs meeting necessary bioequivalence requirements.

BC: Drugs in extended-release dosage forms with bioequivalence issues.

BP: Active ingredients and dosage forms with potential bioequivalence problems.

B: Drugs for which no determination of therapeutic equivalence will be made until certain questions have been resolved.

Refills

The number of refills or length of time the prescription is valid is legislated by the states. The number of refills will be limited by federal law, depending on whether the medication is a controlled substance. If it is a schedule III, IV, or V drug (21 C.F.R. § 1306.22), it can only be refilled a maximum of five times in a 6-month period from the day it was written, if so indicated by the practitioner. A schedule II medication cannot be refilled under any conditions (21 C.F.R. § 1306.12).

Although schedule II prescriptions cannot be refilled, and the total amount is to be dispensed at the time it is presented at the pharmacy, there are certain circumstances when the prescription may have to be partially filled. For example, when the pharmacist is presented a prescription for 60 meperidine tablets and he or she has only 30 on hand, what is the proper procedure? It is permissible to supply the quantity that the pharmacy has available and then fill the balance within 72 hours [21 C.F.R. § 1306.13(a)]. If the balance of the prescription cannot be filled within the 72-hour period, the pharmacist is to notify the prescriber and, if needed, have the patient obtain a new prescription. The pharmacist is not allowed to supply any more from the first prescription. There are two other situation where partial filling of a schedule II prescription is allowed, and that is for patients in long-term care facilities (LTCF) or patients with a documented terminal illness. Then individual dosage units may be dispensed, however, only up to a 60-day supply from the date of issuance [21 C.F.R. § 1306.13(b)], and no partial fillings can exceed the original quantity prescribed. The pharmacist must document that the patient is either terminally ill or a LTCF patient, and it must be recorded on the prescription. If it is not recorded, the pharmacist is considered to be in violation of the Controlled Substance Act.

Labeling of the Prescription Vial

The label of the prescription vial must contain certain information according to federal law. The information to be included on the label is the Pharmacy's name and address, serial number or prescription number, date the prescription is written or dispensed, prescriber's name, and, if stated in the prescription, the patient's name, directions for use, and cautionary statements, if any. State law may require other additional information to be on the label. That added information may include the drug name, strength, and quantity, expiration date, and pharmacy's telephone number. The labeling requirements apply only to prescriptions dispensed in a community setting; they do not apply to medications dispensed to an institutionalized patient [21 U.S.C. § 356 (b)(2)].

SUMMARY

The pharmacist may be held criminally and/or civilly liable if any laws are violated and harm comes to a patient. The physician who prescribes the medicine must perform risk assessment on the patient to determine what is the best course of treatment for the particular disease. The physician will perform a risk versus benefit analysis on all possible treatment for a patient and determine which is the best for the patient. As long as the treatment that the physician decides on is an accepted medical treatment, he is generally safe from civil liability. The pharmacist, on the other hand, must perform risk management. The pharmacist must help the patient manage the risk of the treatment. For example, if the treatment requires a medication that may cause drowsiness, the pharmacist needs to council the patient about this possibility and ways to control it or to avoid situations that may cause harm. In this way, the pharmacist is helping the patient manage the risk of this treatment.

This chapter has covered the functions of the FDA and DEA agencies and the federal rules and regulations for filling prescriptions. You should now work to learn more about the rules and regulations upheld by these federal agencies. The federal laws discussed here are only a portion of the information you need to practice pharmacy, but they are a good start for your early career. As you advance through the pharmacy program, each piece of information you learn about the laws regulating the practice of pharmacy will add to the basic premises discussed in this chapter. Filling a prescription requires more than putting the right drug in the right bottle. As a pharmacy student/intern you must practice according to the law now, so that when you alone are responsible, you will be able to make the right decisions.

QUESTIONS

1. A patient enters your pharmacy and requests that her prescriptions be dispensed in containers with no lids. Is it legal to do this, and if not what could you as the pharmacist do?
2. A gentleman walks into your pharmacy and tells you he has a product that can cure the common cold and wants you to sell it in your pharmacy. Should you do this? Why or why not?
3. A patient bring a prescription for Tylox (A schedule II controlled substance) into your pharmacy with just the patient's name, the medication's name, the quantity to dispense, and the prescriber's signature. What additional information do you need if any?
4. A new patient brings a prescription into your pharmacy. What types of information do you need to perform a prospective DUR?
5. Is informing a patient that a medication may cause drowsiness risk assessment or risk management, and why?

REFERENCES

1. Code of Federal Regulations. Washington DC: Office of the Federal Register, National Archives and Records Administration, US Government Printing Office, annual.
2. Pharmacist's Manual: An Informational Outline of the Controlled Substance Act of 1970. Washington DC: Drug Enforcement Agency, 1995.
3. Food and Drug Administration. Approved Drug Products with Therapeutics Equivalence Evaluations. Washington DC: Government Printing Office, 1979 and annual updates.

INTERPRETATION OF CLINICAL LABORATORY DATA

Karen Daniel

Goals: After reviewing the information in this chapter, you should be able to:

1. Recognize normal ranges for common laboratory values.
2. Identify common causes for abnormal laboratory values.
3. List circumstances that may produce false-negative or false-positive laboratory results.
4. Interpret the clinical significance of abnormal laboratory values.
5. Utilize clinical laboratory data to monitor various disease states.

INTRODUCTION

This chapter is designed to provide an overview of common laboratory tests used in clinical practice. The most frequently used tests such as complete blood count (CBC), electrolytes and blood chemistries, and urinalysis (UA) are provided first, followed by other clinical and diagnostic tests grouped by organ system.

CLINICAL PEARLS WHEN INTERPRETING LAB DATA

- Normal values may vary from lab to lab depending on techniques and reagents used.
- Normal values may also vary depending on the patient's age, gender, weight, height, and other factors.
- Laboratory error is a fairly uncommon occurrence; however, it can happen. The following are some potential causes of laboratory error:[1,2]
  — Technical error
  — Spoiled specimen
  — Specimen taken at the wrong time (improper sample timing)
  — Incomplete specimen
  — Faulty reagents

— Diet; e.g., red meat consumption may cause a false-positive hemoccult stool test
— Medications; e.g., iron supplements may cause a false-positive hemoccult stool test
- If laboratory error is suspected, the test should be repeated.
- Remember: always treat the patient, not the lab value!

HEMATOLOGY

Complete Blood Count

The complete blood count is an extremely common laboratory test that provides values for hemoglobin (Hgb), hematocrit (Hct), white blood cells (WBCs), red blood cells (RBCs), and red cell indices—mean corpuscular volume (MCV), mean corpuscular hemoglobin (MCH), and mean corpuscular hemoglobin concentration (MCHC).[1,3] In addition, some laboratories may also include platelet count and WBC differential.

Hemoglobin (Hgb)

Normal Range

Male	14–18 g/dL	SI 8.7–11.2 mmol/L
Female	12–16 g/dL	SI 7.4–9.9 mmol/L

Description

Hemoglobin is the oxygen-carrying compound found in the RBCs. Hemoglobin level is a direct indicator of the oxygen-carrying capacity of the blood.[4,5] Adaptation to high altitudes, extreme exercise, and pulmonary conditions may cause variations in hemoglobin values.[2]

Clinical Significance

Increased Hemoglobin

Hemoglobin values may be increased in diseases such as polycythemia vera and chronic obstructive lung disease. Hgb may also be increased in chronic smokers and individuals who engage in regular vigorous exercise or live at high altitudes.[2,5]

Decreased Hemoglobin

Hemoglobin is decreased in anemia of all types, particularly iron-deficiency anemia (IDA). Hgb is also reduced with blood loss, hemolysis, pregnancy, fluid replacement, or increased fluid intake.[1,5]

Hematocrit (Hct)

Normal Range

Male	42–52%	SI 0.42–0.52
Female	37–47%	SI 0.37–0.47

Description

The hematocrit describes the volume of blood that is occupied by RBCs. It is expressed as a percentage of total blood volume. Another name for hematocrit is packed cell volume. As a rule of thumb, the Hct value is generally about three times the value of hemoglobin.[4]

Clinical Significance

Increased Hematocrit

Similar to increases in Hgb, increases in Hct are associated with polycythemia vera, chronic obstructive lung disease, and individuals who live at high altitudes. Increased hematocrit may also be seen in cases of dehydration and shock.[1,2,5]

Decreased Hematocrit

Hematocrit is decreased in all types of anemias, blood loss, hemolysis, pregnancy, cirrhosis, hyperthyroidism, and leukemia.

Red Blood Cell (RBC) Count or Erythrocyte Count

Normal Range

Male	$4.3–5.9 \times 10^6$ cells/mm^3	SI $4.3–5.9 \times 10^{12}$ cells/L
Female	$3.5–5.5 \times 10^6$ cells/mm^3	SI $3.5–5.5 \times 10^{12}$ cells/L

Description

RBCs are produced in the bone marrow. They are released into the systemic circulation and serve to transport oxygen from the lungs to the body tissues. After circulating for a life span of approximately 120 days, the RBCs are cleared by the reticuloendothelial system.[1,2]

Clinical Significance

Increased RBCs

Increased red blood cell counts are associated with polycythemia vera, high altitudes, and strenuous exercise.

Decreased RBCs

Red blood cell counts are decreased in various types of anemias.

Mean Corpuscular Volume or Mean Cell volume (MCV)

Normal Range

76–96 μm^3/cell   SI 76–96 fL

Description

The MCV provides an estimate of the average volume of the erythrocyte. The higher the MCV, the larger the average size of the RBC. Cells with an abnormally large MCV are classified as *macrocytic*. Conversely, cells with a low MCV are referred to as *microcytic*. *Normocytic* RBCs have an MCV that falls within the normal range.

Clinical Significance

Increased MCV

An increase in MCV is associated with folate deficiency, B_{12} deficiency, alcoholism, chronic liver disease, hypothyroidism, and use of medications such as valproic acid, AZT, stavudine, and antimetabolites.[2,5,6]

Decreased MCV

Decreased MCV may result from iron deficiency anemia, hemolytic anemia, lead poisoning, and thalassemia.

Mean Corpuscular Hemoglobin or Mean Cell Hemoglobin (MCH)

Normal Range

27–33 pg/cell   SI 27–33 pg/cell

Description

The MCH indicates the average weight of hemoglobin in the RBC. Cells with a low MCH are pale in color and are referred to as *hypochromic*. Cells with an increased MCH are *hyperchromic*.

Clinical Significance

Increased MCH

Elevated MCH may be caused by folate deficiency. In hyperlipidemia patients, MCH may be falsely elevated because of specimen turbidity.[4]

Decreased MCH

Decreased MCH is associated with iron deficiency anemia.

Mean Corpuscular Hemoglobin Concentration or Mean Cell Hemoglobin Concentration (MCHC)

Normal Range

32–36 g/dL   SI 320–360 g/L

Description

MCHC is a measure of average hemoglobin concentration in the RBC.

Clinical Significance

Increased MCHC

Increased MCHC is associated with hereditary spherocytosis.[5]

Decreased MCHC

MCHC may be decreased in iron deficiency anemia, hemolytic anemia, lead poisoning, and thalassemia.

Reticulocytes

Normal Range

0.5–2% of RBC   SI 0.005–0.02 RBC

Description

Reticulocytes are immature RBCs formed in the bone marrow. An increase in reticulocytes usually indicates an increase in RBC production, but may also be indicative of a decrease in the circulating number of mature erythrocytes.[4]

Clinical Significance

Increased Reticulocytes

Increased reticulocyte counts are associated with hemolytic anemia, hemorrhage, and sickle cell disease. Increased reticulocytes are also indicative of response to treatment of anemias secondary to iron deficiency, B_{12} deficiency, or folate deficiency.[4,5]

Decreased Reticulocytes

Reticulocytes may be decreased as a result of infectious causes, renal disease (from decreased erythropoietin), toxins, iron deficiency anemia, and drug-induced bone marrow suppression.[2,4,5]

White Blood Cell (WBC) or Leukocyte Count

Normal Range

3,200–10,000 cells/mm^3 SI 3.2–10.0 $\times$ 10^9 cells/L

Description

The WBC count represents the total number of WBCs in a given volume of blood. Mature white blood cells exist in many forms, including neutrophils, lymphocytes, monocytes, eosinophils, and basophils. A WBC count with differential provides a breakdown of the percentage of each type of WBC.

Clinical Significance

Increased WBCs

An increase in WBC count is referred to as *leukocytosis*. Leukocytosis may be caused by infection, leukemia, trauma, and corticosteroid use. Emotion, stress, and seizures may also increase WBC count.[2]

Decreased WBCs

A decrease in WBC count is referred to as *leukopenia*. Decreased WBCs may be seen in viral infection, aplastic anemia, and use of chemotherapy or anticonvulsants.

Neutrophils (Polys, Segs, PMNs)

Normal Range

Segs	36–73%	SI 0.36–0.73
Bands	3–5%	SI 0.03–0.05

Description

Neutrophils are the most common type of WBC. Their primary function is to fight bacterial and fungal infections by phagocytizing foreign particles. Neutrophils may also be involved in the pathogenesis of some inflammatory disorders, e.g., rheumatoid arthritis and inflammatory bowel disease.[1] Bands are immature neutrophils. An increase in bands, often referred to as a "shift to the left" or "left shift," may occur during infection or leukemia.

Clinical Significance

Increased Neutrophils

An increase in circulating neutrophils is called *neutrophilia*. Neutrophilia is associated with infection, metabolic disorders (e.g., diabetic ketoacidosis), uremia, response to stress, emotional disturbances, burns, acute inflammation, and use of medications such as corticosteroids.[1,2]

Decreased Neutrophils

A decrease in the number of circulating neutrophils is called *neutropenia*. Neutropenia may result from viral infections (e.g., mononucleosis, hepatitis), septicemia, overwhelming infection, and use of chemotherapy agents.

Absolute neutrophil count (ANC) is the total number of circulating segs and bands[1] and is calculated from the equation:

$$ANC = [WBC \times (segs + bands)]/100$$

The risk of infection increases dramatically as the ANC decreases. An ANC less than $500/mm^3$ is associated with a substantial risk of infection.

Lymphocytes

Normal Range

20–40%

Description

Lymphocytes are the second most common type of circulating WBC. They are important in the immune response to foreign antigens.

Clinical Significance

Increased Lymphocytes

An elevated lymphocyte count is called *lymphocytosis*. Lymphocytes may be elevated in hepatitis, mononucleosis, chickenpox, herpes simplex, herpes zoster, and other viral infections. Some bacterial infections (e.g., syphilis, brucellosis), leukemia, and multiple myeloma are also associated with lymphocytosis.[1,2,5]

Decreased Lymphocytes

A decreased lymphocyte count is referred to as *lymphopenia*. Lymphopenia may result from acute infections, burns, trauma, lupus, HIV, and lymphoma.

Monocytes

Normal Range

2–8%

Description

Monocytes are synthesized in the bone marrow, released into the circulation, and subsequently migrate into lymph nodes, spleen, liver, lung, and bone marrow. In these tissues, monocytes mature into macrophages and serve as scavengers for foreign substances.[2,4]

Clinical Significance

Increased Monocytes

An elevated monocyte count is referred to as *monocytosis*. Monocytosis may be observed in the recovery phase of some infections, subacute bacterial endocarditis (SBE), tuberculosis (TB), syphilis, leukemia, lymphoma, lupus, rheumatoid arthritis, and cirrhosis.[4,5]

Decreased Monocytes

A reduced monocyte count is called *monocytopenia*. Monocytopenia is usually not associated with a specific disease but may be seen with use of bone marrow suppressive agents or severe stress.

Eosinophils

Normal Range

0–4%

Description

Eosinophils are phagocytic white blood cells that assist in the killing of bacteria and yeast. They are also involved in allergic reactions and in the immune response to parasites.[1,2,4]

Clinical Significance

Increased Eosinophils

An increased eosinophil count, or *eosinophilia*, is associated with allergic disorders, allergic drug reactions, collagen vascular disease, parasitic infections, and some malignancies.

Basophils

Normal Range

0–1%

Description

Basophils are phagocytic white blood cells present in small numbers in the circulating blood. They contain heparin, histamine, and leukotrienes and are probably associated with hypersensitivity reactions.

Clinical Significance

Increased basophils *(basophilia)* may be seen in hypersensitivity reactions to food or medications, certain leukemias, and ulcerative colitis.[2,4]

Platelets

Normal range

150,000–400,000/μL   SI 150–400 $\times$ 10^9/L

Description

Platelets are a critical element in blood clot formation. The risk of bleeding is low unless platelets fall below 20,000–50,000/μL.

Clinical Significance

Increased Platelets

Increased platelets (*thrombocytosis, thrombocythemia*) may be caused by infection, malignancies, splenectomy, chronic inflammatory disorders (e.g., rheumatoid arthritis), polycythemia vera, severe stress, surgery, or trauma.[2,5]

Decreased Platelets

Decreased platelet counts (*thrombocytopenia*) may occur in autoimmune disorders such as idiopathic thrombocytopenic purpura (ITP) and also with aplastic anemia, radiation, chemotherapy, space-occupying lesion in the bone marrow, and use of heparin or valproic acid.[2,5,7]

Aspirin and NSAIDs do not affect platelet count but impair the platelet function.

URINALYSIS

Description

Urinalysis (UA) is a useful laboratory test that enables the clinician to identify patients with renal disorders, as well as some nonrenal disorders. Common elements included in the UA are gross appearance, pH, specific gravity, protein, glucose, ketones, blood, bilirubin, leukocyte esterase, and nitrites.

Appearance

On visual examination, the normal urine color should range from clear to dark yellow. Some cloudiness is normal and may be caused by phosphates or urate, which precipitate as the urine cools to room temperature.[5,8] Abnormal appearances of urine include the following:[2,8]

- *Red-orange* may be caused by presence of myoglobin (from muscle breakdown from seizures, cocaine, or injuries), hemoglobin, medications (rifampin, phenazopyridine, phenolphthalein, phenothiazines), or foods (beets, carrots, blackberries).
- *Blue-green* may result from methylene blue or ingestion of beets.
- *Brown-black* may be associated with presence of myoglobin or porphyrins from porphyria or sickle cell.
- *Foamy urine* indicates the presence of protein or bile acids.

Specific Gravity (SG)

Normal Range

1.010–1.025

Description

Specific gravity is an indication of the ability of the kidney to concentrate urine. Unusually low specific gravity would suggest that the kidneys are not able to concentrate urine appropriately.

Clinical Significance

Low Specific Gravity

Low specific gravity may occur in chronic renal failure or diabetes insipidus.[8]

High Specific Gravity

High specific gravity may be associated with dehydration, excretion of radiologic contrast media, or SIADH. In addition, increased excretion of glucose or protein greater than 2 g per day may also increase urine specific gravity.

pH

Normal Range

4.5–8

Description

Normal urine specimens are acidic. The normal urine pH is approximately 6.

Clinical Significance

Alkaline urine may be found in certain urinary tract infections (UTIs caused by urea-splitting organisms E. coli, Proteus, Klebsiella), renal tubular acidosis, and with use of acetazolamide or thiazide diuretics.[2,5,8]

Protein

Normal Range

0 (<30 mg/dL) to 1+ (30–100 mg/dL)

Description

Trace protein in the urine is a common clinical finding and often has no clinical significance.

Clinical Significance

Repeated positive tests or proteinuria of greater than 150 mg/dL may be a marker of renal disease.[1]

Causes of protein in the urine include diabetic nephropathy, hypertension, fever, exercise, pyelonephritis, multiple myeloma, lupus, and severe CHF.[8]

Glucose and Ketones

Normal Range

Glucose negative; ketones negative

Description

Glucose begins to spill into urine when serum blood glucose is greater than 180.

Clinical Significance

Glucose in the urine suggests diabetes mellitus or, in a known diabetic, suggests the need for improved glucose control.[2,5,8] Glucose in the urine may also be associated with Cushing's disease, pancreatitis, and use of thiazide diuretics, steroids, or oral contraceptives.

Diabetic ketoacidosis (DKA), starvation, the Atkins diet, and alcoholism may produce ketones in the urine.

Blood

Normal Range

Negative to trace

Description

Blood in the urine (*hematuria*) may indicate urinary tract damage.

Clinical Significance

Common causes of hematuria are infection, nephrolithiasis, malignancies, and benign prostatic hypertrophy (BPH).[9]

False-positive results for blood in the urine may occur when povidone iodine is used as a cleansing agent before urine specimen collection.[5,8]

False-negative results may occur in patients taking high doses of vitamin C.

Bilirubin

Normal Range

Zero to trace

Description

Bilirubin in the urine usually produces a dark yellow or brown color.

Clinical Significance

Bilirubin in the urine may be associated with liver disease (e.g., hepatitis) or obstructive biliary tract disease.

Phenazopyridine or phenothiazines may cause a false-positive result for bilirubin in the urine.[8]

Leukocyte Esterase

Normal Range

Zero to trace

Description

Positive leukocyte esterase provides an indication of WBCs in the urine.

Clinical Significance

Leukocyte esterase in the urine is associated with infections and/or inflammation of the urinary tract.

Nitrites

Normal Range

Negative

Description

Gram-negative bacteria are capable of converting dietary nitrates to nitrites.

Clinical Significance

Presence of nitrites in the urine suggests colonization or infection with gram-negative organisms.[8]

ELECTROLYTES AND BLOOD CHEMISTRY

Sodium (Na$^+$)

Normal Range

135–147 mEq/L   SI 135–147 mmol/L

Description

Sodium is the most prevalent cation in the extracellular fluid. Sodium is important in regulating serum osmolality, fluid balance, and acid–base balance.[10] In addition, sodium also assists in maintaining the electric potential necessary for transmission of nerve impulses.[2,10]

Clinical Significance

Increased Sodium

Increased sodium (*hypernatremia*) may result from increased sodium intake or increased fluid loss. Thirst is the primary mechanism to prevent hypernatremia, and, therefore, hypernatremia usually occurs in individuals who are unable to obtain adequate fluid intake. Fluid loss from gastroenteritis, diabetes insipidus, Cushing's disease, hyperaldosteronism, and administration of hypertonic saline solution are causes of hypernatremia.[1,5]

Decreased Sodium

Decreased sodium (*hyponatremia*) may be caused by a decrease in total body sodium but is more commonly attributed to excess accumulation of body water (*dilutional hyponatremia*).[1,2]

Common causes of dilutional hyponatremia include CHF, cirrhosis, and nephrotic syndrome.[1,5] Sodium depletion may also be seen in SIADH, cystic fibrosis, mineralocorticoid deficiency, or fluid replacement with solutions that do not contain sodium.

SIADH may be associated with the use of medications, including chlorpropamide, thiazide diuretics, and carbamazepine.

Potassium (K^+)

Normal Range

3.5–5.0 meq/L   SI 3.5–5.0 mmol/L

Description

Potassium is the main intracellular cation. Serum concentrations of potassium are not always an accurate indicator of potassium levels because potassium is an intracellular ion. Potassium plays a key role in many bodily functions, including regulation of nerve excitability and muscle function. Cardiac function and neuromuscular function can be significantly affected by either an increase or decrease in potassium levels.[2]

Clinical Significance

Increased Potassium

Causes of increased potassium (*hyperkalemia*) include metabolic or respiratory acidosis, renal failure, Addison's disease, and massive cell damage from burns, injuries, and surgery.[2,5] Medications such as ACE inhibitors, potassium supplements, and potassium-sparing diuretics are also contributing factors to hyperkalemia.

It is important to remember that a high potassium value may be reported if the specimen was hemolyzed when the laboratory test was performed.

Decreased Potassium

Causes of decreased potassium (*hypokalemia*) include severe diarrhea and/or vomiting, alkalosis, hyperaldosteronism, Cushing's disease, and use of amphotericin B or thiazide, loop, or osmotic diuretics.[1,5]

If a patient is hypokalemic and potassium supplements have not helped to correct the low potassium, check to see if the magnesium is also low. Decreased potassium is difficult to correct while magnesium remains low.[2]

Chloride

Normal Range

95–105 mEq/L   SI 95–105 mmol/L

Description

Chloride is the principal extracellular anion. Chloride primarily serves a passive role in the maintenance of fluid balance and acid–base balance. Serum chloride values are useful in identifying fluid or acid–base balance disorders.[2,5]

Clinical Significance

Increased Chloride

Increased chloride (*hyperchloremia*) may be seen in metabolic acidosis, respiratory alkalosis, dehydration, and renal disorders.[5]

Decreased Chloride

Decreased chloride (*hypochloremia*) may be associated with prolonged vomiting, gastric suctioning, metabolic alkalosis, CHF, SIADH, and Addison's disease.

Carbon Dioxide (CO_2) Content

Normal Range

22–28 mEq/L   SI 22–28 mmol/L

Description

The majority of CO_2 in the plasma is present as bicarbonate ions, and a small percentage is dissolved CO_2. The CO_2 content is the sum of both bicarbonate ions and dissolved CO_2. CO_2 and bicarbonate are extremely important in regulating physiologic pH.[1,2]

Clinical Significance

Increased CO_2

Increased CO_2 is seen in metabolic alkalosis.

Decreased CO_2

Decreased CO_2 is associated with metabolic acidosis and hyperventilation.[2,5]

Anion Gap

Normal Range

3–11 mEq/L   SI 3–11 mmol/L

Description

The anion gap is calculated using the following formula:

$$Anion\ gap = [Na^+ - (Cl^- + HCO_3^-)]$$

Anion gap is reflective of unmeasured anions. An increase in anion gap suggests an increase in the number of negatively charged weak acids in the plasma.[11] Anion gap is useful in evaluating causes of metabolic acidosis.

Clinical Significance

Anion gap may be increased in conditions such as renal failure, lactic acidosis, ketoacidosis, and salicylate, methanol, or ethylene glycol toxicity.[5,11]

Glucose

Normal Range

Fasting   70–110 mg/dL   SI 3.9–6.1 mmol/L

Description

Glucose is an important energy source for most cellular functions. Blood glucose regulation is achieved through a complex set of mechanisms that involves insulin, glucagon, cortisol, epinephrine, and other hormones.

Clinical Significance

Increased Glucose

The most common cause of increased glucose (*hyperglycemia*) is diabetes mellitus. A fasting blood sugar greater than 126 mg/dL on two occasions or a random blood sugar greater than 200 mg/dL on two occasions is consistent with a diagnosis of diabetes mellitus.[12] Other causes of hyperglycemia include Cushing's disease, sepsis, pancreatitis, shock, trauma, myocardial infarction, and use of corticosteroids or niacin.[2,5]

Decreased Blood Glucose

Decreased blood glucose (*hypoglycemia*) may result from missing a meal, oral hypoglycemic agents, insulin overdose, or Addison's disease.[2,5]

Blood Urea Nitrogen (BUN)

Normal Range

8–18 mg/dL   SI 3.0–6.5 mmol/L

Description

Urea nitrogen is an end product of protein catabolism.[1,2] It is produced in the liver, transported in the blood, and cleared by the kidneys. BUN concentration serves as a marker of renal function.

Clinical Significance

Increased BUN

Increased BUN may be associated with acute or chronic renal failure, CHF, gastrointestinal bleeding (gut flora metabolizes blood to ammonia and urea nitrogen), high-protein diet, shock, dehydration, and nephrotoxic medications.[1,5,8]

Decreased BUN

Decreased BUN is seen in liver failure because of inability of the liver to synthesize urea.

Creatinine

Normal Range

0.6–1.3 mg/dL   SI 53–115 μmol/L

Description

Muscle creatine and phosphocreatine break down to form creatinine. Creatinine is released into the blood and excreted by glomerular filtration in the kidneys. As long as muscle mass remains fairly constant, creatinine formation remains constant. An increase in serum creatinine in the face of unchanged creatinine formation suggests a diminished ability of the kidneys to filter creatinine. Thus, serum creatinine is used as a tool to identify patients with renal dysfunction.[1,2]

Clinical Significance

Increased Creatinine

Increased creatinine is associated with renal dysfunction, dehydration, urinary tract obstruction, increased exercise, hyperthyroidism, myasthenia gravis, and use of nephrotoxic drugs such as cisplatin and amphotericin B.[8]

Decreased Creatinine

Serum creatinine may be reduced in cachexia, inactive elderly or comatose patients, and spinal cord injury patients.

BUN/Creatinine Ratio

Calculating the BUN/creatinine ratio may suggest an etiology for renal dysfunction.[7,8] A BUN/creatinine ratio greater than 20 suggests a prerenal cause such as GI bleeding. A BUN/creatinine ratio between 10 and 20 indicates intrinsic renal disease.

Calcium (Ca^{++})

Normal Range

8.5–10.5 mg/dL   SI 2.1–2.6 mmol/L

Description

The majority of calcium in the body (98–99%) is found in the skeletal bones and teeth. The remainder is found in the blood, muscle, and other tissues. In addition to playing a role in bone mineralization, calcium is important in cardiac and skeletal muscle contraction, blood coagulation, enzyme activity, glandular activity, and transmission of nerve impulses.[2,7,10] In the blood, approximately half of the calcium is in the ionized "free" state, and the other half is bound to proteins or complexed with anions. Only calcium in the free state may be utilized in physiologic functions.[2,7] Calcium levels are regulated by a complex system that involves the skeleton, kidneys, intestines, parathyroid hormone, vitamin D, and serum phosphate.

Clinical Significance

Increased Calcium

The most common causes of increased calcium (*hypercalcemia*) are malignancies and primary hyperparathyroidism. Other causes include Paget's disease, sarcoidosis, vitamin D intoxication, milk alkali syndrome, Addison's disease, and use of thiazide diuretics and lithium.[2,7]

Decreased Calcium

Causes of decreased calcium (*hypocalcemia*) include hypoparathyroidism, vitamin D deficiency, hyperphosphatemia, pancreatitis, alkalosis, renal disease, and use of loop diuretics.[7]

Pseudohypocalcemia

Approximately one-half of serum calcium circulates bound to plasma proteins such as albumin. A decreased albumin concentration may lead to a decreased total serum calcium concentration, and calcium levels may appear falsely low in the presence of low albumin. Serum calcium levels may be corrected for low albumin as follows:

Corrected calcium = Reported serum calcium + 0.8 (4.0 − patient's albumin)

Inorganic Phosphorus

Normal Range

2.6–4.5 mg/dL   SI 0.84–1.45 mmol/L

Description

Phosphate is an intracellular anion involved in several critical physiologic functions. Phosphate is necessary for formation of the cellular energy source adenosine triphosphate (ATP) and the synthesis of phospholipids. Phosphate also plays a role in protein, fat, and carbohydrate metabolism, as well as acid–base balance.[2,10]

Clinical Significance

Increased Phosphate

Increased phosphate (*hyperphosphatemia*) can result from renal dysfunction, increased vitamin D intake, increased phosphate intake, hypoparathyroidism, and bone malignancy.[2,5,10]

Decreased Phosphate

Decreased phosphate (*hypophosphatemia*) can be associated with overuse of aluminum- and calcium-containing antacids (these bind phosphorus in the GI tract), alcoholism, malnutrition, and respiratory alkalosis.[2,5]

Magnesium (Mg^{++})

Normal Range

1.7–2.4 mg/dL   SI 0.85–1.2 mmol/L

Description

Magnesium is a necessary cofactor in physiologic functions utilizing ATP.[2,10] It is also vital in protein and nucleic acid synthesis, as well as neuromuscular function.

Clinical Significance

Increased Magnesium

Increased magnesium (*hypermagnesemia*) may result from renal failure or Addison's disease. In addition, the administration of Mg supplements or Mg-containing antacids or laxatives to patients with renal dysfunction may also result in hypermagnesemia.

Decreased Magnesium

Reduced magnesium (*hypomagnesemia*) may be associated with diarrhea, vomiting, malabsorption, alcoholism, hyperaldosteronism, pancreatitis, and use of diuretics, amphotericin B, or cisplatin.

Uric Acid

Normal Range

Male   3.6–8.5 mg/dL   SI 214–506 μmol/L
Females   2.3–6.6 mg/dL   SI 137–393 μmol/L

Description

Uric acid is the main metabolic end product of the purine bases of DNA.[7,13]

Clinical Significance

Increased Uric Acid

Increased uric acid (*hyperuricemia*) may be caused by excessive production of purines or inability of the kidney to excrete urate. Common causes of hyperuricemia are renal dysfunction, tumor lysis syndrome, high-protein diet, and use of furosemide, thiazide diuretics, and niacin.

Hyperuricemia may be associated with the development of gouty arthritis, nephrolithiasis, and gouty tophi.[13]

Decreased Uric Acid

Decreased uric acid levels (*hypouricemia*) are usually of little clinical significance but may occur with a low-protein diet or use of allopurinol, probenecid, or high doses of aspirin or vitamin C.[13]

Osmolality

Normal Range

280–295 mOsm/kg   SI 280–295 mmol/kg

Description

Plasma osmolality describes the osmotic concentration or number of osmotically active particles in the plasma. Sodium, glucose, and blood urea nitrogen are the main components that determine serum osmolality. The serum osmolality may be calculated as follows:[2,14]

$$\text{Serum osmolality} = 1.86\,[Na^+] + \text{glucose}/18 + \text{BUN}/2.8$$

Clinical Significance

Increased Serum Osmolality

Increased serum osmolality may occur with dehydration, diabetic ketoacidosis (DKA), diabetes insipidus, and ethanol, methanol, or ethylene glycol toxicity.

Decreased Serum Osmolality

Decreased serum osmolality may be caused by overhydration or SIADH.

Total Serum Protein

Normal Range

6.0–8.5 g/dL   SI 60–85 g/L

Description

The total serum protein is the sum of albumin, globulins, and other circulating proteins in the serum.[2,5] Albumin and globulins are indicators of nutritional status.

Clinical Significance

Increased Protein

Increased protein (*hyperproteinemia*) may be associated with collagen vascular diseases (lupus, rheumatoid arthritis, scleroderma), sarcoidosis, multiple myeloma, and dehydration.

Decreased Protein

Decreased serum protein may result from a decreased ability to synthesize protein (liver disease) or an increased protein wasting as seen in renal disease, nephrotic syndrome, and third-degree burns.[2,5]

Cholesterol

For a complete discussion of cholesterol, please see the section on cardiac diagnostic tests.

CARDIAC DIAGNOSTIC TESTS

Creatine Kinase (CK)

Normal Range

The normal range may vary with the assay used.

Total CK

Male	40–200 IU/L
Female	35–150 IU/L

CK-MB

<12 IU/L or <4% of total CK

Description

Creatine kinase is an enzyme that is found primarily in skeletal muscle and in smaller fractions in the brain and cardiac muscle.[15] CK levels may be fractionated into isoenzymes to distinguish CK from muscle (CK-MM), brain (CK-BB), and cardiac tissue (CK-MB). CK-MB is an important marker in the diagnosis of acute myocardial infarction (AMI).[2,15,16]

Clinical Significance

The CK-MB levels begin to rise 4 to 8 hours after onset of acute myocardial infarction.[5,15,16] The concentration usually peaks between 12 and 24 hours, and levels return to normal 2 to 3 days after AMI. Serial CK-MB tests are useful in the diagnosis of AMI. An elevated CK-MB level or a CK-MB fraction greater than 4–5% of total CK is suggestive of AMI.[5,16]

An elevation of total CK may be seen with trauma, surgery, shock, tonic–clonic seizures, muscular dystrophy, cerebrovascular accident, polymyositis, dermatomyositis, chronic alcoholism, and malignant hyperthermia.

Troponin

Normal Range

Troponin I	<1.5 ng/mL (varies with assay)
Troponin T	0.1–0.2 ng/mL

Description

Troponin I and T are sensitive markers of cardiac injury.[15,17]

Clinical Significance

Troponin levels begin to rise within 4 hours of onset of chest pain.[15] Levels should be drawn on admission and within 8 to 12 hours thereafter.[17] Patients with elevated troponin levels are considered at high risk for a significant cardiac event.

Approximately 30% of patients with no elevation in CK-MB may demonstrate elevated troponin and thus be diagnosed with a non-Q-wave myocardial infarction.[17]

LIPOPROTEIN PANEL

Total Serum Cholesterol

Blood Levels

Desirable Level	<200 mg/dL	SI <5.17 mmol/L
Borderline High	200–239 mg/dL	SI 5.2–6.21 mmol/L
High Cholesterol	≥ 240 mg/dL	SI 6.22 mmol/L

Description

Cholesterol is an important component of cell membranes and is necessary for the synthesis of many hormones and bile acids.[18] Elevated total serum cholesterol is well known to be associated with an increased risk of developing coronary heart disease (CHD).[21] Total serum cholesterol is a useful screening test to determine CHD risk.

Clinical Significance

Adults over 20 years of age should have a baseline cholesterol profile, and testing should be repeated at least every 5 years thereafter.[19,21] Cholesterol levels should be performed after the patient has fasted for at least 12 hours.

In cases of elevated cholesterol, the need for diet or drug therapy should be based on the individual components of the lipid profile (LDL, HDL, and triglycerides) and the number of CHD risk factors.

Decreased cholesterol levels may be seen in malabsorption, malnutrition, hyperthyroidism, chronic anemia, or severe liver disease.[2,5,21]

Low-Density Lipoproteins (LDL)

Desired Range[19,20]

No CHD and <2 CHD risk factors	< 160 mg/dL (4.11 mmol/L)
No CHD and ≥ 2 CHD risk factors	< 130 mg/dL (3.36 mmol/L)
With CHD or diabetes	< 100 mg/dL (2.6 mmol/L)

Description

Low-density lipoprotein is a major cholesterol transport protein. LDL is considered the "bad" cholesterol and has been linked to atherogenesis.

Clinical Significance

When the triglycerides are less than 400 mg/dL, LDL may be calculated as follows:

$$LDL = total\ cholesterol - HDL - (TG/5)$$

LDL levels should be interpreted in conjunction with CHD risk factors (see desired ranges above), which include:[19]

- Male ≥ 45 or female ≥ 55 years (or premature menopause without estrogen replacement)
- Family history of premature CHD
- Current cigarette smoking
- Hypertension (BP ≥ 140/90 or on antihypertensive medication)
- HDL cholesterol <40 mg/dL

An HDL greater than or equal to 60 mg/dL is considered a negative risk factor, and one CHD risk factor may be subtracted.

Dietary therapy should be initiated when LDL is above the desired range. Drug therapy should be considered when LDL is 30 mg/dL or more above the desired range. In patients with two or more CHD risk factors and a 10-year risk of CHD of 10–20%, drug therapy may be initiated when the LDL is greater than 130 mg/dL.

In addition to lipid disorders, elevated LDL may also be associated with diabetes mellitus, hypothyroidism, and nephrotic syndrome.[2]

High-Density Lipoproteins (HDL)

Blood Levels

Normal Range	30–70 mg/dL	SI 0.78–1.81 mmol/L
Desired Range	>40 mg/dL	SI >1.04 mmol/L

Description

High-density lipoproteins are responsible for transport of 20% to 30% of serum cholesterol. HDL removes excess cholesterol from peripheral tissues. It is considered the "good" cholesterol, and elevated HDL levels are associated with a decreased risk for CHD.

Clinical Significance

Decreased HDL may be associated with cigarette smoking, diabetes mellitus, lack of exercise, and use of anabolic/androgenic steroids or β-blockers.[2,5]

It is estimated that CHD risk increases by 2–3% with each 1 mg/dL decrease in HDL. Elevated HDL may be seen with moderate alcohol intake or in patients taking estrogen, oral contraceptives, or nicotinic acid.[2]

Triglycerides

Blood Levels

Normal range[19]	<150 mg/dL	SI 1.7 mmol/L
Borderline High	150–199 mg/dL	SI 1.7–2.26 mmol/L
High	200–499 mg/dL	SI 2.26–5.64 mmol/L
Very High	≥500 mg/dL	SI >5.64 mmol/L

Description

Triglycerides are the main storage form of fatty acids.

Clinical Significance

Triglycerides may be significantly elevated in the nonfasting state and should be measured after a fast of at least 12–14 hours.

In addition to lipid disorders, elevated triglycerides may be associated with a nonfasting sample, diabetes mellitus, pancreatitis, nephrotic syndrome, chronic renal failure, alcoholism, gout, and use of oral contraceptives or intravenous lipid infusion.[2,5,21]

ENDOCRINE DIAGNOSTIC TESTS: THYROID FUNCTION TESTS

Thyroid-Stimulating Hormone (TSH)

Normal Range

0.3–5 μU/mL   SI 0.3–5 mU/L

Description

Thyroid-stimulating hormone is a sensitive screening test used to detect hypothyroidism or hyperthyroidism.

Clinical Significance

Elevated TSH

Elevated TSH levels are indicative of hypothyroidism. TSH may be falsely elevated in the first trimester of pregnancy.[14]

Low TSH

Abnormally low TSH levels (<0.10) are associated with hyperthyroidism. Medications with dopaminergic activity (e.g., dopamine, levodopa, bromocriptine) can decrease TSH levels.[2,14]

TSH is also a useful test in monitoring therapy for hypothyroidism or hyperthyroidism. Abnormal TSH levels should be followed up with the appropriate thyroid hormone test (free T_4 or T_3). TSH should be monitored 6 to 8 weeks after initiation or a change in therapy. A desirable TSH in the normal range indicates a return to euthyroid state.

Thyroxine (T_4)

Normal Range

4–12 μg/dL   SI 51–154 nmol/L

Description

T_4 is the predominant circulating thyroid hormone. Total serum thyroxine measures both free thyroxine and thyroxine bound to albumin and prealbumin. Only the unbound thyroxine is active. T_4 levels are a measure of the functional status of the thyroid gland.[14] T_4 may also be used to monitor thyroid therapy. T_4 levels may be affected by conditions that increase or decrease the thyroxine-binding proteins.

Clinical Significance

Increased T_4

T_4 can be increased in hyperthyroidism, pregnancy, hepatitis, and with the use of estrogen replacement therapy or oral contraceptives.[2,5,14]

Decreased T_4

Decreased T_4 is most commonly seen in hypothyroidism but may also be associated with renal failure, malnutrition, cirrhosis, and use of medications that compete for T_4 binding sites on T_4 binding proteins (e.g., high-dose salicylates, phenytoin).

Free Thyroxine (Free T_4)

Normal Range

0.8–2.7 ng/dL   SI 10–35 pmol/L

Description

Because total T_4 levels can be affected by conditions that alter the amount of thyroxine binding proteins, free T_4 is the most accurate reflection of clinical thyroid status.

Clinical Significance

Free T_4 is a diagnostic test that may be used to confirm the diagnosis of hypothyroidism (decreased free T_4) or hyperthyroidism (increased free T_4).[2,14] Free T_4 levels may be increased or decreased by amiodarone and iodides and decreased with sulfonamides and lithium.[14]

Total Triiodothyronine (T_3)

Normal Range

80–160 ng/dL   SI 1.2–2.5 nmol/L

Description

Although T_3 is not the predominant circulating thyroid hormone, T_3 is three to four times more potent than T_4. The majority of T_3 is formed from deiodination of T_4 in the kidney and liver. Total T_3 measures both bound and unbound T_3. T_3 is usually used in the diagnosis of hyperthyroidism or T_3 toxicosis, but has little utility in the diagnosis of hypothyroidism.[2,14]

Clinical Significance

Increased T_3

Increased T_3 is seen in hyperthyroidism, T_3 toxicosis, high doses of levothyroxine, and other conditions that also increase T_4 (e.g., pregnancy, oral contraceptive use).

Decreased T_3

Decreased T_3 may be associated with hypothyroidism and malnutrition. Glucocorticoids and propranolol decrease peripheral conversion of T_4 to T_3 and may result in reduced T_3 levels.[2,14]

ENDOCRINE DIAGNOSTIC TESTS: DIABETES MELLITUS

Hemoglobin A_{1c} (HbA$_{1c}$)

Normal Range

4–6%

Description

The HbA$_{1c}$ measures the percentage of hemoglobin molecules that are bound to glucose. During the life span of a RBC, glucose binds irreversibly to hemoglobin in the RBC. As the serum glucose becomes more elevated, more glucose binds to the hemoglobin. Because the RBC has a life span of approximately 120 days, the HbA$_{1c}$ reflects blood glucose control for the 2 to 3 months preceding the test.[2,14]

Clinical Significance

The HbA$_{1c}$ may be used to assess blood sugar control over the 2 to 3 months preceding the test.

The American Diabetes Association recommends a target HbA$_{1c}$ of less than 7% for diabetic patients.[20] A HbA$_{1c}$ greater than 7% indicates the need for improved diabetic control through adjustment of diet, exercise, or medication regimen.

From the HbA$_{1c}$, the average blood glucose may be calculated as follows:

$$\text{Mean blood glucose} = 33.3\,(\text{HbA}_{1c}) - 86$$

ENDOCRINE DIAGNOSTIC TESTS: ADRENAL GLAND TESTS

Cortisol

Normal Range

Morning	6–25 μg/dL	165–690 nmol/L
Evening	3–12 μg/dL	83–331 nmol/L

Description

Cortisol is a hormone produced by the adrenal cortex. It plays a critical role in carbohydrate metabolism and response to stress. Cortisol plasma levels undergo a normal diurnal variation and are highest in the early morning hours.[2,5]

Clinical Significance

Increased Cortisol

Increased cortisol levels are associated with Cushing's syndrome, Cushing's disease, hyperthyroidism, oral contraceptive use, pregnancy, stress, and morbid obesity.[2,5,7]

Decreased Cortisol

Decreased cortisol may be secondary to Addison's disease, hypothyroidism, or decreased pituitary function.

Dexamethasone Suppression Test

Normal Range

Cortisol <5 μg/dL at 8:00 a.m.

Description

In the dexamethasone suppression test, 1 mg of dexamethasone is given at midnight, and plasma cortisol levels are drawn at 8:00 a.m. In a normal patient, the administration of exogenous steroid (dexamethasone) should suppress the release of cortisol from the adrenal gland. The dexamethasone suppression test is useful in the diagnosis of Cushing's syndrome.[2,5]

Clinical Significance

A plasma cortisol level > 5 μg/dL suggests the diagnosis of Cushing's syndrome. Elevated cortisol levels may also be seen in patients who are under various types of stress, including acute illness, pregnancy, and psychiatric disorders. Results should be interpreted with caution in these populations.[2,5]

Adrenocorticotropic Hormone (ACTH)

Normal Range

<60 pg/mL   SI <13.2 pmol/L

Description

Adrenocorticotropic hormone is a hormone secreted from the anterior pituitary. It controls the release of cortisol from the adrenal gland.

Clinical Significance

Increased ACTH

Increased ACTH may be associated with Cushing's disease, adrenal hyperplasia, Addison's disease, or ectopic ACTH production.[5]

Decreased ACTH

Decreased ACTH may be seen in adrenal malignancy or states of pituitary insufficiency.[5]

ACTH Stimulation Test (Cosyntropin)

Description

In the ACTH stimulation test, a baseline cortisol level is drawn. Then synthetic ACTH (cosyntropin) is administered, and cortisol levels are collected 30 and 60 minutes postadministration.

Clinical Significance

Normal

A normal response is doubling of the baseline cortisol level. A rise in cortisol greater than 10 μg/dL above baseline may also be considered a normal response.[2,5,7]

Abnormal

If plasma cortisol remains low and fails to rise greater than 10 μg/dL above baseline, this is indicative of adrenal insufficiency. Further testing (e.g., aldosterone level) is necessary to determine if the cause of the adrenal insufficiency is related to failure of the adrenal (primary adrenal insufficiency) or malfunction of the pituitary (secondary adrenal insufficiency). [2,5,7]

GASTROINTESTINAL/HEPATIC/PANCREATIC DIAGNOSTIC TESTS

Alanine Aminotransferase (ALT)

Formerly called serum glutamic pyruvic transaminase (SGPT).

Normal Range

0–35 U/L   SI 0–0.58 μkat/L (varies with assay)

Description

ALT is an intracellular enzyme present in liver tissue. It is also located in myocardial, muscle, and renal tissue.[5,22]

Clinical Significance

High serum ALT concentrations are indicative of hepatocellular disease. Elevations greater than two times the upper limit of normal are considered significant.

ALT is much more concentrated in liver tissue than the aminotransferase AST and is considered a more specific marker for liver disease.[22]

Increased levels of ALT may occur with hepatitis, alcoholic liver disease, CHF, mononucleosis, and cholestasis.[5,22] Elevated ALT may be caused by a number of medications including HMG-CoA reductase inhibitors and niacin.

Aspartate Aminotransferase (AST)

Formerly called serum glutamic oxolacetic transaminase (SGOT).

Normal Range

0–40 U/L   SI 0–0.67 μkat/L (varies with assay)

Description

AST is another intracellular aminotransferase found in the liver. It is also present in the heart, kidney, pancreas, lungs, and skeletal muscle.[1,5,22] Injury to these tissues will release AST into the systemic circulation and result in serum AST elevation.

Clinical Significance

Elevated AST is associated with hepatitis, alcoholic liver disease, cholestasis, pericarditis, acute myocardial infarction, trauma, CHF, mononucleosis, severe burns, renal infarction, pulmonary infarction, pulmonary embolus, and acute pancreatitis.[5,22]

In alcoholic liver disease, the ratio of AST to ALT is usually greater than 2:1.

Elevations of AST may also be seen with drug toxicity. Erythromycin, levodopa, methyldopa, and tolbutamide may falsely elevate AST by interfering with the assay.[22]

Alkaline Phosphatase (Alk Phos)

Normal Range

This varies with age and assay used.

Description

Alkaline phosphatases are a group of isoenzymes located in bone, liver, intestine, and the placenta.

Clinical Significance

Elevated concentrations of alkaline phosphatase may be seen in a variety of conditions, including obstructive liver disease, cholestasis, cirrhosis, healing bone fractures, Paget's disease, bone metastases, hyperthyroidism, pregnancy, and sepsis.[1,2,5,22]

If the source of elevated alkaline phosphatase is unclear, the isoenzyme may be fractionated to discern if the cause is liver, bone, or other. Alternatively, an increased γ-glutamyl transpeptidase (GGT) with an elevated alkaline phosphatase is highly suggestive of a liver source for the increased alkaline phosphatase (see section on GGT).

Ammonia (NH$_3$)

Normal Range

30–70 μg/dL   SI 17–41 μmol/L

Description

Ammonia is generated through metabolism of protein by intestinal bacteria. Usually, ammonia is absorbed into the systemic circulation, metabolized by the liver, and the by-product urea is excreted by the kidneys.[2,22] Ammonia concentration is most often used in the diagnosis and monitoring of hepatic encephalopathy.

Clinical Significance

Elevated concentrations of ammonia are associated with cirrhosis, other liver diseases, Reye's syndrome, and inherited disorders of the urea cycle.

Bilirubin (Bili)

Normal Range

Total bili	0.1–1.0 mg/dL	SI 2–18 μmol/L
Indirect	0.2–0.7 mg/dL	SI 3.4–12 μmol/L
Direct	0–0.2 mg/dL	SI 0–3.4 μmol/L

Description

Bilirubin is a breakdown product of hemoglobin. The bilirubin produced from hemoglobin metabolism is referred to as unconjugated or indirect bilirubin. Unconjugated bilirubin is converted to conjugated or direct bilirubin by the liver through the process of glucuronidation. Conjugated bilirubin is excreted into the bile and subsequently into the intestine. In the intestine, some bilirubin is excreted in the feces, and the remainder is broken down to urobilinogen. Urobilinogen is later excreted renally.[1,22]

Clinical Significance

Increased levels of indirect bilirubin may result from hemolysis, large hematomas, and the inherited disorder Gilbert's syndrome.[1,2,22]

Elevated direct bilirubin may be associated with hepatocellular disease, hepatitis, cirrhosis, and cholestasis.[1] Jaundice is a classic sign of hyperbilirubinemia that usually occurs when total bilirubin exceeds 2–4 mg/dL. Other signs of hyperbilirubinemia include scleral icterus and dark urine.[22]

γ-Glutamyl Transpeptidase (GGT, GGTP)

Normal Range

Male	0–65 U/L	SI 0–1.08 μkat/L
Female	0–40 U/L	SI 0–0.67 μkat/L

Description

γ-Glutamyl transpeptidase is an enzyme found in the liver, kidney, and prostate. GGT levels are useful in the diagnosis and monitoring of alcoholic liver disease.

Clinical Significance

Increased GGT activity may be seen in alcoholic liver disease, metastatic liver disease, obstructive jaundice, cholelithiasis, pancreatitis, myocardial infarction, and CHF.[5,22]

Enzyme inducers that cause microsomal proliferation such as phenobarbital, rifampin, phenytoin, and carbamazepine may also increase GGT levels.[2,22]

As mentioned previously, an elevated GGT associated with an increased alkaline phosphatase suggests a hepatic source for the abnormal alkaline phosphatase. Conversely, a normal GGT in the face of an elevated alkaline phosphatase points to a nonhepatic cause of the elevated alkaline phosphatase.

Elevations of GGT without elevations of other hepatic enzymes may not be indicative of liver damage.

Lactate Dehydrogenase (LDH)

Normal Range

100–210 IU/L   SI 1.67–3.5 μkat/L (may vary with assay)

Description

Lactate dehydrogenase is an enzyme involved in the interconversion of lactate and pyruvate. It is found in many tissues, including heart, brain, liver, skeletal muscle, kidneys, and RBCs. Elevated LDH is not a very specific finding, as it may occur with damage to any of the aforementioned tissues. If LDH is elevated, it may be fractionated into five isoenzymes to better determine the source of the abnormality.[2,22]

Clinical Significance

Elevated levels of LDH_5 are indicative of liver disease and may be seen in hepatitis, cirrhosis, and biliary tract obstruction. LDH_1 and LDH_2 may be used to confirm the diagnosis of myocardial infarction. After an acute MI, levels of LDH begin to rise within 8 to 12 hours, and the ratio of LDH_1: LDH_2 will be greater than 1 (referred to as a "flip" because levels of LDH_2 normally exceed LDH_1).[2,15]

Other conditions associated with an increased LDH include hemolysis, trauma, muscular dystrophy, pulmonary embolism, pulmonary infarction, acute renal infarction, malignancy, and myocarditis.[5]

Amylase

Normal Range

20–128 IU/L (may vary with assay)

Description

Amylase is an enzyme that aids in digestion by breaking down starch into glucose. The majority of amylase originates from the pancreas and salivary glands, and lesser amounts are secreted by the fallopian tubes, lungs, thyroid, and tonsils.[22] Serum amylase levels are most often used in the diagnosis of acute pancreatitis. The amylase level begins to rise 2 to 6 hours after the onset of acute pancreatitis.

Clinical Significance

Increased concentrations of amylase may be seen in acute pancreatitis, exacerbation of chronic pancreatitis, cholecystitis, appendicitis, ruptured ectopic pregnancy, mumps, alcoholism, and diabetic ketoacidosis.[2,5]

Alcohol abuse and cholecystitis are the two most common causes of pancreatitis in adults.[5] Some medications associated with a risk for pancreatitis include cimetidine, didanosine, estrogens, pentamidine, sulfonamides, tetracycline, and valproic acid.[22]

Lipase

Normal Range

<15 U/dL (may vary with assay)

Description

Lipase is an enzyme that aids in the digestion of fat. It is primarily secreted by the pancreas. Lipase is also useful in the diagnosis of pancreatitis and is considered a more specific marker for pancreatitis than amylase. Like amylase, the lipase level begins to rise within 2 to 6 hours of onset of acute pancreatitis.[5]

Clinical Significance

Elevations of lipase are most often associated with acute pancreatitis. A lipase level greater than three times the upper limit of normal is highly predictive of acute alcoholic pancreatitis.[5,22] Lipase may also be elevated with cholecystitis, cirrhosis, pancreatic cancer, and small bowel obstruction; however, it is usually to a lesser extent than that seen with acute pancreatitis.[2,22]

If lipase is normal and amylase is elevated, this suggests a nonpancreatic origin for the increased amylase.

Helicobacter pylori IgG

Normal Value

Negative

Description

Helicobacter pylori is a curved gram-negative rod that is responsible for the majority of cases of peptic ulcer disease. *H. pylori* can be detected in 90% to 100% of patients with duodenal ulcers and 70% to 80% of patients with gastric ulcers. *H. pylori* IgG is a serologic test that detects antibodies to *H. pylori*. A positive test indicates the presence of *H. pylori*.

Clinical Significance

A positive *H. pylori* IgG in the presence of dyspeptic symptoms is highly suggestive of peptic ulcer disease, and a course of antibiotic therapy is warranted. *H. pylori* IgG may remain positive for many months after treatment of the infection.

   H. pylori has been linked to some types of gastric lymphoma and gastric cancer.[22]

Hemoccult

Normal Value

Negative

Description

The hemoccult test is most commonly used to detect the presence of occult blood in the stool.

Clinical Significance

A positive hemoccult test indicates blood loss in the gastrointestinal tract and deserves further work-up.

   A false-positive result may be obtained if the patient is receiving iron supplementation or has eaten read meat, broccoli, turnips, or radishes within 3 days of the test.[2,23] False negatives may occur in patients taking high doses of vitamin C.

   A hemoccult test should be performed yearly in all patients more than 50 years of age.[24]

HEMATOLOGIC DIAGNOSTIC TESTS

Iron

Normal Range

Male	50–160 μg/dL	SI 9–29 μmol/L
Female	40–150 μg/dL	SI 7–27 μmol/L

Description

The serum iron measures the concentration of iron bound to the iron transport protein transferrin.[2,4,25] Under normal circumstances, approximately one-third of transferrin molecules are bound to iron.

Clinical Significance

Increased Serum Iron

Increased iron may be associated with excessive iron therapy, frequent transfusions, pernicious anemia, hemolytic anemia, thalassemia, and hemochromatosis (iron overload).[2,4]

Decreased Serum Iron

Reduced serum iron is most commonly associated with iron deficiency anemia, a microcytic, hypochromic anemia. Causes include poor dietary intake, pregnancy, blood loss associated with menses, peptic ulcer disease, gastrointestinal bleeding, and inflammatory bowel disease. Other causes of decreased iron are malignancies, anemia of chronic disease, chronic renal disease, hemodialysis, and some infections.[2,4,5]

In iron deficiency anemia, serum iron levels may remain within the lower limit of normal. Thus, serum iron levels are best interpreted along with total iron-binding capacity (TIBC).[25]

Ferritin

Normal Range

Male	15–200 ng/mL	SI 15–200 μg/L
Female	12–150 ng/mL	SI 12–150 μg/L

Description

Ferritin is the storage form of iron. The serum ferritin level provides an accurate reflection of total body iron stores.[2,25]

Clinical Significance

Increased Serum Ferritin

Increased ferritin may result from hemochromatosis, malignancies, inflammation, acute hepatitis, and liver disease.[5]

Decreased Serum Ferritin

Decreased serum ferritin is associated with iron deficiency anemia.[2,25]

Total Iron-Binding Capacity (TIBC)

Normal Range

250–400 μg/dL   SI 44.8–71.6 μmol/L

Description

Total iron-binding capacity is an indirect measurement of serum transferrin. The test is performed by adding an excess of iron to a plasma sample. Any excess unbound iron is removed from the sample, and the serum iron concentration in the sample is measured. This serum iron concentration reflects the TIBC of serum transferrin.

Clinical Significance

Increased TIBC

Increased TIBC may be associated with iron deficiency anemia, pregnancy, and oral contraceptive use.[5]

Decreased TIBC

Decreased TIBC may be caused by anemia of chronic disease, malignancy, infections, uremia, and hemochromatosis.

Vitamin B_{12} (Cyanocobalamin)

Normal Range

100–900 pg/mL   SI 74–664 pmol/L

Description

This test measures serum levels of vitamin B_{12}. Vitamin B_{12} is important in DNA synthesis, neurologic function, and maturation of RBCs.[4,25] Deficiency of vitamin B_{12} produces a macrocytic anemia. Patients may also present with glossitis, paresthesias, muscle weakness, gastrointestinal symptoms, loss of coordination, tremors, and irritability.

Clinical Significance

Decreased vitamin B_{12} may be caused by inadequate dietary intake (rare), decreased production of intrinsic factor, or decreased absorption of B_{12}.[4,25] Decreased levels of B_{12} are associated with pernicious anemia, gastrectomy, Crohn's disease, small bowel resection, intestinal infections, and use of colchicine or neomycin.[4,5,25]

Folate

Normal Range

3.1–12.4 ng/mL   SI 7.0–28.1 nmol/L

Description

This test measures serum folate. Like vitamin B_{12}, folic acid is a vitamin necessary for synthesis of DNA. Deficiency of folic acid results in a megaloblastic anemia.

Clinical Significance

Inadequate intake, decreased absorption, or inability to convert folic acid to the active form tetrahydrofolic acid may cause decreased folic acid. Folate deficiency is associated with alcoholism, poor nutrition, pregnancy, hyperthyroidism, Crohn's disease, small bowel resection, celiac disease, and the use of medications such as trimethoprim-sulfamethoxazole, methotrexate, and sulfasalazine.[4,25]

COAGULATION TESTS

Prothrombin Time (PT)

Normal Range

11–13 seconds (varies)

Description

The prothrombin test is sensitive to changes in the levels of clotting factors prothrombin (factor II), factor VII, and factor X.[26] It is performed by adding thromboplastin and calcium to a plasma sample. After addition of these reagents, the time it takes the blood to clot is measured.

Clinical Significance

The PT is used to monitor warfarin therapy. Because the PT may vary according to the thromboplastin used to test the sample, the international normalized ratio (INR) is a better monitoring tool.[1,26,27]

The normal PT in a person not on anticoagulation therapy is 11–13 seconds. An increased PT may be seen with anticoagulation therapy, liver disease, vitamin K deficiency, and clotting factor deficiencies.[2,5]

International Normalized Ratio (INR)

Desired Range

Depends on indication for anticoagulation (see below)

Description

Because the PT may vary due to the thromboplastin used, the INR is used to standardize the PT.[1,26,27] The INR adjusts the PT ratio based on the sensitivity of the thromboplastin used to perform the test.

The INR may be calculated as follows:

$$INR = [(Patient\ PT)/(Mean\ Normal\ PT)]^{ISI}$$

ISI is the international sensitivity index rating assigned to a particular thromboplastin.

Desired ranges for the INR are as follows:[26]

INR 2.0–3.0	Atrial fibrillation
	DVT treatment
	PE treatment
	Prophylaxis of venous thrombosis
	Tissue heart valves
	Valvular heart disease
INR 2.5–3.5	Mechanical prosthetic valve

Clinical Significance

An INR below the desired range indicates suboptimal anticoagulation and a need to increase warfarin dosage. Conversely, an INR above the desired range indicates a need to reduce the warfarin dosage.

To appropriately interpret an INR value and decide on the need for dosage adjustments, patients should be questioned regarding dosage of warfarin, missed doses, dietary intake, alcohol intake, and concomitant medications.

Activated Partial Thromboplastin Time (aPTT)

Normal Range

20–45 seconds (varies)

Description

The aPTT is sensitive to changes in the clotting factors thrombin (factor IIa), factor Xa, and factor IXa. It is used to monitor heparin therapy.

Clinical Significance

The normal value above represents a control range for patients not on anticoagulation therapy. Patients on heparin therapy will have an elevated aPTT. Much like the prothrombin time, the aPTT can vary depending on the reagent (partial thromboplastin) used to test the sample. Therefore, a therapeutic range should be established for each institution based on the partial thromboplastin used at that laboratory.[28]

IMMUNOLOGIC DIAGNOSTIC TESTS

Antinuclear Antibodies (ANA Titer)

Normal Value

<1:20 or <1:40 (varies)

Description

Antinuclear antibodies (ANA) are antibodies directed against nucleic acids and other nucleic proteins.[13] The ANA test is used as a diagnostic tool for autoimmune and connective tissue diseases, particularly systemic lupus erythematosus (SLE).[13]

Clinical Significance

High titers may be associated with SLE, rheumatoid arthritis, scleroderma, Sjögren's syndrome, polymyositis, dermatomyositis, and drug-induced lupus (hydralazine, procainamide).[5,13]

False-positive ANA test results may occur in 2–5% of healthy patients. False-positive results may be caused by use of certain medications, including carbamazepine, chlorpromazine, methyldopa, and phenytoin.[5]

Rheumatoid Factor (RF)

Normal Value

< 1:160

Description

Rheumatoid factor is an immunoglobulin whose activity is directed against IgG. Thus, a positive RF test (titer 1:160 or greater) is indicative of an autoimmune process.

Clinical Significance

A positive rheumatoid factor test is most commonly associated with rheumatoid arthritis but may also be seen with SLE, scleroderma, Sjögren's syndrome, malignancy, and infectious diseases such as tuberculosis, syphilis, and endocarditis.[5,13]

Erythrocyte Sedimentation Rate (ESR)

Normal Range

Male	1–15 mm/hr (increases with age)
Female	1–20 mm/hr (increases with age)

Description

The erythrocyte sedimentation rate measures the rate of erythrocyte settlement in anticoagulated blood. In the presence of proteins known as acute phase reactants, erythrocytes settle much more quickly. Acute phase reactants are often associated with infectious or inflammatory disorders. Thus, the ESR is a nonspecific diagnostic test that may be used to support a diagnosis or monitor the progress of an inflammatory or infectious process.[2,5,13]

Clinical Significance

The ESR may be elevated in bacterial infections such as tuberculosis and syphilis, malignancies, ulcerative colitis, polymyalgia rheumatica, temporal arteritis, rheumatoid arthritis, SLE, scleroderma, and other collagen vascular diseases.

INFECTIOUS DISEASE DIAGNOSTIC TESTS

Enzyme-Linked Immunosorbent Assay (ELISA) for HIV

Description

The ELISA test for HIV detects antibodies to HIV. It is a highly sensitive and specific test and is the most commonly used screening test for HIV.[29]

Clinical Significance

False Positive

False-positive results may occur in patients with lupus, syphilis (with positive RPR), influenza, hepatitis B vaccine, chronic hepatitis, and malaria. Positive tests should be repeated to assure positive results. Repeatedly positive samples should be confirmed with the Western blot test.[29]

False Negative

False negatives may be seen in early HIV infection, malignancy, and bone marrow transplant.

Western Blot

Description

The Western blot is a confirmatory test used following a positive ELISA result. It detects antibodies to specific HIV proteins and glycoproteins.[2,30]

Clinical Significance

Positive Result

A positive result following a positive ELISA test confirms the diagnosis of HIV.

False Negative/Indeterminate

False-negative or indeterminate results may occur if seroconversion is not complete. Individuals should be retested at a later date.

CD$_4$ (T$_4$ Lymphocytes)

Normal Range

400–1185/mm^3

Description

CD$_4$ cells are a subset of lymphocytes also known as "helper" cells. CD$_4$ cells are responsible for cell-mediated immunity and are a good marker of immune function.

Clinical Significance

As the CD$_4$ cell count decreases, the patient is at increased risk of acquiring opportunistic infections. When the absolute CD$_4$ cell count falls to less than 200, the diagnosis is no longer just HIV but AIDS.

CD$_4$ cell counts are used as indicators for starting prophylaxis in HIV patients (e.g., PCP prophylaxis is initiated at a CD$_4$ <200). With appropriate medication and adherence to treatment the CD$_4$ count may increase.

HIV Viral Load

Range of Assay

HIV-1 RNA by PCR   400–750,000 copies/mL (varies)

Description

HIV viral load testing measures the amount of HIV virus detectable per milliliter of plasma. Higher viral loads are associated with a poorer prognosis and
progression of disease. Viral loads are measured at baseline, 2 to 4 weeks after
initiation of therapy, and approximately every 3 months thereafter.

Clinical Significance

Desirable viral loads are below the limit of detection; e.g., "undetectable" is
<400 copies/mL for HIV-1 RNA by PCR.
    Increasing viral loads may indicate viral resistance or nonadherence to ther-
apy. Patients with undetectable viral loads may be followed up with an ultrasen-
sitive assay that is capable of detecting viral loads as low as 50 copies/mL.

RPR (Rapid Plasma Reagin)

Normal Value

Nonreactive

Description

Syphilis is caused by the spirochete *Treponema pallidum*. The RPR is a nontreponemal serologic test used to screen for syphilis. It may also be used to assess
response to syphilis therapy.

Clinical Significance

A positive RPR titer is suggestive of syphilis and should be followed up with a
confirmatory treponemal test such as the fluorescent treponemal antibody absorbed test (FTA-abs).[31]

False Positive

False-positive results may occur with other infectious diseases such as measles,
chickenpox, malaria, mononucleosis, hepatitis, early HIV infection, and conditions such as pregnancy, lupus, and connective tissue disease.

False Negative

False-negative results may been seen early in infection, and in late infection the test may also be nonreactive.

Most patients revert to a nonreactive test following successful treatment. A fourfold decline in the RPR titer after 1 year may also be considered an adequate response to treatment.[5]

Venereal Disease Research Laboratory Test (VDRL)

Normal Value

Nonreactive

Description

The VDRL is a nontreponemal serologic test used to screen for syphilis. It may also be used to assess response to syphilis therapy.

Clinical Significance

A positive VDRL titer is suggestive of syphilis and should be followed up with a confirmatory treponemal test such as the fluorescent treponemal antibody absorbed test (FTA-abs).[31]

False Positive

False-positive results may be caused by other infectious diseases such as measles, chickenpox, malaria, mononucleosis, hepatitis, early HIV infection, and other conditions such as pregnancy, lupus, and connective tissue disease.

False Negative

False-negative results may been seen early in infection, and in late infection the test may also be nonreactive.

Most patients revert to a nonreactive test following successful treatment. A fourfold decline in the VDRL titer after 1 year may also be considered an adequate response to treatment.[5]

HEPATITIS A

Anti-HAV IgM

Normal Value

Negative

Description

Hepatitis A IgM antibodies may be detected in the serum 4–6 weeks after exposure to hepatitis A and often coincide with the onset of jaundice.

Clinical Significance

The presence of anti-HAV IgM indicates acute hepatitis A.[2,5,22] Anti-HAV IgM
becomes negative within 2–3 months after acute hepatitis.[2,22,32]

Anti-HAV IgG

Normal Value

Negative

Description

Anti-HAV IgG can be detected 6–12 weeks after exposure to hepatitis A.

Clinical Significance

Presence of anti-HAV IgG indicates previous infection with HAV and immunity
to the virus.[2,22,32]

HEPATITIS B

HBsAg (Hepatitis B Surface Antigen)

Normal Value

Negative

Description

HBsAg is a protein coat that surrounds the hepatitis B virus. It can be detected
in the serum 4–12 weeks after infection.[2,22]

Clinical Significance

A positive test for HBsAg indicates acute hepatitis B. Persistence of HBsAg for
20 weeks or more after acute infection is indicative of chronic hepatitis B.[5,22,33]

Hepatitis B "e" Antigen (HBeAg)

Normal Value

Negative

Description

HBeAg is used to assess the degree of infectivity of patients with hepatitis B.

Clinical Significance

Presence of HBeAg is associated with active viral replication and a high degree of infectivity. HBeAg is usually present for 2–6 weeks after acute infection. Persistence of HBeAg is indicative of chronic hepatitis B.[2,5,22]

Hepatitis B Core Antibody (Anti-HBc)

Normal Value

Negative

Description

Anti-HBc may be detected in the blood a few weeks after the appearance of HBsAg.

Clinical Significance

Positive results for anti-HBc indicate past infection with hepatitis B. These antibodies seem to persist for life.[2,5,33]

Hepatitis B Surface Antibody (Anti-HBs)

Normal Value

Negative

Description

Anti-HBs is usually detected in the blood 5 to 6 months after infection.

Clinical Significance

Presence of anti-HBs indicates recovery and immunity to hepatitis B.

Individuals who have been vaccinated for hepatitis B will test positive for anti-HBs. Because anti-HBs levels may decline and/or disappear over time, revaccination at 5 to 7 years is recommended.[5,33]

HEPATITIS C

Hepatitis C Antibody (Anti-HCV)

Normal Value

Negative

Description

Anti-HCV is used as a screening test for hepatitis C virus.

Clinical Significance

Presence of anti-HCV indicates prior exposure to or chronic infection with hepatitis C. Unlike antibodies to hepatitis A and hepatitis B, antibodies to hepatitis C do not confer immunity.

Antibodies may not be present until 6–12 weeks after acute infection.

A positive test for Anti-HCV should be followed by a confirmatory test such as the radioimmunoblot assay (RIBA) or hepatitis C viral load (HCV RNA by PCR).[22,34]

QUESTIONS

1. Which of the following would be considered an abnormal laboratory value?
   A. A red blood cell count of $5.0 \times 10^6/mm^3$
   B. A urine specific gravity of 1.012
   C. A magnesium level of 1.2 mg/dL
   D. A total iron binding capacity (TIBC) of 300 $\mu g/dL$
   E. An alanine aminotransferase level of 30 U/L
2. Which of the following is *not* a common cause of hyperkalemia?
   A. Renal failure
   B. Cushing's disease
   C. Metabolic acidosis
   D. ACE inhibitors
   E. Severe burns
3. Which of the following may cause a false-positive rapid plasma reagin (RPR)?
   A. Pregnancy
   B. Mononucleosis
   C. Hepatitis
   D. HIV infection
   E. All of the above may cause a false-positive RPR
4. Which of the following abnormal laboratory values would be considered clinically significant?
   A. A potassium of 6.0 meq/L in a patient taking a potassium-sparing diuretic
   B. A positive hemoccult in a patient taking iron supplements
   C. A uric acid level of 2.2 mg/dL in a patient taking Vitamin C
   D. A red-orange urine specimen in a patient taking phenazopyridine
   E. A calcium of 8.0 mg/dL in a patient with a serum albumin of 3.0 g/dL

5. Which of the following laboratory values would suggest the need for a change in pharmacotherapy to better achieve treatment goals?

A. A hemoglobin A_{1c} of 5.8% in a diabetic patient

B. An LDL level of 122 mg/dL in a patient with three risk factors for coronary heart disease

C. An international normalized ratio (INR) of 2.8 in a patient with atrial fibrillation

D. A thyroid-stimulating hormone (TSH) level of 7.5 μU/mL in a patient with hypothyroidism

E. A mean corpuscular volume (MCV) of 90 μm^3/cell in a patient with a history of vitamin B_{12} deficiency

REFERENCES

1. Holland EG, Young LY. Interpretation of clinical laboratory tests. In: Koda-Kimble MA, Young LL, eds. Applied therapeutics: the clinical use of drugs, 7th ed. Baltimore, MD: Lippincott Williams & Wilkins, 2001:2-1–2-22.
2. Christopherson RC, Vick Smith KE. Clinical laboratory tests. In: Boh LE, ed. Clinical clerkship manual. Vancouver, WA: Applied Therapeutics, 1993:5-1–5-63.
3. Speicher CE. A physician's guide to laboratory medicine, 2nd ed. Philadelphia: WB Saunders, 1993.
4. Jordan NS. Hematology: red and white blood cell tests. In: Traub SL, ed. Basic skills in interpreting laboratory data, 2nd ed. Bethesda, MD: American Society of Health-System Pharmacists, 1996:297–319.
5. Bakerman S, Bakerman P, Strausbach P. ABC's of interpretive laboratory data, 3rd ed. Myrtle Beach, SC: Interpretive Laboratory Data, 1994.
6. Kenna WF. Macrocytosis as an indicator of human disease. J Am Board Fam Pract 1989;2:252–256.
7. Vaughn G. Understanding and evaluating common laboratory tests. Stamford, CT: Appleton & Lange, 1999.
8. Traub SL. The kidneys. In: Traub SL, ed. Basic skills in interpreting laboratory data, 2nd ed. Bethesda, MD: American Society of Health-System Pharmacists, 1996:131–157.
9. Sutton JM. Evaluation of hematuria in adults. JAMA 1990;263:2475–2480.
10. Ateshkadi A, Pelter MA. Electrolytes, other minerals, and trace elements. In: Traub SL, ed. Basic skills in interpreting laboratory data, 2nd ed. Bethesda, MD: American Society of Health-System Pharmacists, 1996:93–130.
11. Hall TG. Arterial blood gases and acid–base balance. In: Traub SL, ed. Basic skills in interpreting laboratory data, 2nd ed. Bethesda, MD: American Society of Health-System Pharmacists, 1996:159–174.
12. Report of the expert committee on the diagnosis and classification of diabetes mellitus. Diabetes Care 2002;25(Suppl 1):S5–S20.
13. Marble DA. Rheumatic diseases. In: Traub SL, ed. Basic skills in interpreting laboratory data, 2nd ed. Bethesda, MD: American Society of Health-System Pharmacists, 1996:371–396.
14. Traub SL. Endocrine disorders. In: Traub SL, ed. Basic skills in interpreting laboratory data, 2nd ed. Bethesda, MD: American Society of Health-System Pharmacists, 1996:245–280.
15. Geraets DR. The heart and myocardial infarction. In: Traub SL, ed. Basic skills in interpreting laboratory data, 2nd ed. Bethesda, MD: American Society of Health-System Pharmacists, 1996:187–211.
16. Stringer KA, Lopez LM. Myocardial infarction. In: DiPiro JT, Talbert RL, Yee GC, et al, eds. Pharmacotherapy: a pathophysiologic approach, 4th ed. Stamford, CT: Appleton & Lange, 1999:211–231.
17. Antman EM, Fox KM. Guidelines for the diagnosis and management of unstable angina and non-Q-wave myocardial infarction: proposed revisions. Am Heart J 2000;139:461–475.

18. Talbert RL. Hyperlipidemia. In: DiPiro JT, Talbert RL, Yee GC, et al, eds. Pharmacotherapy: a pathophysiologic approach, 4th ed. Stamford, CT: Appleton & Lange, 1999:350–373.
19. Executive summary of the third report of the National Cholesterol Education Program (NCEP) expert panel on detection, evaluation, and treatment of high blood cholesterol in adults (Adult Treatment Panel III). JAMA 2001;285:2486–2497.
20. Standards of medical care for patients with diabetes mellitus. Diabetes Care 2002;25(Suppl 1): S33–S49.
21. Traub SL. Metabolic disorders. In: Traub SL, ed. Basic skills in interpreting laboratory data, 2nd ed. Bethesda, MD: American Society of Health-System Pharmacists, 1996:281–295.
22. Farkas P, Hyde D. Liver and gastroenterology tests. In: Traub SL, ed. Basic skills in interpreting laboratory data, 2nd ed. Bethesda, MD: American Society of Health-System Pharmacists, 1996:213–244.
23. Willis J. Gastrointestinal diseases. In: Carey CF, Lee HH, Woeltje KF, eds. The Washington manual of medical therapeutics, 29th ed. Philadelphia: Lippincott-Raven, 1998:302–328.
24. Whelan AJ, Mutha S. Patient care in internal medicine. In: Carey CF, Lee HH, Woeltje KF, eds. The Washington manual of medical therapeutics, 29th ed. Philadelphia, Lippincott-Raven, 1998:1–25.
25. Sproat TT. Anemias. In: DiPiro JT, Talbert RL, Yee GC, et al, eds. Pharmacotherapy: a pathophysiologic approach, 4th ed. Stamford, CT: Appleton & Lange, 1999:1531–1548.
26. Hirsh J, Dalen JE, Anderson JR, et al. Oral anticoagulants: mechanism of action, clinical effectiveness, and optimal therapeutic range. Chest 2001;119(Suppl):8S–21S.
27. Groce JB, Carter BL. Hematology: blood coagulation tests. In: Traub SL, ed. Basic skills in interpreting laboratory data, 2nd ed. Bethesda, MD: American Society of Health-System Pharmacists, 1996:321–346.
28. Hirsh J, Warkentin TE, Shaughnessy SG, et al. Heparin and low-molecular weight heparin: mechanisms of action, pharmacokinetics, dosing, monitoring, efficacy, and safety. Chest 2001;119 (Suppl):64S–94S.
29. Schleupner CJ. Detection of HIV-1 infection. In: Mandell GL, Bennett JE, Dolin R, eds. Mandell, Douglas, and Bennett's principles and practice of infectious diseases, 4th ed. Philadelphia: Churchill Livingstone, 1995:1253–1267.
30. Jordan NS. Infectious diseases. In: Traub SL, ed. Basic skills in interpreting laboratory data, 2nd ed. Bethesda, MD: American Society of Health-System Pharmacists, 1996:347–369.
31. Tramont EC. Treponema pallidum (syphilis). In: Mandell GL, Bennett JE, Dolin R, eds. Mandell, Douglas, and Bennett's principles and practice of infectious diseases, 4th ed. Philadelphia: Churchill Livingstone, 1995:2117–2133.
32. Battegay M, Gust ID, Feinstone SM. Hepatitis A virus. In: Mandell GL, Bennett JE, Dolin R, eds. Mandell, Douglas, and Bennett's principles and practice of infectious diseases, 4th ed. Philadelphia: Churchill Livingstone;1995:1636–1656.
33. Robinson WS. Hepatitis B and hepatitis D virus. In: Mandell GL, Bennett JE, Dolin R, eds. Mandell, Douglas, and Bennett's principles and practice of infectious diseases, 4th ed. Philadelphia: Churchill Livingstone, 1995:1406–1439.
34. Lemon SM, Brown EA. Hepatitis C virus. In: Mandell GL, Bennett JE, Dolin R, eds. Mandell, Douglas, and Bennett's principles and practice of infectious diseases, 4th ed. Philadelphia: Churchill Livingstone, 1995:1474–1486.

C H A P T E R 6

A BRIEF LOOK AT THE CONSTRUCTION OF MEDICAL TERMINOLOGY, DEFINITIONS INCLUDED

Pat Parteleno and Ruth E. Nemire

Goals: After reviewing the information in this chapter, you should be able to:

1. Identify the four elements of a medical word.
2. Combine a prefix, root, and/or suffix to form a medical term.
3. Given a medical terminology word, analyze the meaning of the word by defining the prefix, root word, and suffix.

INTRODUCTION

This chapter is included to assist you in understanding the medical terminology you hear. You will find medical jargon used in your microbiology courses, anatomy, physiology, and as you start your rotations early in the course of your pharmacy education. Many of the medical words we use are derived from Greek and Latin languages. You do not have to speak either of these languages to understand the terminology spoken on a daily basis. Once you learn a few common root words, prefixes, and suffixes, you will be able to sound out a word for pronunciation and determine its meaning.

This chapter is not meant to be inclusive of all terms; it is included to help you begin to find your way around medical terminology. This manual contains two tables, one listing prefixes and root words with their meaning and one that names common suffixes. Following the tables is a list of words, many which are used in this textbook and some that are not. If you are looking for the meaning of a term, refer to the alphabetical list of terminology. If you do not find the word there, see if you can piece together the meaning from the word parts listed in the tables. Putting the words together yourself will help you remember the meaning later. In the beginning check a dictionary to make sure you are correct.

We suggest for in-depth study that you invest in a good medical terminology text, as it will include pictures and many exercises to aid in improving your vocabulary.

WHAT'S IN A WORD?

Each medical term used has a *root* word. It establishes the basic meaning and is the part to which the prefix and/or suffix are added. You must be always mindful, for a root word can have more than one meaning in different fields of study. Not all roots are complete words; for example, *"cardi"* is a root word meaning heart. You will not use the word "cardi" alone, but, when combined with the suffix "logy," the word becomes *cardiology* and means the study of the heart. You might wonder why it is spelled with an extra letter "o"; it is to make the word easier to say. A vowel that is inserted between a root and a suffix to ease pronunciation is called a *combining vowel*. In many medical terms this is the letter "o." If you are trying to put word parts together and you can't say it, or it doesn't sound right, try adding an "o" or other vowel. The example of "cardi" and "logy" is a perfect use for the combining vowel.

A *prefix* is added to the beginning of a word to modify the meaning. For example, if you add the prefix "pre," meaning *before,* to the word surgical, you get presurgical, meaning before surgery.

You will find a list of prefixes and root words with combining vowels and examples of their use in Table 6.1.

The *suffix* is added at the end of the root word to modify the meaning or enhance the meaning. The suffix "itis" means inflammation. When added to the root word "arthr," meaning *joint*, you form the word arthritis, meaning inflammation of the joint (Table 6.2).

With a little practice identifying word parts and putting them together, you will soon be speaking the language of the health care professional.

DEFINITIONS

Accreditation.   Accreditation programs give an official authorization or approval to an organization by comparing it with a set of industry-derived standards.

Adherence.   Formerly referred to as compliance. The patient taking the prescribed dose of medication at the prescribed frequency for the prescribed length of time.

Adjudication.   The process of completing all validity, process, and file edits necessary to prepare a claim for final payment or denial.

Adjustment.   A credit or debit amount appearing at the carrier/group level on claims and administrative fee invoices sent to plan sponsors or at a claim level on adjustment advice sent to pharmacies. An adjustment can result from claims processing and/or billing errors (e.g., incorrect dispensing fee paid, incorrect pharmacy paid, incorrect administration fee billed, wrong carrier/group billed).

(*Definitions continue on page 144*)

TABLE 6.1. PREFIX AND ROOT WORDS

ROOT	MEANING	EXAMPLE
A/an~	Without, out	Aphonia (without word or speech)
Ab,apo,de~	Away from	Abnormal (pertaining to away from normal)
Abdomin~	Abdomen	Abdominal (pertaining to abdomen)
Actino~	Radiated structure, ray	Actinodermatitis (skin inflammation caused by exposure to radiation)
Ad~	To, toward, near	Adhesion (to sick to)
Adip/o~	Fat	Adiposis (abnormal condition pertaining to fat)
Aer~o	Air, gas	Aerobic (pertaining to air)
Alb, albumin, leuk~o	White	Albumen (white of egg) Leukocyte (white blood cell)
Alge~	Pain	Algesia (supersensitivity to pain)
Allo~	Not normal	Allophasis (incoherent speech)
Alveo~	Hollow	Alveolus (small hollow socket of a tooth; air sac of the lungs)
Amaur~	Dark	Amaurosis (complete loss of vision)
Ambi, amphi, ampho~	Both	Ambidextrous (dexterity in both hands)
Ambly~	Dim, dull	Amblyacousia (dullness of hearing)
Ambulo~	Walk about	Ambulatory (able to walk)
Aneurysm/o~	Localized abnormal dilatation of a vessel	Aortic aneurysm (an aneurysm affecting any part of the aorta from the aortic valve to the iliac arteries)
Aniso~	Unequal, dissimilar	Anisocoria (Inequality of the size of the pupils)
Ankyl~	Attached, crooked	Ankylodactylia (adhesion of two or more fingers or toes)
Ante,fore,pre, pro~	Before, forward	Antepartum (before labor)

(continued)

133

TABLE 6.1. PREFIX AND ROOT WORDS (*Cont.*)

ROOT	MEANING	EXAMPLE
Anter/o~	In front of	Anterograde (moving frontward)
Anti,contra, counter~	Against, opposite	Anticoagulant (against clotting), contraception (opposed to becoming pregnant)
Astro~	Combining form indicating relationship to a star	Astrocyte (a neuroglial cell of the central nervous system that supports neurons and contributes to the blood–brain barrier.)
Atel~	Imperfect	Atelocephaly (incomplete development of the head)
Auto~	Self	Autocytolysis (self-digestion or self-destruction of cells)
Bi, bin, di, diplo, dis~	Two, twice	Bilateral (pertaining to two or both sides)
Bio~	Life	Biology (science of life)
Blast~	Germ	Blastolysis (destruction of a germ cell)
Brachy, brevi~	Short	Brachydactylia (abnormal shortness of the fingers and toes)
		Brevicollis (shortness of the neck)
Brady~	Slow	Bradycardia (condition of slow heart)
Bucc~	Cheek	Buccinator (muscle of the cheek)
Caco~	Bad, ill	Cacosmia (unpleasant odor)
Calori~	Heat	Calorie (unit of heat)
Cardio~	Heart	Cardiologist (one who specializes in treatment of the heart)
Cata~	Down	Catatropia (condition in which both eyes are turned downward)
Centi~	One one-hundredth	Centigram (one hundredth of a gram)
Cervico~	Neck	Cervicodynia (pain or cramp of the neck)
Chir~	Hand	Chiroplasty (plastic surgery on the hand)
Chlor, verdin~	Green	Chloroplast (green cell organelle found in the leaves of plants)

(continued)

134

TABLE 6.1. PREFIX AND ROOT WORDS (*Cont.*)

Chroma~	Color	Chromatism (unnatural pigmentation)
Chron~	Time	Chronological (occurring in natural sequence according to time)
Ciner, glauc, polio~	Gray	Cinerea (gray matter of the brain or spinal cord)
Circum,peri~	Around	Circumvascular (pertaining to around a vessel)
Cirrh, flav, lute, xanth~	Yellow	Cirrhosis (a chronic liver disease), xanthoderma (yellowness of the skin)
Clas~	Break, smash	Clastogenic (capable of breaking chromosomes)
Clin~	Bedside	Clinician (a healthcare professional with expertise in patient care rather than research or administration)
Co, com, con, sym, syn~	Together, with	Congenital (pertaining to being born with)
Cry~	Cold	Crymodinia (pain from cold)
Cryo~	Cold	Cryogenic (pertaining to low temperatures)
Crypt~	Hidden	Cryptic (having a hidden meaning)
Cyano~	Blue	Cyanopia (vision in which all objects appear to be blue)
Cycl~	Round, circular	Cyclooxygenase (one of several enzymes that make prostaglandins from arachidonic acids)
Cyt~	Cell	Cytology (study of cell)
Deca~	Ten	Decagram (mass equal to ten grams)
Deci~	One tenth	Decimeter (one tenth of a meter)
Demi, hemi, semi~	Half	Hemiplegia (paralysis of one side of the body)
Dextro~	To the right	Dextrocardia (condition of the heart on the right side)
Di, dis~	Apart from	Disinfect (to free from infection)

(continued)

135

TABLE 6.1. PREFIX AND ROOT WORDS (*Cont.*)

ROOT	MEANING	EXAMPLE
Dia, per, trans~	Across, through	Dialysis (dissolution across or through a membrane transmission to send across or through)
Dolicho~	Long	Dolichofacial (having a long face)
Dorsi, dorso~	Back	Dorsosacral (pertaining to the lower back)
Dys~	Difficult, painful	Dysphonia (condition of difficult voice or speeh, hoarseness)
E, ec, ex~	Out from	Edentia (condition of teeth out)
		Eccentric (pertaining to away from center)
		Excise (to cut out)
Ecto, extra, extro~	Outside	Ectopic (pertaining to a place outside)
		Extravascular (pertaining to outside vessel)
Em, en, im, in~	In	Encapsulate (within little box)
Endo, ento, intra~	Within	Endoscope (instument for examination within)
		Entotic (pertaining to the interior of the ear)
		Intracardiac (within the heart)
Epi~	Over, upon	Epidermal (pertaining to upon the skin)
Erythr, rube~	Red	Erythrocyte (red cell)
Eso~	Inward	Esophoria (inward turning of the eye)
Eu~	Easily, well	Eugenic (pertaining to good production)
Eury~	Broad	Eurycephalic (having a broad or wide head)
Extra, hyper, per, pleo, super~	Outside of, Excessive, more	Extracellular (outside the cell)
		Hyperalgesia (an excessive sensitivity to pain)
Febri~	Fever	Febrifacient (producing fever)
Gen~	Producing	Generation (act of reproducing offspring)
Gero~	Aged	Gerontology (the scientific study of the effects of aging)

(*continued*)

TABLE 6.1. PREFIX AND ROOT WORDS (*Cont.*)

Glyco~	Sweet, sugar	Glycogeusia (a sweet taste)
Gony~	Knee	Gonyoncus (tumor of the knee)
Gust~	Taste	Gustation (the sense of taste)
Haplo~	Single, simple	Haplopia (single vision)
Hecto~	Hundred	Hectoliter (one hundred liters)
Hept, sept~	Seven	Heptaploidy (having seven sets of chromosomes)
Heter~	Different, other	Heterography (writing different words from those that the writer intended)
Hex, sex~	Six	Sextuplet (one of six children born of a single gestation)
Hidro~	Sweat	Hidrosis (excessive sweating)
Histo~	Tissue	Histoblast (tissue cell)
Holo~	Entire, complete	Holophytic (having plantlike characteristics)
Homo~	Same	Homoblastic (developing from a single type of tissue)
Hydro~	Water	Hydrophobia (exaggerated fear of water)
Hyper~	Above, over	Hyperlipemia (excessive fat in the blood)
Hypno~	Sleep	Hypnogenic (producing sleep)
Hypo~	Below, beneath, under	Hypothermia (condition of below the normal temperature)
Ictero~	Jaundice	Icterogenic (causing jaundice)
Im, in, ir, non, un~	In, within, not	Nondominant (in neurology, the hemisphere that does not control the speech or preferential use of hand)
Infra, sub~	Deficient, less	Infraumbilical (pertaining to under the naval)
		Sublingual (pertaining to under the tongue)
Inter~	Between	Inercostal (pertaining to between ribs)
Intra~	Within	Intraabdominal(within the abdomen)
Ipsi, iso~	Equal, same	Ipsitaleral (on the same side)

(continued)

TABLE 6.1. PREFIX AND ROOT WORDS (*Cont.*)

ROOT	MEANING	EXAMPLE
Iso~	Equal	Isopia (equal vision in the eyes)
Juxta~	Near	Juxtaarticular (situated close to a joint)
Kilo~	Thousand	Kilogram (1000 g)
Kinesio~	Movement	Kinesia (sickness caused by motion)
Lapar~	Flank, loin	Laparocele (abdominal hernia)
Latero~	To the side	Lateroposition (displacement to one side)
Leio~	Smooth	Leiodermia (dermatitis characterized by abnormal glossiness and smoothness of the skin)
Lepto~	Slender, thin	Leptophonia (weakness of the voice)
Levo, sinistro~	To the left	Sinistromanual (left-handed)
Lip~	Fat	Lipoid (resembling fat)
Litho~	Stone	Lithiasis (presence of a stone)
Lysis	Suffix: dissolving or loosen Combining form: relief of or reduction	Cardiolysis (an operation that seperates adhesions constricting the heart)
Macro~	Large, long	Macrocyte (large cell)
Mal~	Bad, ill, poor	Malignant (growing worse)
Malaco~	Soft	Malacosteon (softening of the bones)
Medi, mes, mid~	In the middle	Midline (line that bisects a structure that is bilaterally symmetrical)
Medule~	Marrow	Medullitis (inflammation of marrow)
Megalo~	Large	Megalencephaly (abnormally large size of the brain)
Melan, nigro~	Black	Melanoma (black tumor)

(continued)

TABLE 6.1. PREFIX AND ROOT WORDS (*Cont.*)

Mero~	Part	Meromelia (partial absence of a limb)
Meta~	After, changes, over	Metastasis (beyond stopping or standing, spread of disease from one part of the body to another)
Micro~	Small	Microlith (small stone)
Micro~	One one-millionth	Microgram (one millionth of a gram)
Milli~	One one-thousandth	Milliliter (one thousandth of a liter)
Mis~	Bar, improper, wrong	Misinformation (data or information concerning a patient that may be assumed erroneously to be accurate)
Mono, uni~	One	Monochromatic (pertaining to one color), unilateral (pertaining to one side)
Muco, myx~	Mucus	Mucocele (mucous cyst), myxadenitis (inflammation of mucous gland)
Multi, poly~	Many	Polyphobia (condition of many fears), multicellular (pertaining to many cells)
Myco~	Fungi	Mycoid (fungus-like)
Necro~	Death	Necrocytosis (condition of cell death)
Noct~	Night	Nocturia (excessive or frequent urination after going to bed, typically caused by excessive fluid intake, etc.)
Noso~	Disease	Nosophyte (disease-causing plant microorganism)
Octa~	Eight	Octaploid (having eight pairs of chromosomes)
Oligo~	Few	Oligospermia (condition of deficient sperm)
Omo~	Shoulders	Omodynia (pain in the shoulder)
Omphalo~	Umbilicus	Omphalorrhexis (rupture of the umbilicus)
Oneir~	Dream	Oneirodynia (painful dreaming)
Opistho, poster, reto~	Backward, behind	Opisthotic (located behind the ear)

(continued)

TABLE 6.1. PREFIX AND ROOT WORDS (*Cont.*)

ROOT	MEANING	EXAMPLE
Oxy~	Keen, sharp	Oxyecoia (abnormal sensitivity to noises)
Pachy~	Thick	Pachycephally (pertaining to thick head)
Paleo~	Old	Paleontology (branch of biology dealing with ancient plant and animal life)
Pan~	All	Panacea (a cure-all)
Papilla~	Pustule, a small protuberance or elevation	Papillomavirus (any group of viruses that cause papillomas or warts in humans and animals)
Para~	Beside, near	Paramedic (pertaining to alongside of medicine)
Patho~	Disease	Pathology (study of disease)
Pedia~	Child	Pediatrics (treatment of child)
Pedo~	Foot	Pedal (pertaining to the foot)
Penta, quinqu, quinti~	Five	Quintuplet (one of five children born to one mother during the same birth), quintapara (a woman who has had five pregnancies that have gone beyond the 20th week of gestation)
Pero~	Deformed	Peropus (individual with congenitally deformed feet)
Phago~	Devour, eat	Phagocytosis (a three staged process where neutrophils, monocytes, and eosinophils engulf and destroy microorganisms, other foreign cell debris, and antigens)
Photo~	Light	Photalgia (pain produced by light)
Phren~	Diaphragm	Phrenospasm (spasm of the diaphragm)
Physio~	Nature	Physiological (concerning body function)
Phyt~	Plant	Phytoid (plantlike)

(continued)

140

TABLE 6.1. PREFIX AND ROOT WORDS (*Cont.*)

Prefix/Root	Meaning	Example
Platy~	Flat	Platycephaly (flattening of the skull)
Pod~	Foot	Podiatry (treatment of the foot)
Poly~	Many, much	Polyadenous (involving or relating to many glands)
Post~	After, behind	Postoperative [after operation (surgery)]
Presby~	Old	Presbyatric (geriatric)
Primi, prot~	First	Primordial (existing first)
Proso~	Anterior, forward	Prosoplegia (facial paralysis)
Prosop~	Face	Prosopectasia (abnormal enlargement of the face)
Proto~	First	Protoplasia (primary formation of tissue)
Pseudo~	False	Pseudocyst (dilation resembling a cyst)
Psychr~	Cold	Psychralgia (painful sensation of cold)
Puri~	Pus	Puriform (resembling pus)
Purpur~	Purple	Pupupura (any rash in which the blood cells leak into the skin or mucous membranes)
Pyro~	Fever, heat	Pyrogenic (producing fever)
Quad, tetra~	Four	Quadrilateral (having four sides)
Radio~	Ray	Radiolucent (penetrable by x-rays)
Re~	Again	Reactivate (to make active again)
Schisto~	Divide, split	Schistoglossia (a cleft tongue)
Sclero~	Hard	Sclerosis (a condition of hardness)
Scoli~	Crooked, curved	Scoliosis (lateral curvature of the spine)
Somni~	Sleep	Somniferous (sleep-producing)
Sphygmo~	Pulse	Sphygmomanometer (an instrument for measuring aterial blood pressure indirectly)
Splanchna~	Viscera	Splanchnic (pertaining to the viscera)
Staphylo~	Grapelike structure	*Staphylococcus* (gram-positive bacteria; under a microscope it looks round and clustered like grapes)

(continued)

TABLE 6.1. PREFIX AND ROOT WORDS (*Cont.*)

ROOT	MEANING	EXAMPLE
Stear/steat~	Fat	Steatosis (fatty degeneration)
Steno~	Contracted, narrow	Stenosis (a condition of narrow)
Strepto~	Curved, twisted	*Streptococcus* (gram-positive cocci occuring in chains)
Super, supra, ultra~	Above, excessive	Supernumerary (excessive numbers, too small to count), suprarenal (pertaining to above the kidney)
Tachy~	Fast	Tachycardia (a condition of fast heart)
Tel, tele, telo~	Distance, end	Teleceptor (distance receptor)
Ter, tri~	Three, third	Tertiary (third in order or stage)
		Triangular (having three sides)
Thermo~	Heat	Thermotherapy (therapeutic application of heat)
Thrombo~	Clot	Thrombosis (formation or presence of a blood clot within the vascular system)
Top/topo~	Topical	Toponarcosis (local anesthesia)
Torsi~	Twist	Torsive (twisted)
Trachy~	Rough	Trachyphonia (roughness or hoarseness of the voice)
Trans~	Across, through	Transocular (across the eye)
Ul~	Gingiva, scar	Ulitis (gingivitis)
Varico~	Swollen, twisted	Varicose (distended, swollen, knotted veins)
Ventro~	Anterior	Ventrodorsal (in a direction from the front to the back)
Viscer~	Organ	Viscera (internal organs inclosed within a cavity)
Vita~	Life	Vitality (state of being alive)
Xeno~	Foreign,strange	Xenogeneic (obtained from a different species)
Xero~	Dry	Xeroderma (dryness of the skin)

TABLE 6.2. SUFFIXES

SUFFIX	DEFINITION	EXAMPLE
~algia, dynia	Pain	Myalgia or myodynia (muscle pain)
~ac	Means pertaining to and forms an adjective when combined with a root	Cardiac (pertaining to the heart)
~al	Means pertaining to or concerning and forms and adjective when combined with a root	Pedal (pertaining to the foot)
~an, ar, ic, ical, ory, tic, ~eal	Pertaining to	Cyanotic (pertaining to blue), toxic (pertaining to poison)
~oid	Like or resembling	Toxoid (resembling a toxin)
~e, er, icing, ist, or	Agent or noun maker or one who specializes in	Pharmacist
~ia, iasis, id, ism, ity, osis, tia, tion	Abnormal condition, state	Abnormal condition
~cle, cule, culum, culus, et, ium, ole, olum, olus	Small	Ventricle (small belly or pouch) Bronchiole (small airway) Macula (small spot)
~lysis	Breaking down or dissolution	Hemolysis (breakdown of blood)
~megaly	Enlargement	Splenomagaly (enlarged spleen)
~spasm	Involuntary condition	Vasospasm

An adjustment can also be processed against a general ledger account (e.g., bad debt or error).

Administrative Costs.   The costs assumed by a managed care plan for administrative services such as claims processing, billing, and overhead costs.

Adverse Selection.   A particular health plan, whether indemnity or managed care, is selected against by the enrollee, and thus, an inequitable proportion of enrollees requiring more medical services are found in that plan.

Agency for Health Care Policy and Research (AHCPR).   Created by Congress in 1989 to conduct federal research into technology assessment and outcomes management and to develop practice guidelines for public dissemination. The AHCPR is perhaps best known for funding the patient outcomes-based research trials that form the basis for its practice guideline efforts.

Alkylate.   Drugs used to treat certain kinds of malignancies.

American Association of Preferred Provider Organizations (AAPPO).   The national trade association for PPOs, founded in 1983. There are currently over 1200 members. The mission statement of the AAPPO is "to provide direction and assistance to and for PPOs and their partners in managed care through education, information, research, and advocacy."

Analgesic.   Relieves pain. Tylenol (APAP), aspirin (ASA), nonsteroidal anti-inflammatory drugs, and narcotics are examples of analgesics.

Angiography.   1. A description of blood vessels and lymphatics. 2. Diagnostic or therapeutic radiography of the heart and blood vessels using a radiopaque contrast medium. Types include magnetic resonance, interventional, and computed tomography.

Antibiotic.   Inhibits growth or destroys microorganisms whose overgrowth causes infection. Penicillins, quinolones, β-lactams and cephalosporins are all examples.

Anticoagulant.   1. Delaying or preventing blood coagulation. 2. An agent that prevents or delays blood coagulation. Warfarin sodium.

Antidepressant.   Any medicine or other mode of therapy that acts to prevent, cure, or alleviate mental depression.

Antihistamine.   A drug that opposes the action of histamine. Although there are two classes of histamine-blocking drugs, the term antihistamine is typically used to describe agents that block the action of histamines on the H_1 receptors. These agents are used to treat allergies, hives, etc.

Antiinflammatory.   Counteracting inflammation. An agent that counteracts inflammation.

Apparent Volume of Distribution (V_z).   A hypothetical volume calculated using the elimination rate constant. It is considered to be equivalent to V_{ss} in most cases.

Arthroscopy.   Direct joint visualization by means of an arthroscope, usually to remove tissue such as cartilage fragments or torn ligaments.

Aspiration.   Withdrawal of fluid from a cavity by suctioning with an aspirator. The purpose of aspiration is to remove fluid or air from an affected area or to obtain specimens.

Astringent. Drawing together, constricting, binding. An agent that has a constricting or binding effect.

Audiometry. Testing of the hearing sense.

Authorization. As it applies to managed care, authorization is the approval of care, such as hospitalization. Preauthorization may be required before admission takes place or care is given by non-HMO providers.

Average Wholesale Price (AWP). The published average "cost" of a drug product paid by the pharmacy to the wholesaler. This price is specific to drug strength or concentrating dosage form, package size, and manufacturer or labeler. The average wholesale price of each drug is maintained on the National Drug Code (NDC) master file. This price is used to calculate the upper limit of payment available under a plan.

Average Wholesale Price Discount. A cost-containment program implemented to reduce drug program costs for plan sponsors without influencing cardholders. The AWP no longer always equals the actual cost of a drug to the pharmacy, so applying a discount to AWP allows a new upper limit of payment to be established, and savings are realized by the plan sponsors. An example is a plan sponsor with a plan that allows average wholesale price less 10% (AWP − 10%).

Beneficiary (Insured). The primary person receiving the benefit coverage. This information is maintained on the eligibility file of the plan sponsor. If the client can provide the information, dependent names are also maintained.

Benefit Package. Services an insurer, government agency, health plan, or an employer offers under the terms of a contract.

Bioavailability (F). The fraction of given drug that reaches the systemic circulation. It will be reported as a percentage or fraction.

Brand–Brand Interchange. Dispensing one brand name product for another brand name product marketed by another manufacturer.

Brand Drug. The drug manufacturer whose name is listed on the application to the FDA for approval of a new drug.

Brand Name. The trademarked name of the drug that appears on the package label.

Bronchoscopy. Examination of the bronchi through a bronchoscope.

Cardiac Catheterization. Percutaneous intravascular insertion of a catheter into any chamber of the heart or great vessels for diagnosis, assessment of abnormalities, interventional treatment, and evaluation of the effects of pathology on the heart.

Capitation. A per-member monthly payment to a provider that covers contracted services and is paid in advance of its delivery. In essence, a provider agrees to provide specified services to HMO members for this fixed, predetermined payment for a specified length of time (usually a year), regardless of how many times the member uses the service. The rate can be fixed for all members, or it can be adjusted for the age and sex of the member, based on actuarial projections of medical utilization.

Cardholder (Insured or Beneficiary). The primary person receiving the benefit coverage in whose name the card is issued. This information is maintained in the eligibility file. If the client can provide the information, dependent names are also maintained.

Carrier/Group. The combination used to signify both the plan sponsor (carrier) and the specific group under it. An example of a carrier/group would be 0007/0023: 0007, Carrier, ABZ Insurance Co.; 0023, Group, The Marley Company.

Carrier Name. This term is used to identify any plan sponsor—the underwriter of an insured account or the company name of a self-administered account. This name is often used on management reports sent to the plan sponsor.

Carrier Number. An assigned four-digit number that identifies the plan sponsor (insurance company, self-administered account, third-party administrator, multiple employer trust, health maintenance organization). A plan sponsor may have more than one carrier number.

Case Management. The process whereby a health care professional supervises the administration of medical or ancillary services to a patient, typically one who has a catastrophic disorder or who is receiving mental health services. Case managers are thought to reduce the costs associated with the care of such patients while providing high-quality medical services.

Central Volume of Distribution (Vc). The volume of blood and highly perfused tissues where a drug will initially distribute. It is used to calculate loading doses.

Certification. Certification is the official authorization for use of services.

Claim. Information submitted by a provider or covered person to establish that medical services were provided to a covered person, from which processing for payment to the provider or covered person is made.

Claims Adjudication. See Adjudication.

Claims Review. The method by which an enrollee's health care service claims are reviewed before reimbursement is made. The purpose of this monitoring system is to validate the medical appropriateness of the provided services and to be sure the cost of the service is not excessive.

Clearance (CL). The amount of blood that can have all the drug eliminated from it per unit time. Therefore, the units for clearance are volume per time. It is a determinant of $C_{ss,avg}$, k, $t\frac{1}{2}$ and peak-to-trough ratio.

COBRA (Consolidated Omnibus Budget Reconciliation Act of 1985). Legislation that requires group health plans of covered employers to give employees and family members the opportunity to continue their health care coverage at their own expense at group rates in circumstances where coverage would otherwise end.

Coinsurance. The percentage of the costs of medical services paid by the patient. This is a characteristic of indemnity insurance and PPO plans. The coinsurance usually is about 20% of the cost of medical services after the deductible is paid.

Compliance. More accurately referred to as adherence. The ability of a patient to take medication or follow treatment protocol according to the directions for which it was prescribed; patient taking prescribed dose of medication at the prescribed frequency for the prescribed length of time.

Continuous Quality Improvement (CQI).   A comprehensive philosophy of continuously improving the quality of a product or service by constantly monitoring operations, correcting problems, and implementing systems to better assist customers. It is a comprehensive approach for improving overall organizational performance and challenges the traditional way of doing business. It contends that most quality problems involve procedures and strategies (i.e., the process) and are not the fault of individuals.

Contraceptive.   Any process, device, or method that prevents conception. Categories of contraceptives include, steroids, chemical, physical, or barrier or combinations of these.

Copayment.   A nominal fee charged to an insured member to offset costs of paperwork and administration for each office visit or pharmacy prescription filled.

Corticosteroid.   Any of several steroid hormones secreted by the cortex of the adrenal gland or manufactured synthetically for use as a drug.

Cost Benefit.   Cost–benefit analysis expresses the outcomes of therapies (e.g., the benefits) in monetary rather than physical units.

Cost Containment.   A program to decrease the overall costs of a drug, medical benefit, or health care.

Cost-Effectiveness.   Usually considered as a ratio, the cost-effectiveness of a drug or procedure, for example, relates the cost of that drug or procedure to the health benefits resulting from it. In health terms, it is often expressed as the cost per year per life-year saved or as the cost per quality-adjusted life-year saved.

Cost Shifting.   The redistribution of payment sources. Typically, cost shifting occurs when a discount on provider services is obtained by one payer and the providers increase costs to another payer to make up the difference.

CPT.   Physician's Current Procedural Terminology.

Cytochrome P450 Enzymes (CYP).   Phase I enzymes responsible for much of the intestinal and hepatic metabolism of drugs.

DAW (Dispense as Written).   A notation used by a physician, pharmacy, or cardholder that will determine whether or not generic substitution occurs. There are ten DAW codes defined as follows (numeric values are assigned to each code for computer entry for on-line claims adjudication systems):

0,   No Product Selection Indicated.
This is the field default value used for prescriptions when product selection is not an issue. Examples include prescriptions written for single-source brand products and prescriptions written using the generic name, and a generic product is dispensed.

1,   Substitution Not Allowed by Prescriber.
This value is used when the prescriber indicates, in a manner specified by prevailing law, that the product is to be dispensed as written.

2,   Substitution Allowed, Patient-Requested Product Dispensed.

This value is used when the prescriber has indicated, in a manner specified by prevailing law, that generic substitution is permitted, and the patient requests the brand product. This situation can occur when the prescriber writes the prescription using either the brand or generic name and the product is available from multiple sources.

3,   Substitution Allowed, Pharmacist-Selected Product Dispensed.

This value is used when the prescriber has indicated, in a manner specified by prevailing law, that generic substitution is permitted, and the brand product is dispensed because a currently marketed generic is not stocked in the pharmacy. This situation exists as a result of the buying habits of the pharmacist, not because of the unavailability of the generic product in the marketplace.

4,   Substitution Allowed, Generic Drug Not in Stock.

This value is used when the prescriber has indicated, in a manner specified by prevailing law, that generic substitution is permitted, and the brand product is dispensed because a currently marketed generic is not stocked in the pharmacy. This situation exists as a result of the buying habits of the pharmacist, not because of the unavailability of the generic product in the marketplace.

5,   Substitution Allowed, Brand Drug Dispensed as a Generic.

This value is used when the prescriber has indicated, in a manner specified by prevailing law, that generic substitution is permitted, and the pharmacist is utilizing the brand product as the generic entity.

6,   Override.

This value is used by various claims processors in very specific instances as defined by that claims processor and/or its client(s).

7,   Substitution Not Allowed, Brand Drug Mandated by Law.

This value is used when the prescriber has indicated, in a manner specified by prevailing law, that generic substitution is permitted, but prevailing law or regulation prohibits the substitution of a generic product even though generic versions of the product may be available in the marketplace.

8,   Substitution Allowed; Generic Drug Not Available in Marketplace.

This value is used when the prescriber has indicated, in a manner specified by prevailing law, that generic substitution is permitted, and the brand product is dispensed because the generic is not currently manufactured or distributed or is temporarily unavailable.

9,   Other.

This value is reserved and currently not in use. NCPDP does not recommend use of this value at the present time. Please contact NCPDP if you intend to use this value and document how it will be utilized by your organization.

Decongestant.   Reducing congestion or swelling, or any agent that reduces congestion or swelling.

Deductible.   A fixed amount of health care dollars of which a person must pay 100% before his or her health benefits begin. Most indemnity plans feature a $200 to $500 deductible and then pay up to 100% of money spent for covered services above this level.

Dependent Coverage Code.   Allows the plan sponsor to control the type of coverage each cardholder receives.

DESI (Drug Efficacy Study Indicator).   A study of drugs by the Food and Drug Administration (FDA) that rates certain drugs as not safe and effective and experimental or investigational in nature.

Diagnostic-Related Groups (DRGs).   A program in which hospital procedures are rated in terms of cost, taking into account the intensity of services delivered. A standard flat rate per procedure is derived from this scale, which is paid by Medicare for its beneficiaries, regardless of the cost to the hospital to provide that service.

Direct Costs.   Direct costs are those that are wholly attributable to the service in question, for example, the services of professional and paraprofessional personnel, equipment, and materials.

Disease Management.   A philosophy toward the treatment of the patient with an illness (usually chronic) that seeks to prevent recurrence of symptoms, maintain high quality of life, and prevent future need for medical resources by using an integrated approach to health care. Pharmaceutical care, continuous quality improvement, practice guidelines, and case management all play key roles in this effort, which should result in decreased healthcare costs as well.

Dispensing Fee.   Contracted rate of compensation paid to a pharmacy for the processing/filling of a prescription claim. The dispensing fee is added to the negotiated formula for reimbursing ingredient cost.

Diuretic.   Increasing urine secretion, An agent that increases urine output.

Doppler Ultrasonography.   The use of ultrasound to produce an image or photograph of an organ or tissue. Doppler effect is the shift in frequency produced when an ultrasound wave is echoed from something in motion. The use of the Doppler effect permits measuring the velocity of that which is being studied.

Dose Interval (τ or Tau).   How often the patient is receiving the drug. The units are in time. It is a determinant of peak-to-trough ratio.

Dose Rate (DR).   The amount of drug the patient is receiving per time. The units will be amount/time. It is a determinant of $C_{ss,avg}$.

Drug Utilization Evaluation (DUE).   An evaluation of prescribing patterns of physicians to specifically determine the appropriateness of drug therapy.

DUR (Drug Utilization Review).   A system of drug use review that can detect potential adverse drug interactions, drug–pregnancy conflicts, therapeutic duplication, drug–age conflicts, etc. There are three forms of DUR: prospective (before dispensing), concurrent (at the time of prescription dispensing), and retrospective (after the therapy has been completed). Appropriate use of an integrated DUR program can curb drug misuse and abuse and monitor quality of care. DUR can reduce hospitalization and other costs related to inappropriate drug use.

Echocardiogram.   The graphic record produced by echocardiography.

Electrocardiograph.   A device for recording changes in the electrical energy produced by the action of heart muscles.

Electroencephalography.   Amplification, recording, and analysis of the electrical activity of the brain. The record obtained is called the electroencephalogram (EEG).

Elimination Rate Constant (k).   Represents the fraction of drug eliminated per time. The units are inverse time. It is a dependent variable determined by clearance (CL) and volume of distribution (V_d).

Endoscopy.   Inspection of body organs or cavities by use of an endoscope.

Employee Retirement Income Security Act of 1974 (ERISA).   This law mandates reporting and disclosure requirements for group life and health plans.

Enterohepatic Cycling.   A cycle through which absorbed drug is reintroduced to the intestine. After absorption and exposure to the liver, the drug is stored in the gallbladder and then secreted into the bile to reenter the intestine.

Exclusive Provider Organization (EPO).   The EPO is a form of a preferred provider organization in which patients must visit a caregiver who is on its panel of providers. If a visit to an outside provider is made, the EPO will offer limited or no coverage for the office or hospital visit.

Expectorant.   An agent, such as guaifenesin, that promotes the clearance of mucus from the respiratory tract.

Fee for Service.   Traditional provider reimbursement, in which the physician is paid according to the service performed. This is the reimbursement system used by conventional indemnity insurers.

Fee Schedule.   A comprehensive listing of fees used by either a healthcare plan or the government to reimburse physicians and other providers on a fee-for-service basis.

First-Dollar Coverage.   A feature of an insurance plan in which there is no deductible, and therefore, the plan's sponsor pays a proportion or all of the covered services provided to a patient as soon as he or she enrolls.

Formulary.   A specific list of drugs that are included with a given plan for a client. Types include closed formulary, negative formulary, and open formulary.

Fraction Absorbed (f_a).   The fraction of orally administered drug that is absorbed from the gut lumen to the gut wall.

Fraction Escaping Gut Metabolism (f_g).   The fraction of orally administered drug not metabolized or effluxed from the gut wall back into the gut lumen.

Fraction Escaping Hepatic First Pass (f_{fp}).   The fraction of drug presented to the liver that is not metabolized. It has an inverse relationship with hepatic extraction ratio.

Free Average Concentration at Steady State ($C_{ss,avg,free}$).   The average concentration of only the pharmacologically active unbound drug during a dosing interval at steady state. It is often the parameter that we are trying to maintain within a given therapeutic range. The units are amount per volume.

Gatekeeper.   Most HMOs rely on the primary-care physician, or "gatekeeper," to screen patients seeking medical care and effectively eliminate costly and sometimes needless referral to specialists for diagnosis and management. The gatekeeper is responsible for the administration of the patient's treatment, and this person must coordinate and obtain authorization for all medical services, laboratory studies, specialty referrals, and hospitalizations. In most HMOs, if an enrollee visits a specialist without prior authorization from his or her designated primary-care physician, the enrollee must pay for medical services.

Generic Substitution.   In cases in which the patent on a specific pharmaceutical product expires and drug manufacturers produce generic versions of the original branded product, the generic version of the drug (which is theorized to be identical to the product manufactured by a different firm) is dispensed even though the original product is prescribed. Some managed care organizations and Medicaid programs mandate generic substitution because of the generally lower cost of generic products. There are state and federal regulations regarding generic substitutions.

Half-Life ($t\frac{1}{2}$).   The time required for the serum concentration to decrease by 50%. It is in units of time. Half-life also is important in determining time to steady state and P:T ratio. Volume of distribution (V_d) and clearance (CL) determine half-life.

HCFA (Health Care Financing Administration).   The federal agency responsible for administering Medicare and overseeing states' administration of Medicaid.

Health Alliances.   Also known as regional health alliances, these entities are purchasing pools that are responsible for negotiating health insurance for employers and employees. Alliances use their leverage as large healthcare purchasers to negotiate contracts.

HEDIS.   Health Education Data Information System.

HMO (Health Maintenance Organization).   A form of health insurance in which its members prepay a premium for the HMO's health services, which generally include inpatient and ambulatory care. For the patient, it means reduced out-of-pocket costs (i.e., no deductible), no paperwork (i.e., insurance forms), and only a small copayment for each office visit to cover the paperwork handled by the HMO. There are several different types of HMOs.

• *Group Model.* In the group-model HMO, the HMO contracts with a physician group, which is paid a fixed amount per patient to provide specific services. The administration of the group practice then decides how the HMO payments are distributed to each participating physician. This type of HMO is usually located in a hospital or clinic setting and may include a pharmacy. These physicians usually do not have any fee-for-service patients.

- *Hybrid Model.* A combination of at least two managed care organizational models that are melded into a single health plan. Because its features do not uniformly fit one model, it is called a hybrid.
- *Individual Practice Association (IPA) Model.* The individual practice association contracts with independent physicians who work in their own private practices and see fee-for-service patients as well as HMO enrollees. They are paid by capitation for the HMO patients and by conventional means for their fee-for-service patients. Physicians belonging to the IPA guarantee that the care needed by each patient for whom they are responsible will fall under a certain amount of money. They guarantee this by allowing the HMO to withhold an amount of their payments (usually about 20% per year). If, by the end of the year, the physician's cost for treatment falls under this set amount, then the physician receives his entire "withhold fund." If the opposite is true, the HMO can then withhold any part of this amount, at its discretion, from the fund. Essentially, the physician is put "at risk" for keeping down the treatment cost. This is the key to the HMO's financial viability.
- *Network Model.* A network of group practices under the administration of one HMO.
- *Point-of-Service (POS) Model.* Sometimes referred to as an "open-ended" HMO. The point-of-service model is one in which the patient can receive care either by physicians contracted with the HMO or by those not contracted. Physicians not contracted with the HMO who see an HMO patient are paid according to the services performed. The patient is incentivized to utilize contracted providers through the fuller coverage offered for contracted care.
- *Staff Model.* The staff-model HMO is the purest form of managed care. All of the physicians in a staff-model HMO are in a centralized site, in which all clinical and perhaps inpatient services and pharmacy services are offered. The HMO holds the tightest management reigns in this setting because none of the physicians traditionally practices on an independent fee-for-service basis. Physicians are more likely to be employees of the HMO in this setting because they are not in a private or group practice.

Holter Monitor. A portable device small enough to be worn by a patient during normal activity. It consists of an electrocardiograph and a recording system capable of storing up to 24 hours of the individual's ECG record.

Horizontal Integration. Affiliation of firms (e.g., drug manufacturers) or providers (e.g., physicians, pharmacists, etc.) on the same level to expand distribution systems, or multichannel systems in which manufacturers diversify in selecting channels to cover different markets.

Hospice. A healthcare facility that provides supportive care for the terminally ill.

ICD-9. International Classification of Diseases, ninth edition.

Indemnity Insurance.   Traditional fee-for-service medicine in which providers are paid according to the service performed.

Indirect Costs.   Indirect costs are usually termed overhead costs; they are the costs shared by many services concurrently. For example, maintenance, administration, equipment, electricity, and water.

Insulin.   A hormone secreted by the β cells of the pancreas that controls the metabolism and cellular uptake of sugars, proteins, and fats. As a drug it is used principally to treat diabetes mellitus.

Insurance Company (Plan Sponsor).   A client, also referred to as a carrier, who underwrites the insurance for individual groups. The insurance company signs the contract and is financially responsible for all bills incurred by groups insured by them. Each insurance company is assigned a unique insurance code and can generally tailor the program for their individual groups.

Integrated Healthcare Systems.   Healthcare financing and delivery organizations created to provide a "continuum of care," ensuring that patients get the right care at the right time from the right provider. This continuum of care from primary care provider to specialist and ancillary provider under one corporate roof guarantees that patients get cared for appropriately, thus saving money and increasing the quality of care.

Intervention.   Educational, directive (e.g., formulary or prior authorization), or consultative communications between providers, especially pharmacists to physicians.

Intradermal.   Drug route of administration by injection into the skin.

Intramuscular.   Drug route of administration by injection into a muscle.

Intrathecal.   Drug route of administration by injection into the meninges around the spinal cord.

Laryngoscopy.   Visual examination of the interior of the larynx to determine the cause of hoarseness, obtain cultures, manage the upper airways, or take biopsies.

Long-Term Care.   Services ordinarily provided in a skilled nursing, intermediate-care, personal-care, supervisory-care, or eldercare facility.

MAC (Maximum Allowable Cost).   A cost management program that sets upper limits on the payment for equivalent drugs available from multiple manufacturers. It is the highest unit price that will be paid for a drug and is designed to increase generic dispensing, to ensure the pharmacy dispenses economically, and to control future cost increases.

Magnetic Resonance Imaging (MRI).   A type of diagnostic radiography that uses the characteristic behavior of protons (and other atomic nuclei) when placed in powerful magnetic fields to make images of tissues and organs.

Managed Health Care.   The sector of health insurance in which healthcare providers are not independent businesses run by, for example, the private practitioner, but by administrative firms that managed the allocation of healthcare benefits. In contrast with conventional indemnity insurers, which did not govern the provision of medical services but simply paid for them, managed care firms have a significant say in how the services are administered so that they may better control health care costs. HMOs and PPOs are examples of managed care organizations.

Managed Services Organization (MSO). A type of integrated healthcare plan in which the hospital provides administrative services to a physician group, and the physician group provides patients to the hospital.

Medicaid. An entitlement program run by both the state and federal government for the provision of healthcare insurance to patients younger than 65 years of age who cannot afford to pay private health insurance. The federal government matches the states' contribution on a certain minimal level of available coverage. The states may institute additional services, but at their own expense.

Medicaid Prudent Pharmaceutical Purchasing Act (MPPPA). Enacted as part of the Omnibus Budget Reconciliation Act of 1990, MPPPA provides that Medicaid must receive the best discounted price of any institutional purchaser of pharmaceuticals. Thus, drug companies provide rebates to Medicaid that are the difference between the discounted price and the price at which the drug was sold.

Medical Protocols. Medical protocols are the guidelines physicians are asked to follow to achieve an acceptable clinical outcome. The protocol provides the caregiver with specific treatment options or steps to follow when faced with a particular set of clinical symptoms or signs or laboratory data.

Medicare. An entitlement program run by the Health Care Financing Administration of the federal government by which people aged 65 years or older receive healthcare insurance. Medicare Part A covers hospitalization and is a compulsory benefit. Medicare Part B covers outpatient services and is a voluntary service.

Member. A participant in a health plan who makes up the plan's enrollment.

Miotic. An agent that causes the pupil to contract, such as pilocarpine.

Mydriatic. Causing pupillary dilation. A drug that dilates the pupil such as atropine, cocaine, and ephedrine.

Mucolytic. Pertaining to a class of agents that liquefy sputum or reduce its viscosity.

NCPDP (National Council for Prescription Drug Programs). An organization that promotes standardization and efficiency within the third-party prescription drug program industry and provides accurate and reliable information as to third-party prescription drug programs.

NDC (National Drug Code). A unique seven-digit character code given to a drug that identifies the labeler, product, and package size.

Nitrates. Salts of nitric acid. Agents in the class include isosorbide dinitrate or monhydrate and nitroglycerin. They are arteriovenous dilators and are used to treat angina, hypertension, and congestive heart failure.

Outcomes Management. A clinical outcome is the result of medical or surgical intervention or nonintervention. Managed care is now attempting to better manage the clinical outcomes of their enrollees to increase patient and payer satisfaction while holding down costs. It is thought that a database of outcomes experience will help caregivers see which treatment modalities result in consistently improved outcomes for patients. Outcomes management will, as a natural consequence, lead to medical protocols.

Outcomes Research. Studies that evaluate the effect of a given product, procedure, or medical technology on health or costs. Outcomes research information is vital to the development of practice guidelines.

Out-of-Pocket Costs. The share of health services payments paid by the enrollee.

P-glycoprotein (P-gp). A drug efflux system that is a member of the ABC cassette family of transporters. P-gp has been found in the cells lining the blood–brain barrier, kidney, adrenal glands, and lungs as well as the gut.

Palpation. Examination by application of the hands or fingers to the external surface of the body to detect evidence of disease or abnormalities in the internal organs.

Parenteral. Drug administration by other than the oral route, specifically by injection.

PBM (Pharmacy Benefit Management Companies). Firms used by plan sponsors to design and administer pharmaceutical benefit plans.

Peak-to-Trough Ratio (P:T). Ratio describing the variation between the highest and lowest achieved concentrations within a dosing interval.

Per Diem Reimbursement. Reimbursement of an institution, usually a hospital, based on a set rate per day rather than on charges. Per diem reimbursement can be varied by service (e.g., medical/surgical, obstetrics, mental health, and intensive care) or can be uniform regardless of intensity of services.

Performance Measures. Methods or instruments used to estimate or monitor how a health care provider's actions conform to criteria and standards of quality.

Pharmaceutical Care. A fairly new concept in providing health care defined by Hepler and Strand in 1990; it is a strategy that attempts to utilize drug therapy more efficiently to achieve definite outcomes that improve a patient's quality of life. A pharmaceutical care system requires a reorientation of physicians, pharmacist, and nurses toward effective drug therapy outcomes. It is a set of relationships and decisions through which pharmacist, physicians, nurses, and patients work together to design, implement, and monitor a therapeutic plan that will produce specific therapeutic outcomes.

Pharmacy Services Administrative Organization (PSAO). An organization that is dedicated to providing prescription benefits to enrollees of managed care plans by using existing community pharmacies. The PSAO contracts as a provider group with the managed care organization so that the individual pharmacies receive negotiating representation in numbers and the prepaid health plan does not have to provide the capital necessary to start, own, and operate its own pharmacy department.

Physician–Hospital Organization (PHO). A type of integrated healthcare system that in its simplest form is an organization that collectively commits both physicians and the hospital to payer contracts. They sometimes use existing

IPA structures or individual physician contracting. In its most effective form, the PHO must commit the entire physician and hospital panel, without an opt-out, to the PHO organization.

Plan Sponsor. The company that assumes financial responsibility for an insured group. A plan sponsor can be an insurance company, third-party administration, or the company itself, if the company is self-insured.

PMPM. Per member per month. Often used in the context of pharmacy or medical costs.

POS. Point of sale or point of service.

Preadmission Certification. The practice of reviewing claims for hospital admission before the patient actually enters the hospital. This cost-control mechanism is intended to eliminate unnecessary hospital expenses by denying medically unnecessary admissions.

Preferred Provider Organization (PPO). A managed care organization in which physicians are paid on a fee-for-service schedule that is discounted, usually about 10% to 20% below normal fees. PPOs are often formed as a competitive reaction to HMOs by physicians who contract out with insurance companies, employers, or third-party administrators. A patient can use a physician outside of the PPO providers, but he or she will have to pay a greater portion of the fee.

Preferred Providers. Physicians, hospitals, and other healthcare providers who contract to provide health services to persons covered by a particular health plan.

Premium. The amount paid to a carrier for providing coverage under a contract.

Preventive Care. Health care emphasizing priorities for prevention, early detection, and early treatment of conditions, generally including routine physical examination, immunization, and wellness care.

Primary Care Physician (PCP). Sometimes referred to as a "gatekeeper," the primary care physician is usually the first doctor a patient sees for an illness. This physician then treats the patient directly, refers the patient to a specialist (secondary care), or admits the patient to a hospital when necessary. Often, the primary care physician is a family physician or internist.

Prior Authorization. The process of obtaining certification or authorization from the health plan or pharmacy benefit manager for specified medications or specified quantities of medications. Often involves appropriateness review against preestablished criteria. Failure to obtain prior authorization often results in a financial penalty to the subscriber.

Private-Sector Health Care Programs. Signifies healthcare companies not directly affiliated with any federal, state, or local government. Normally, they are enterprises that perform services for a profit.

Provider. Any supplier of services (i.e., physician, pharmacist, case management firm, etc.).

Pulmonary Function Tests (PFT). One of several different tests used to evaluate the condition of the respiratory system. Measures of expiratory flow and lung volumes and capacities are obtained.

Pyelogram. A radiograph of the ureter and radial pelvis. IVP, a pyelogram in which a radiopaque material is given intravenously. Multiple radiographs of the urinary tract are taken.

Quality-Adjusted Life-Year (QALY). This unit of measure is one way to quantify health outcomes resulting from some types of intervention. The number of quality-adjusted life-years is the number of years at full health that would be valued equivalently to the number of years of life experienced in a less desirable health state.

Quality Assurance (QA). Quality assurance or quality assessment is the activity that monitors the level of care being provided by physicians, medical institutions, or any healthcare vendor in order to ensure that health plan enrollees are receiving the best care possible. The level of care is measured against preestablished standards, some of which are mandated by law.

Quality Improvement (QI). A continuous process that identifies problems in healthcare delivery, examines solutions to those problems, and regularly monitors the solutions for improvement.

Quality of Life (QOL). A patient's perceptions of how he or she deals with a disease or with everyday life when suffering from a particular condition. It is subjective because information cannot be measured objectively; however, it has been in the health care literature for at least 20 years.

Quality-of-Life Measures. An assessment of the patient's perceptions of how he or she is dealing with a disease or with everyday life when suffering from a particular condition.

Radiography, Roentgenography. The process of obtaining an image for diagnosis using a radiologic modality.

Risk Contract. Also known as a Medicare risk contract. A contract between an HMO or CMP and the HCFA to provide services to Medicare beneficiaries under which the health plan receives a fixed monthly payment for enrolled Medicare members and then must provide all services on an at-risk basis. This type of contract may be between physicians and an HMO, placing the physician at risk for costs of services provided.

Screening. The method by which managed care organizations limit access to health care for unnecessary reasons. In most HMOs, a phone call to the physician or his or her medical office staff is required before an office visit can be arranged. "Gatekeepers" and concurrent review are other methods of screening patients.

Self-Insured. Clients who obtain benefits on a self-funded basis. The company assumes all of the financial risk and liability that would normally be covered by an insurance company.

Skilled Nursing Facility (SNF). Typically an institution for convalescence or a nursing home, the skilled nursing facility provides a high level of specialized care for long-term or acute illnesses. It is an alternative to extended hospital stays or difficult home care.

Standards of Quality. Authoritative statement of minimum levels of acceptable performance, excellent levels of performance, or the range of acceptable performance.

Subcutaneous. A drug route of administration in which it is injected just beneath the skin.

Sublingual. Under the tongue.

Surgicenter. A separate, free-standing medical facility specializing in outpatient or same-day surgical procedures. Surgicenters drastically reduce the costs associated with hospitalizations for routine surgical procedures because extended inpatient care is not required for specific disorders.

Tertiary Care. Tertiary care is administered at a highly specialized medical center. It is associated with the utilization of high-cost technology resources.

Therapeutic Substitution. A drug that is believed therapeutically equivalent (i.e., will achieve the same outcome) to the exact drug prescribed by a physician is substituted. Therapeutic substitution is generally mandated by formulary compliance programs.

Third-Party Administrator (TPA). Clients who handle the administration of the program for a group or insurance company. The TPA is considered the plan sponsor and is therefore financially responsible.

Third-Party Payer. A public or private organization that pays for or underwrites coverage for healthcare expenses.

Total Average Concentration at Steady State ($C_{ss,avg,tot}$). The average concentration of both bound and unbound drug during a dosing interval at steady state. It is often the parameter that we are trying to maintain within a given therapeutic range. The units are amount per volume.

Transdermal. Absorbed through the skin.

Triage. The evaluation of patient conditions for urgency and seriousness, and establishment of a priority list for multiple patients. In the setting of managed care, triage is often performed after office hours on the telephone by a nurse or other health professional to screen patients for emergency treatment.

Triple Option. A type of health plan in which employees may choose from an HMO, a PPO, and an indemnity plan, depending on how much they are willing to contribute to cost.

U&C (Usual and Customary) Pricing. The amount that a pharmacist would charge a cash-paying customer for a prescription.

UCR. Usual, customary, and reasonable.

Ultrasonography. The use of ultrasound to produce an image or photograph of an organ or tissue. Ultrasonic echoes are recorded as they strike tissues of different densities.

UPIN (Unique Physician Identification Number). A unique identification number assigned to a physician that is used for prescribed drug claims.

Utilization Review (UR). Performed by the HMO to discover if a particular physician-provider or other provider (e.g., pharmacy) is spending as much of the HMO's money on treatment or any specific portion thereof (e.g., specialty referral, drug prescribing, hospitalization, radiologic or laboratory services) as his or her peers.

Volume of Distribution (V_d).   Parameter that relates the amount of drug in the body to the measured plasma concentration. The larger the volume of distribution, the higher the amount of tissue binding and the slower the elimination from the body. Elimination rate is dependent on the volume of distribution and the clearance of a drug.

Volume of Distribution at Steady-State (V_{ss}).   A physiologic volume describing the determinants of distribution. It is very difficult to measure and is reported in units of volume. It is primarily dependent on plasma and tissue protein binding.

QUESTIONS

For the following terms, separate prefixes, combining forms, and suffixes. Define each term.

1. Acrodynia
2. Pediatrics
3. Microscope
4. Orthopedic
5. Epigastrum
6. Hemodialysis
7. Vasospasm
8. Podiatry
9. Angiomegaly
10. Tachycardia
11. Cardiograph
12. Dysphonic
13. Urologist
14. Oliguria
15. Gastrostomy
16. Laparotomy
17. Ultrasonography
18. Pancytopenia
19. Cyanosis
20. Pyretic

Select the combining form that matches the meaning of each of the following terms:

glia	phasia	a	myel/o
itis	thromb/o	oma	dys
mening/o	vascul/o	osis	rrhagia
scler/o	oid		

A. without
B. abnormal condition
C. blood clot
D. blood vessel
E. glue or gluelike
F. hardening
G. inflammation
H. resembling
I. softening
J. speech
K. spinal cord, bone marrow
L. tumor

Write the meaning of each word part

1. –dynia
2. –ectomy
3. –edema
4. –logist
5. –malacia
6. –ptosis
7. –scope
8. –spasm
9. –stenosis
10. –aden/o
11. blephar/o
12. dipl/o
13. ophthalmo
14. retin/o
15. scler/o
16. encephal/o
17. neuro/o
18. a
19. adip/o
20. holo

REFERENCES

1. Cohen BJ. *Medical terminology: an illustrated guide.* Philadelphia: Lippincott Williams & Wilkins, 1998.
2. Gylys BA, Masters RM. *Medical terminology simplified: a programmed learning approach by body systems.* Philadelphia: FA Davis, 1998.
3. Medical Interface: Managed Care. A–Z managed care terms. Bronxville, NY: Medicom International, Merck-Medco Managed Care.
4. Multilingual glossary of technical and popular medical terms in nine European languages. http://allserv.rug.ac.be/~rvdstich/eugloss/welcome.html
5. Venes D, ed. *Tabers cyclopedic medical dictionary.* Philadelphia: FA Davis, 1997.

PHARMACY CALCULATIONS

A. Timothy Eley

Goals: After reviewing the information in this chapter, you should be able to:

1. Interpret a prescription or medication order.
2. Convert between the metric and common systems of measurement.
3. Calculate an appropriate dose.
4. Prepare, concentrate, or dilute compounded medications accurately.
5. Interpret osmolarity, isotonicity, and milliequivalents.
6. Prepare isotonic solutions.
7. Reconstitute dry powders to appropriate concentration.
8. Utilize the aliquot method for solids and liquids.

INTRODUCTION

The profession of pharmacy is one in which mathematics is used extensively. With the exception of some pharmacokinetic expressions, most of the calculations you will be expected to perform will be simple arithmetic. That being said, *the importance of not making errors in your arithmetic cannot be overemphasized.* An error in a calculation by a pharmacist could easily be the difference between life and death. You should develop several methods to check your work as you go. Estimate the final answer before beginning the work. Anything quite different from your approximation should cause you to reexamine your work. As you progress further into your pharmacy education and your career, you will become more comfortable with estimating what these answers should be in a given situation and for a given patient, such that you can identify an unreasonable solution relatively easily. If you are interested in reviewing this subject in more detail, there are several texts available. The latest edition of *Pharmaceutical Calculations* by M. J. Stoklosa and H. C. Ansel[1] is a valuable resource, as this text could be considered the apparent gold standard for this material. The latest edition of *Remington's Pharmaceutical Sciences*[2] has a chapter on calculations that includes information about the history of different weights and measures that pharmacists are expected to be able to use.

162 Pharmacy Clerkship Manual

Assumptions and Expectations

In order for this chapter to be brief, basic math is not reviewed. There are a multitude of reliable resources for such material, including those mentioned previously. You are expected to be able to perform basic arithmetic (addition, subtraction, division, and multiplication) and to do so not only with whole numbers or integers but with fractions as well. Last, you are expected to be able to interpret Roman numerals.

Dimensional Analysis and Ratio/Proportion

In everyday practice you will be expected to convert a value expressed in a certain way (more formally a "denomination") into a value expressed a different way because circumstances dictate it. For instance, a physician has ordered an administration rate for an intravenous drug to be 5 mg/min. You have prepared an intravenous (IV) solution of that drug to have a concentration of 2 mg/mL. The nursing staff needs to know how to administer the IV solution in terms of flow rate (i.e., volume per unit time) in order to achieve the administration rate desired by the physician. In order to provide the nursing staff with this answer, you need to determine the volume of the solution you have prepared that contains 5 mg of the drug and direct the nursing staff to administer that volume every minute. You could do this computation by using ratio and proportion or dimensional analysis, but dimensional analysis allows you to do the same calculation in a stepwise approach and be more cautious in the process. Dimensional analysis tends to be safer for the beginner. The calculation would be as follows:

$$\frac{5 \text{ mg}}{\text{min}} \times \frac{1 \text{ ml}}{2 \text{ mg}} = \frac{2.5 \text{ ml}}{\text{min}}$$

Most of the conversions you have to deal with are rather simple, like the one above. Frequently we have somewhat uncomplicated problems to solve, e.g., "What amount of active ingredient X will give us a 5% ointment when incorporated into ointment base Y," and so on. Prescriptions requiring compounding with several ingredients tend to be more difficult.

Significant Figures

In short, the purpose of significant figures is to indicate how exact a measurement is. For example, the *absolute number* 54,021.3 has a value of exactly 54,021.3, but the *measurement* 54,021.3 g means exactly 54,021 and approximately 3/10 of a gram. The measurement has six significant figures. If you **add or subtract** a number with more or fewer significant figures, what you need to be worried about is how many digits there are behind (i.e., to the right of) the decimal place. For instance, if I want to add 3.222 g to 54,021.3 g, the answer cannot have more than one digit behind the decimal place because 54021.3 g has only one (the three). The sum cannot be reported as 54,024.522 g, rather it is reported as 54,024.5 g. Because the 0.3 in 54021.3 g was only approximate, that means that now the 0.5 at the end of 54024.5 g is only approximate. When **multiplying or dividing**, the answer will have the same number of significant figures as the value with the fewest significant figures in the problem. For example, if you multiply 3.222 by 54021.3, the answer will have only four significant figures even though the number of digits in the answer may exceed that value. The product of these two numbers is 17410 to the nearest ten, which has only four significant figures (the zero is not significant in this case). The only exception to this rule is when you multiply or divide by an absolute number, such as 3. If you are compounding three suppositories that each need to have 125 mg of active ingredient, the quantity you need to prepare them properly is not 400 to the nearest 100 (one significant figure) but 375 mg to the nearest 1 because all three significant figures are retained. The absolute number 3 is not an approximate figure; it is treated as three followed by the decimal place and an infinite number of zeroes, so the number of significant figures in the other number are the only ones of importance. Significant figures in the practice of pharmacy are primarily related to how much accuracy we need to have when measuring out one or more ingredients for compounding in a prescription. If multiple ingredients are listed, each measurement is expected to have the same accuracy as the ingredient listed with the greatest number of significant figures. For example, you need to compound a cough preparation with 0.125 g of active ingredient A and 0.5 g of active ingredient B. It is implied that the amount of ingredient B that is required is 0.500 g because three significant figures were used to signify the desired amount of ingredient A. Furthermore, it is implied for *any* prescription requiring compounding that ingredients be measured to at least three-figure accuracy. To summarize, you should be prepared to measure anything to three-figure accuracy unless greater accuracy is required. Now that you are aware of the accuracy required, you have to assess whether you are able to measure with that level of accuracy, and if not, find ways to work around those limitations.

THE PRESCRIPTION OR MEDICATION ORDER

Interpretation of prescriptions is a skill that most students pick up rapidly. It is usually more difficult to read the physician's handwriting than it is to interpret what is written. Nevertheless, if you can decipher the physician's handwriting, you will likely find several abbreviations. These abbreviations tell you what medication is requested by the physician and the directions to pass along to the patient. Selected abbreviations that are in frequent use appear in Table 7.1.

TABLE 7.1. EXAMPLES OF PHARMACY ABBREVIATIONS AND INTERPRETATIONS

ABBREVIATION	MEANING	ABBREVIATION	MEANING
aa.[a]	Of each	o.d.	Right eye
a.c.	Before meals	o.s. or o.l.	Left eye
ad	Up to	o.u.	Each eye
a.d.	Right ear	o_2	Both eyes, oxygen
a.s. or a.l.	Left ear	p	After
a.u.	Each ear	p.c.	After meals
b.i.d.	Twice a day	p.o.	By mouth
c[a]	With	p.r.n.	As needed
dil.	Dilute	q.d.	Every day
disp.	Dispense	q.h.	Every hour
div.	Divide	q.i.d.	Four times a day
d.t.d.	Give of such doses	q.o.d.	Every other day
et	And	q.s.	A sufficient quantity
ft.	Make	q.s. ad	A sufficient quantity to make
gr or gr.	Grain	s[a]	Without
gtt.	Drop or drops	ss[a]	One half
h.s.	At bedtime	s/s or s&s	Signs/symptoms
M.	Mix	t.i.d.	Three times a day
mEq	Milliequivalent	u.d. or ut dict	As directed
N&V or N/V	Nausea and vomiting	ung. or oint.	Ointment
non rep or N.R.	Do not repeat	w/a or w.a.	While awake
NPO	Nothing by mouth		

[a]These may appear with or without a horizontal line over them. Either way, the meaning is unchanged.

TABLE 7.2. APOTHECARY WEIGHT				
POUNDS	OUNCES	DRAMS	SCRUPLES	GRAINS
1	12	96	288	5760
	1	8	24	480
		1	3	60
			1	20

COMMON SYSTEMS OF MEASUREMENT AND CONVERSION

In the past, pharmacists were required to use the apothecary and avoirdupois systems of measurement. You are still expected to be able to work with these systems of measurement because you may receive prescriptions written in such terminology. Understanding them will allow you to convert rapidly to the metric system and proceed accordingly. It is not necessary for you to memorize these tables in their entirety to work effectively with these systems of measure. The apothecary and avoirdupois system of weights appear in a useful format in Tables 7.2 and 7.3, respectively.

The grain in either of these systems is equivalent, but obviously the weight of the pound and the ounce differs between the systems. The avoirdupois system of weight is the one in general use in the United States (e.g., at the grocery store). The dram and scruple do not exist in the avoirdupois system. Do your best not to confuse these two systems of weights. Fortunately for you, the apothecary system of volume is one with which you are probably familiar (and there is only one of these systems to learn). The gallon, ounce, pint, and quart have the volumes you see routinely in the United States. One would rarely have occasion to use the fluidram or minim outside the practice of pharmacy. Like the dram and the scruple, these terms are probably new to you. The apothecary system of volume appears in Table 7.4, in the same useful format previously used for weights.

TABLE 7.3. AVOIRDUPOIS WEIGHT		
POUNDS	OUNCES	GRAINS
1	16	7000
	1	437.5

TABLE 7.4. APOTHECARY VOLUME

GALLONS	QUARTS	PINTS	FLUID OUNCES	FLUIDRAMS	MINIMS
1	4	8	128	1024	61,440
	1	2	32	256	15,360
		1	16	128	7,680
			1	8	480
				1	60

Conversion to the Metric System

If you receive a prescription using a common system of measure, you will probably find it easiest to convert to metric units before preparing it. Table 7.5 contains those metric conversions that tend to be most useful.

Conversions of Convenience

For ease of use, several *approximate* conversions are in widespread use by pharmacists and physicians. These are: 1 teaspoonful = 5 mL = 1 fluidram, 1 tablespoonful = 15 mL = $1/2$ fluid ounce, and 30 mL = 1 fluid ounce. Of these, the teaspoonful is the farthest from the fluidram, both in absolute value and in relative value. For the vast majority of drugs, the difference in effect will be negligible because most drugs are safe within a wide range of concentrations in the body.

TABLE 7.5. USEFUL METRIC CONVERSIONS

COMMON WEIGHT/MEASURE	METRIC EQUIVALENT
1 fluid ounce	29.57 mL
1 pint	473 mL
1 gallon (U.S.)	3785 mL
1 pound (avoirdupois)	454 g
1 pound (apothecary)	373 g
1 ounce (avoirdupois)	28.35 g
1 ounce (apothecary)	31.1 g
1 grain	64.8 mg
2.2 pounds (avoirdupois)	1 kg

CALCULATION OF DOSES

Probably the most basic calculation you will perform will be the calculation of a reasonable dose for a patient. The "normal" or "usual" dose for any drug is one that produces the desired response in *most* individuals. It is important to note that the normal dose is not appropriate for everyone. Drug distribution and elimination (covered in more detail elsewhere in this text) can usually be related to a patient's body weight or body surface area such that the most appropriate dose is tied to those patient demographics (e.g., 5 mg/kg or 250 mg/m^2 of drug X). The normal or average adult individual is considered to weigh 70 kg or have 1.73 m^2 of body surface area (BSA). Although calculating a dose using the previous method focuses on body size, a patient's age can further influence the selection of an appropriate dose because body composition (in terms of water, fat, and muscle) and organ function (especially liver and kidney) vary with age. These differences in body composition and organ function can affect drug distribution and elimination, which in turn alters the most appropriate dose. Other factors may affect your final recommendation, depending on your area of practice. You will find yourself considering some or all of these things repeatedly in practice, and your preceptors will familiarize you with any specialized calculations they use when optimizing a dosing regimen.

RATIO STRENGTH AND PERCENTAGE

Several of the active ingredients in products you prepare, dispense, and use will not be pure substances. Rather, they will be diluted in something else (e.g., water, syrup, one inactive ingredient, or more). The strength of these products may be represented as a percentage or ratio strength, i.e., 5% dextrose in water. Percentage is a term that implies "out of a hundred" such that 5% dextrose in water means 5 grams of dextrose in every 100 mL of water. Percentage and ratio strength may be represented as weight/weight (w/w), volume/volume (v/v), or weight/volume (w/v). If it is not obvious which one of these three applies, it should be noted. Weight/weight is probably the most difficult to use. Percentage really is a ratio strength as well, but think of ratio strength as ratios always represented as 1 to some other quantity that is 1 or larger. Examples of these kinds of ratios are 1:1, 1:5, 1:14, 1:1000, 1:15,000. A ratio of 1:1 would indicate equal parts. Ratio strength not represented in percentage terms can be changed to percentage and vice versa. You may find it easier when doing ratio and proportion calculations to alter any ratio strength notations to percentages. For example, the 5% dextrose in water above is 1:20 ratio strength because 5 out of 100 simplifies to 1:20. When you need to convert a ratio strength to percentage, you have to find out how many parts out of 100 it represents. As another example, 1:1000 represents 0.1% because for every 100 total parts, there is 0.1 part of the ingredient that is in this ratio strength.

Dilution/Concentration

If you are not starting "from scratch," you should be able to handle using a concentrated stock solution/compound to make a more dilute solution/compound. Let's say you have an aqueous stock solution that is 25% (w/v) of some drug and we need to dilute it such that the final solution will be 1:2000. We need to know how much of the stock solution and water we need to produce the 1:2000 solution. Basically, you need 1 g in 2 L of water in the final product (1:2000), so you need to figure out how much of the stock solution gives you 1 gram of the drug. The difference between that volume and two liters is the additional water to add to make 1:2000.

$$1g \times \frac{100ml}{25g} = 4 \text{ mL}$$

Therefore, 4 mL of the stock solution contains 1 g of the active ingredient. We should measure out 4 mL of the stock solution and dilute to 2000 mL with water. Another example with an ointment might be that we have a supply of an ointment in which the active ingredient is found to be 10%, and we need to make 60 g of 0.25% (1:400) ointment from that supply. Again the process is that you need to figure out how much of the active ingredient is required to complete the compound and then how much stock ointment contains that amount. After you know the amount of the stock compound to use, make up the remainder with ointment base.

$$60g \text{ final product} \times \frac{0.25g \text{ active ingredient}}{100g \text{ final product}} = 0.15g \text{ active ingredient}$$

$$0.15g \text{ active ingredient} \times \frac{100g \text{ stock ointment}}{10g \text{ active ingredient}} = 1.5g \text{ stock ointment}$$

You would weigh out 1.5 g of the stock ointment and 58.5 g of the ointment base and mix well in an appropriate manner such as geometric dilution. Similar calculations are useful in making a more concentrated stock solution or similar compound. These sorts of calculations can be simplified if we use alligation methods. Alligation is especially useful if we have two stock compounds of different ratio strengths and we need to make a third. Note that an ointment base has a ratio strength of zero. We can use the alligation to tell us how many parts of each are required (relative proportions) to make any quantity of the final product. Once the desired final quantity is known, you divide the total quantity of the final product by the total number of parts required in the alligation to find the weight or volume of one part. Then multiply the number of parts required by that weight or volume. Let's reuse one of the above problems to illustrate this method.

Concentration of drug in ointment	Concentration of drug in final compounded product	Number of parts	Weight of material
10%		0.25	1.5 g
	0.25%		
0% (ointment base)		9.75	58.5 g
		10 parts total	60 g total

Because 60 g of the final product is desired, 60 g is equivalent to 10 parts. Therefore, one part is 6 g. To find the amount of 10% ointment to use, you multiply 0.25 parts by 6 g to get 1.5 g of the 10% ointment, which is the same answer we generated above. For the ointment base, you multiply 9.75 parts by 6 g to get 58.5 g of the ointment base, which, again, is the same answer as before. The number of parts of each component required for the final compound is the difference in percentage concentration between the concentration of drug in the final compound and that of the *other* component. You can see above that the difference between 10% and 0.25% is 9.75, but you represent the answer in parts, not percentages. This answer is the number of parts of the ointment base (0%). The opposite calculation supplies you with the figure 0.25 parts, which is the obvious difference between 0.25% and 0%. This method is extremely useful because of its relative speed once you master the process. In order to make a stock solution/compound or to concentrate one you have, you must know what the desired concentration is and from where you are starting. Suppose you want to make a stock ointment more concentrated, to contain, for example, 40 % (w/w) of active ingredient instead of 30 % (w/w). The final quantity desired is 2000 g. With alligation (illustrated below), the difference between the concentration of pure drug (100 %) and the final stock ointment (40 %) is 60. The difference between concentration in the present stock (30% w/w) and final stock (40 % w/w) ointments is 10. The total number of parts to make 2000 g of ointment is 70, or 28.57 g/part.

Concentration of drug in ointment	Concentration of drug in final compounded product	Number of parts	Weight of material
30%		60	1714.3 g
	40%		
100% (pure drug)		10	285.7 g
		70 parts total	2000 g total

You would use 60 parts × 28.57 g/part or 1714.3 g of the 30% w/w ointment, and 10 parts × 28.57 g/part or 285.7 g of pure drug. Once properly incorporated, you will have 2000 g of the 40 % w/w ointment you wanted.

ALIQUOTS

When you get into a situation where you need to measure an amount of material that is too small to measure accurately with the equipment you have, you may be forced to use the aliquot method. The standard pharmacy balance has a sensitivity requirement of 6 mg, and the maximum acceptable error in our measurement is 5%. These two figures generate the least weighable amount (LWA) of 120 mg on these balances. This amount is a number that will be repeated to you frequently in your pharmaceutics compounding laboratory. The LWA is the smallest quantity that can be measured with acceptable error. When you are faced with this dilemma, you will have to work around the limitations of your equipment. In using the aliquot method, we weigh out an amount of the substance in question that is equal to or in excess of the LWA for the balance. Then, you dilute that amount with a known quantity of inert material, mix well and weigh out the portion of the mixture that contains the desired amount of the substance.

You must remember that everything you weigh on the balance must be equal to or in excess of the LWA. For example, you could not weigh out 120 mg of active ingredient, 120 mg of inert substance, mix well and weigh 80 mg to take the desired quantity of the active ingredient. Eighty milligrams is less than the LWA, so this measurement is not acceptable. There are multiple keys to doing an aliquot properly. First, you have to choose an amount of the active ingredient you want that is at least the LWA. If at all possible, this amount should be a whole-number multiple of the amount you truly need. Second, you must weigh out a quantity of an appropriately chosen inert substance that is $=/>$ the LWA. The inert substance should be compatible with the active ingredient and all other ingredients of the final product. You must weigh out enough inert substance such that the amount of the mixture to be weighed in the end will be at least the LWA. This decision will take some forethought so as to prevent the example given previously in which the final amount to be weighed was not at least the LWA. The advantage of weighing out a whole-number multiple of the desired quantity makes it easier to select this amount and compute the final amount to be weighed. If you need 50 mg of diphenhydramine (Benadryl®), it makes your life much easier to weigh out 150 mg (three times the needed quantity). Here's how: no matter how much inert substance you mix with the 150 mg of diphenhydramine, one-third of it will contain 50 mg of diphenhydramine, assuming uniform mixing (if you had measured out four times the needed amount or 200 mg of diphenhydramine, one-fourth of the eventual mixture will contain 50 mg of diphenhydramine; if you measured out five times what you need, one-fifth of the mixture has the desired quantity and so on). Knowing that you need one-third of the eventual mixture and that this amount must be at least 120 mg, you know that you must make a total quantity of the mixture that is not less than 360 mg. In order to proceed, you could weigh out 210 mg of the inert substance (360 mg − 150 mg), mix well with a mortar and pestle, and 120 mg of the mixture should contain 50 mg of diphenhydramine. Third, the quantity of inert substance selected must be reasonable and typically as little as necessary. For example, you would not make an aliquot with 2 g of inert substance if it could be reasonably performed with 200 mg. In other words, you would not want to have an aliquot that is excessively large. Within reason, conserve the raw materials as best you can and waste only what you must in order to prepare the prescription properly. Costs of compounding are passed along to the consumer (typically including the costs of any waste), so minimize waste, especially when the cost of these materials is high.

Another way to measure a small quantity of a solid could be to measure out a quantity at least the LWA and dissolve it in a suitable solvent. Once it has dissolved, you may be able to measure the solution more reliably, depending on what you have to measure fluids. The proper portion of the solution would contain the right amount of drug. The process is the same. An aliquot method of measuring also exists for volumes that cannot be measured reliably. A good general rule is that one cannot measure accurately a volume that is less than 20% of the total volume of the vessel (e.g., 2 mL is the smallest volume measured reliably in a 10 mL graduate). You should measure any volume in the smallest vessel available so as to minimize the potential error in the measurement. If calibrating a dropper is not a reasonable option, measure out a volume accurately using what volumetric tools you have available and dilute in an inert, miscible fluid that is compatible with all other materials in the prescription. Once the fluids are in solution, an aliquot of the mixture can be measured accurately, if properly prepared. These steps are similar to those used in the aliquot method of weighing. The use of a dropper may be indicated if the dropper is properly calibrated for the liquid in question. Remember that a dropper must be calibrated for every liquid to be used; the volume of one drop will vary based on the liquid. There are several references you could refer to for instructions on how to calibrate a dropper if you have forgotten how.

TONICITY AND OSMOLARITY

Isotonic Solutions

There may come a time when you are asked to prepare an isotonic solution. An isotonic solution has the same osmotic pressure as the body fluid it is to be mixed with. Such a solution will be very easy to tolerate, as hypertonic or hypotonic solutions may cause discomfort or other unwanted effects for the patient. Ophthalmic (for the eye), parenteral (by injection), nasal (for the nose), and some enema (per rectum) preparations are those for which you would most likely see the condition of isotonicity placed on your compounding. Normal saline is 0.9% sodium chloride in water, or 9 g of NaCl in 1000 mL of water. This solution is considered to be isotonic with the body fluids. Through extensive work, a table of relationships of tonicity between other substances and sodium chloride has been established. These relationships are collectively called "sodium chloride equivalents." In short, 1 g of each of the substances listed has the same tonicity as the number of grams of sodium chloride listed. For instance, 1 g of silver nitrate is equivalent to 0.33 g of sodium chloride because in solution silver nitrate does not have the same tonicity as NaCl. Approximately 3 g of silver nitrate would have the same tonicity as 1 g of sodium chloride in solution (3 × 0.33 g = 0.99 g). The availability of these tables enables us to quickly calculate the appropriate preparation of an isotonic solution with the components listed. For example, the physician writes for 1 ounce of 1% pilocarpine nitrate in purified water made isotonic with sodium chloride. If you use 30 mL for 1 ounce to make it easier, we know that we need 0.3 g of pilocarpine nitrate. One gram of pilocarpine nitrate is equivalent to 0.23 g sodium chloride, so

$$0.3 \text{ g pilocarpine nitrate} \times \frac{0.23 \text{ g sodium chloride}}{1 \text{ g pilocarpine nitrate}} = 0.069 \text{ g sodium chloride}$$

So 0.3 g pilocarpine nitrate has the same tonicity as 0.069 g sodium chloride. Now we need to know how much total sodium chloride would make 30 mL isotonic and subtract 0.069 g from that figure to solve for how much NaCl to add to the bottle.

$$30ml \times \frac{9g}{1000ml} = 0.27g \text{ sodium chloride}$$

$$0.27 \text{ g} - 0.069 \text{ g} = 0.201 \text{ g sodium chloride}$$

To properly compound these eye drops, we need to add 0.3 g pilocarpine nitrate and 0.201 g sodium chloride to an eye dropper bottle and dissolve it in enough purified water to make 30 mL of the solution. *Remington's Pharmaceutical Sciences* has an exhaustive list of sodium chloride equivalents, and this reference should be available in most pharmacies. They are not presented here.

Electrolyte Solutions

A discussion of electrolyte solutions is really a continuation of the previous section on isotonicity. Compounds in solution that dissociate to some degree are called electrolytes. Good examples of electrolytes are sodium chloride and hydrochloric acid. This dissociation leads to the presence of ions that have positive (cations) or negative (anions) electric charges. Those compounds that do not dissociate are called nonelectrolytes. A good example of a nonelectrolyte is glucose. For a more comprehensive review of dissociation, electrolytes, and ions, consult your chemistry textbooks from courses past. You should remember from your chemistry background that concentration can be represented in many ways. In chemistry, you are more likely to use molarity or the number of moles of solute per liter of solution. Its formula or molecular weight gives the number of grams in a mole (6.02×10^{23} molecules) of a compound. A millimole is 1/1000 of the molecular or formula weight of the compound in question. For example, the molecular weight of NaCl is 58.5 g. That means that 58.5 g of NaCl makes 1 mole of sodium chloride, and a millimole is 58.5 mg of NaCl. An equivalent weight is the mass of the species in question that is capable of providing 1 mole of positive or negative charge. Like the millimole, the milliequivalent (meq) is 1/1000 of that weight. So in the case of NaCl, 1 mmole of NaCl is 1 meq of NaCl because it is capable of providing 1 mole of positive or negative charge. Furthermore, there is 1 meq of Na^+ and 1 meq of Cl^- in 1 meq of NaCl. To get the number of milliequivalents, you multiply the number of millimoles present by the total number of positive or negative charges, not both. That's why the number of mEq of NaCl is the same as the number of mEq of Na^+ and Cl^- because they are all multiplied by 1. In 1 mmole of Na_2HPO_4 there are 2 meq of Na_2HPO_4 and 2 meq of Na^+ and 2 meq of HPO_4^-. In this case, the number of millimoles of sodium (2) and the number of millimoles of hydrogenphosphate (1) do not match up, but the numbers of milliequivalents do. The total number of positive charges should match up with the total number of negative charges, so the number of milliequivalents will as well. The concentration of electrolytes in the blood is likely to be represented in meq/L or meq/dL.

Next, the terms osmolarity and osmolality are introduced. Their importance to pharmacy is in the preparation of isotonic solutions and the proper addition of a certain number of equivalents to intravenous fluid or nutrition. Osmotic pressure is proportional to the number of particles in solution. Osmolarity refers to the number of *separate* particles in solution. One millimole of NaCl in a liter of solution represents two milliosmoles (mOsm) of NaCl because the sodium and the chloride will dissociate almost completely in solution. One millimole of a nonelectrolyte such as glucose will be 1 mOsm because it does not dissociate. The difference between osmolarity and osmolality is that osmolality is the number of species per kilogram of solution. It is important to remember all of these ways to represent concentration because you may find yourself changing from one to another depending on the situation. As suggested previously, osmolarity will be used frequently when isotonic preparations are being made. For example, you should know that normal saline (0.9% NaCl in water) is isotonic. Assuming complete dissociation, normal saline is 308 mOsm of NaCl per liter of water. The concentration is high enough that at each instant a few NaCl molecules are intact, so the true osmolarity is more like 286 mOsm/L. You should note whether the value being reported on any products you use or prepare is actual or ideal (assuming complete dissociation) osmolarity.

RECONSTITUTION AND INTRAVENOUS ADMIXTURES

In order to increase the shelf life of a product, it may be produced by the manufacture in dry powder form (consituted). If you need to dispense the medication or use it to prepare an intravenous medication for someone, you will be faced with having to reconstitute the drug. Reconstitution may produce a solution or a suspension. The most important factor to consider in reconstitution is the contribution of the dry powder to the volume of the reconstituted preparation. For example, if a vial of drug for intravenous use has a very small amount of drug in it, it will be unlikely that the drug contributes significantly to the volume once reconstituted. Therefore, the concentration of the constituted drug in the vial will simply be the amount of drug in the vial divided by the volume of the appropriate solvent (purified water, sterile water for injection, D_5W, NS, etc.). However, if the amount of drug is large enough that it will displace solvent, the volume you must add cannot be the total volume you want in the end. For example, several oral antibiotics come as dry powders in bottles ready for reconstitution. They have directions on the side indicating how much water to add to make the final volume correct. If 250 mL is the final volume, the amount the pharmacist is expected to add will typically be less than 250 mL and may be on the order of 200 mL. The drug itself increases the volume of the final preparation, and in order to get the appropriate amount of medication per dose, the final volume must be correct. It is imperative that you follow the directions for reconstitution that accompany a medication requiring it.

With intravenous admixtures, you must make every effort to ensure that the correct amount of medication is in the intravenous solution. Not only is it important that you correctly calculate the amount to add to the IV fluid, but you must be sure to correctly make the addition. Suppose you have a 1-g vial of an IV drug that must be reconstituted. To properly reconstitute the drug, 8 mL of sterile water for injection must be added to the vial. Proper mixing produces 10 mL of solution. If you want 250 mg of the drug, you must take one-fourth of the *final volume* of the drug in solution (2.5 mL)—not one-fourth of the volume you added (2 mL).

You have to take extra steps with intravenous admixtures because the drug will be administered into the circulation. Drugs administered IV need to be in solution if at all possible. Precipitation of drug in the veins can be disastrous. You will be faced with compatibility issues repeatedly: Can this drug be reconstituted with solvent A? Is the drug stable in D_5W? Does the addition of potassium cause precipitation? And so on. Rely on your professors, drug information resources, and preceptors to educate you about these incompatibilities. Once an IV solution is prepared, you may be asked to calculate a flow rate based on either the desired rate of drug administration or based on the time over which the entire volume of the IV solution is to be administered. If there is 100 mg of drug in the IV solution and the physician wants the patient to receive 10 mg per hour, then the drug can be administered for 10 hours before a new IV solution is needed to replace this one. Based on that figure, 1/10 of the volume in the solution must be administered per hour to provide the desired administration rate. You may also be asked to convert the flow rate to volume per minute. If that 100 mg is in a 1-L bag of normal saline (assuming no volume expansion by the drug), the flow rate (mL/min) can be calculated as follows:

$$\frac{10mg}{hr} \times \frac{1000ml}{100mg} \times \frac{1hr}{60\ min} = 1.67 \text{ ml/min}$$

If the IV solution with all of its contents is to be given over an 8-hour period, you simply divide the total volume of IV solution by the time period. If it were a 500 mL solution, the flow rate would be 62.5 mL/hour or approximately 1 mL/min. Nurses are frequently responsible for calculating a drip rate that correlates to the desired flow rate. Gravity helps drive the IV solution into the circulation, and a device attached to the IV line can be adjusted to allow a certain number of drops of the IV solution to fall per minute through a small chamber. Just as in calibrating a dropper, you must find out how many drops are in a milliliter using the given equipment and solve accordingly. You may never be asked to do this calculation, but some practice settings may have the pharmacist calculate the drip rate as well.

SUMMARY

The diversity and frequency of the calculations you will be asked to perform will depend greatly on your practice site and any specialty on which you choose to focus. When you chose to become a pharmacist, mathematics became a much larger part of your life. Regardless of the calculation and the presence of devices to assist you (e.g., computer, calculator, PDA), work carefully; someone's life might depend on it.

QUESTIONS

1. Interpret the following prescription or medication orders:
   A. gtts. iv a.u. q.i.d.
   B. M.ft. ung. Disp. 30 g
   C. tab ss b.i.d. u.d.
   D. cap i t.i.d. p.c. et h.s.
2. Convert between the metric and common systems of measurement:
   A. How many milliliters are in a pint?
   B. How many milligrams are in 7 grains?
   C. How many grams are in an apothecary ounce?
   D. When can you interpret the fluidram as 5 mL?
3. Calculate an appropriate dose:
   A. If the normal adult dose is 5 mg/kg/day, how many milligrams will the average adult receive in a day?
   B. If we must compound and dispense 4 fluid ounces of syrup that has 15 mg of drug/tsp, how many milligrams are in 4 ounces?
   C. If an average adult receives 200 mg of a given medication once daily, what dose would be appropriate for a football player who weighs 330 lb (avoirdupois)?
4. Prepare, concentrate, or dilute compounded medications accurately in the following:
   A. An adult patient does not like solid dosage forms and requests an antibiotic suspension from the doctor that is not commercially available. If

500 mg of drug needs to be in each tablespoonful, how many milligrams of drug is needed for the suspension if the directions are to take 1 tablespoonful three times daily for 10 days?

B. How many milligrams of drug are needed to make 200 g of a 30% (w/w) ointment? a 40% (w/w) ointment?

C. Use the alligation method to determine how much of each stock solution is needed to make a 40% (w/v) solution? Stock solution A: 70% (w/v). Stock solution B: 20% (w/v).

D. How many milliliters of water is needed to dilute 100 mL of a 10% (w/v) solution to a ratio strength of 1:200?

5. Interpret osmolarity, isotonicity, and milliequivalents:

A. How many milliosmoles are in one millimole of aluminum chloride?

B. How many milliequivalents of sodium are in 300 mg of sodium chloride?

C. What is the osmolarity of 0.45% NaCl?

D. What is the osmolarity of D_5W (5% dextrose in water)?

6. Prepare isotonic solutions in the following cases:

A. How many grams of sodium chloride are required to make the following prescription?

Physostigmine sulfate	1%
Sodium chloride	q.s.
Purified water	ad 30 mL
M. isotonic solution	
Sig: gtts ii o.d. b.i.d.	

B. How many grams of boric acid is required to make the following prescription?

Cromolyn sodium	2%
Boric acid	q.s.
Purified water	ad 60 mL
M. isotonic solution	
Sig: gtts. iv o.u. q.i.d.	

7. Reconstitute dry powders to appropriate concentration:

A. The directions for reconstitution of an antibiotic are to add 188 mL of water to the bottle in order to achieve 250 mL of a 250 mg/5 mL solution. What volume of water would be required to make a 150 mg/5 mL solution?

B. The directions for reconstitution on a 500-mg injection vial are to add 9 mL of normal saline for injection to make 10 mL of solution. What is the concentration of the drug in the vial after reconstitution?

C. You have appropriately reconstituted 1 g of a drug and placed it in a 500 mL IV bag of normal saline. What rate of flow (in mL/min) will deliver 25 mg/h of the drug?

8. Utilize the aliquot method for solids and liquids:

    A. Explain how you would use the aliquot method of weighing to obtain 10 mg of codeine sulfate is you have a standard pharmacy balance. Use lactose as an inert diluent.

    B. Explain how you would use the aliquot method of weighing to obtain 5 mg of sodium phenobarbital if you have a standard pharmacy balance. Use lactose as an inert diluent.

    C. Explain how you would use the aliquot method for measuring volume if you need 0.5 mL of a 10 mg/mL solution and the smallest graduate cylinder you have is 10 mL (use 20% least measurable volume rule here). Use water as a diluent.

REFERENCES

1. Ansel HC, Stoklosa MJ. Pharmaceutical calculations, 11th ed. Philadelphia: Lippincott Williams & Wilkins, 2001.
2. Gennaro AR. Remington: the science and practice of pharmacy, 20th ed. Philadelphia: Lippincott Williams & Wilkins, 2001.

C H A P T E R 8

DRUG INFORMATION AND DRUG LITERATURE EVALUATION

Karen L. Kier

Goals: After reviewing the information in this chapter, you should be able to:

1. Explain the role that drug information, drug literature evaluation, and professional writing play in establishing a good foundation for a pharmacy professional.
2. Discuss the modified systematic approach to drug information and how it impacts on developing a good search strategy.
3. Specify the differences among primary, secondary, and tertiary literature.
4. Identify essential secondary and tertiary literature used in answering drug information inquiries.
5. Understand the basic concepts of drug literature evaluation and be able to apply them to an article.
6. Recognize and apply key concepts in professional writing.

INTRODUCTION TO DRUG INFORMATION

Drug information is a specialized area of pharmacy focusing on information management. Information management can evolve into many different forms. Drug information can be a verbal answer to a patient's question, or it can involve a detailed monograph presented to the Pharmacy & Therapeutics Committee in order to decide if a drug will be available through a formulary system. Pharmacists and pharmacy students cannot know every potential or possible question or scenario that might be posed to them during their practice. However, they should be prepared to efficiently and effectively answer questions posed to them from consumers or other healthcare professionals. Knowing where to look and how to find the most appropriate information is the basic groundwork for the skills of drug information. Among the skills of drug information is a knowledge of drug literature evaluation, which allows one to provide a critical analysis of the literature and have a better understanding of the studies done in health and medicine. The goal of this chapter is to provide the student with a basic understanding of drug information skills and resources as well as providing the basic tenants of drug literature evaluation. The chapter provides examples of student drug information exercises that could serve as a basic template for written communication.

DRUG INFORMATION SKILLS

In order to provide an accurate and timely answer to a drug information question, one has to ascertain that he or she understands the nature of the question and has asked all necessary questions to get to the "ultimate" question. As with many questions, the first question asked is not necessarily the whole picture or representative of the complete question. Many times the first question asked is a lead to open the conversation, and there is more to the question than first appears. Valuable information can be lost when the pharmacist does not take the time to ask appropriate questions to the requestor. Patients, especially, may not always know the necessary information that is critical for providing a complete and accurate answer. This is why drug information specialists have developed systematic approaches to answering drug information questions. Most specialists today use the modified systematic approach designed by Host and Kirkwood. This approach involves seven steps, which are outlined in Table 8.1.

Looking at each step provides us with a framework for obtaining and answering a drug information request.

Step I. Secure Demographics of Requestor

Know who is requesting the information because this determines the type of response that is given. A response given to a consumer requesting information would involve much less medical terminology, whereas a response to a healthcare professional would involve more technical information including specific medical terminology that would be deemed appropriate. Likewise, it is important to determine the name of the requestor and his or her location (phone, fax, address, e-mail) and affiliation. Some institutions and workplaces have very spe-

TABLE 8.1. MODIFIED SYSTEMATIC APPROACH

Step I	Secure demographics of requestor
Step II	Obtain background information
Step III	Determine and categorize the ultimate question
Step IV	Develop strategy and conduct search
Step V	Perform evaluation, analysis, and synthesis
Step VI	Formulate and provide response
Step VII	Conduct follow-up and documentation

cific policies and procedures for handling information requests. Always ask for a copy of such policies before answering any questions. For example, some institutions will answer only questions requested by employees, and others may not answer consumer questions. Some pharmacies will not handle consumer questions if the patient does not receive his or her medication from that pharmacy. Often this policy is based on not having available profile information that may be needed to answer questions completely and accurately.

Step II. Obtain Background Information

Other demographic information that maybe helpful is knowing if the question is patient specific or if the question is one of general knowledge. Most questions are usually a result of a specific patient need rather than purely academic questions that just arise. Therefore, patient-specific questions require delving into questions related to the patient. These questions can refer to such things as the patient's age, medication profile, disease state profile, past medication history, social history, current laboratory data, and overall health. The better one understands the conditions, health, and demographics of the patient, the better is one's ability to look at the complete picture and provide an appropriate response. Many drug information centers use a standard response form that guides the collection of this information for each request.

Additional information that may be helpful is where the requestors found the information they already have, including the correct spelling of unfamiliar terms, where they have looked, and how quickly they need to know the information. Many times consumers will read or hear information from television, magazines, friends, or other healthcare professionals. They often do not have the correct spelling of information or even accurate descriptions of the information that they heard. Recent advances in using sources such as the internet, Lexis-Nexis (a secondary database that contains television transcripts), and Periodical Abstracts (a secondary database with information from both medical and consumer journals and magazines) have provided additional avenues to identifying the questions posed by consumers.

Step III. Determine and Categorize the Ultimate Question

This step is probably the most critical one in establishing a good search strategy. The first part of this step involves putting the pieces of information together to form the ultimate question. Some interpret the ultimate question as the final iteration of the question. Sometimes the ultimate question is actually more than one distinct question. Once the ultimate question has been determined, the next step is to categorize the question. Many drug information centers have lists of standard categories that they use. A comprehensive list can be found in the textbook called *Drug Information: A Guide for Pharmacists.*[2] Table 8.2 provides some of the most common types. The category is essential to developing the strat-

TABLE 8.2. EXAMPLES OF DRUG INFORMATION CATEGORIES

Adverse Effects	Identification
Availability	Pharmacokinetics
Compatability/Stability	Pharmacology
Compounding	Posioning/Toxicology
Dosing and Administration	Pregnancy and Lactation
Drug Interaction	Therapeutic Use
Herbal	

egy because different references maybe employed for different types or categories of questions. For example, a tablet identification question may require a source such as IDENTIDEX to answer the inquiry, whereas a dosing question may use a standard reference such as *Facts and Comparisons*.

Step IV. Develop Strategy and Conduct Search

Developing an algorithm for searching a question will provide an organized approach to handling the question and assuring that sufficient references and documentation have been acquired to answer the question. A typical algorithm has three essential components, which consist of tertiary, secondary, and primary literature. Primary literature refers to the actual study, case report, or case series. The key to this type of literature is that it refers to the actual subjects whether in a clinical trial or as a case report. The primary literature is considered to be the original study or report. In answering drug information requests, the idea is to be able to identify, evaluate, and report on the primary literature whenever possible. Some types of questions do not require a search this extensive. A good example of that type of question would be a tablet identification code or the availability of a drug in the United States. Secondary literature refers to an indexing or abstracting service. Secondary literature is the indexed primary literature. The secondary sources are an excellent tool in obtaining the primary literature. Secondary sources include such very common databases as the IOWA system, *International Pharmaceutical Abstracts* (IPA), Medline, Lexis-Nexis, Reactions, and InPharma. Some secondary sources will provide an abstract of the primary literature, and others will provide a full text version of the article. The key to secondary systems is to become familiar with the best way to search each system and to identify correct key terms. Often the difference between a mediocre search and a good one is the key words used by the researcher. A better understanding of the nature of the question and the related background information will help in determining key search terms. Tertiary literature refers to compilations or reviews of primary literature done by authors who put the actual studies into their own words. Textbooks are a common example of tertiary literature that involves review of material. One problem with tertiary literature is that it is usually at least 2 years out of date by the time it is published, so its timeliness is limited. Another problem is that the reader is dependent on the interpretation and accuracy of the author who did the review, and this interpretation may differ from what others may have considered appropriate. Tertiary literature can also contain misinformation taken out of context or data that were transformed differently from the primary study. Sometimes this results in mistakes in dosing or administration. Some drug information specialists will often refer to a minimum of two tertiary references to find corroborating information. This provides a level of confidence that the information is accurate and consistent. However, this is not always an absolute.

In designing an algorithm, start the research with tertiary literature. Then proceed to secondary sources, which help to identify the necessary primary literature. Knowing what tertiary and secondary references are useful for the question's category facilitates the algorithm design. Table 8.3 provides some common categories with useful tertiary and secondary sources. This table is by no means comprehensive for all references available but is meant to be a basic guide to establishing an algorithm.

Step V. Perform Evaluation, Analysis, and Synthesis

A good drug information response will demonstrate that the provider took time to evaluate the information, analyze it, and then synthesize it into a good reply. Evaluating the quality of the information is a key. Care should be taken to identify poor data or even controversial data where studies differ on outcomes. Therefore, drug literature evaluation skills become critical to the ability to distinguish good data from poor data. There is no one perfect study, and each study will have some limitations. The professional develops the skills to interpret the merits of a study despite limitations that might be present.

Step VI. Formulate and Provide Response

Establish an outline the helps formulate a response to the drug information request. As with most professional writing, it is important to have an introduction, body, and conclusion. The introduction should provide a comprehensive but concise review of the disease, drug, or situation proposed in the question. The body of the answer should be a review of the pertinent literature that answers the question. The primary literature should be reviewed and discussed in this section. Any controversy or debate among the studies should be addressed. Studies should be

TABLE 8.3. COMMON SECONDARY AND TERTIARY REFERENCES BY CATEGORY

CATEGORY OF INQUIRY	TERTIARY RESOURCES	SECONDARY RESOURCES
Adverse Events	AHFS Drug Information, DRUGDEX, Drug Facts and Comparisons, Drug Information Handbook, USPDI Volume 1	Reactions, IPA, IOWA, MEDLINE
Disease State Information	Cecil Textbook of Medicine, Harrison's Principles of Internal Medicine, The Merck Manual, Pharmacotherapy	IOWA, MEDLINE, InPharma, IPA
Dosage Guidelines (General)	AHFS Drug Information, DRUGDEX, Drug Facts and Comparisons, PDR, Mosby's GenRx, Drug Information Handbook, Pharmacotherapy	IPA, IOWA
Dosage Guidelines (Geriatrics)	Geriatric Dosage Handbook, AHFS Drug Information, DRUGDEX, Drug Facts and Comparisons	IPA, IOWA
Dosage Guidelines (Pediatrics)	Harriet Lane Handbook, Pediatric Dosage Handbook, AHFS Drug Information, DRUGDEX, Drug Facts and Comparisons, Drug Information Handbook	Paediatrics Today, IPA, IOWA, MEDLINE
Drug Administration	AHFS Drug Information, DRUGDEX	IPA, IOWA
Drug Interactions	Drug Facts and Comparisons, Drug Information Handbook Drug Interaction Facts, Evaluation of Drug Interactions, DRUGDEX	Reactions, IPA, IOWA
Drug Use in Pregnancy and Lactation	Drugs in Pregnancy and Lactation, DRUGDEX, Drug Information Handbook	Reactions, IOWA, IPA, MEDLINE
Herbal and Homeopathic Medications	PDR Herbal, Review of Natural Products, Commission E Monographs	IPA, IOWA, MEDLINE

(continued)

TABLE 8.3. COMMON SECONDARY AND TERTIARY REFERENCES BY CATEGORY (*Cont.*)

Category	References	Databases
Identification (Domestic)	American Drug Index, IDENTIDEX, DRUGDEX, Handbook of Nonprescription Drugs, USP Dictionary of USAN & International Drug Names	IPA, IOWA, Lexis-Nexis
Identification (Foreign)	Index Nominum, Martindale: The Extra Pharmacopeia, USP Dictionary of USAN & International Drug Names, DRUGDEX	IPA, InPharma, Lexis-Nexis, MEDLINE
Identification (Imprint Code)	IDENTIDEX, Ident-A-Drug Reference, Clinical Reference Library	
Indications	AHFS Drug Information, DRUGDEX, Facts and Comparisons, Drug Information Handbook, USPDI Volume 1	Lexis-Nexis
Investigational Drugs	USP Dictionary of USAN & International Drug Names, DRUGDEX, Martindale: The Extra Pharmacopeia	InPharma, IOWA, IPA, MEDLINE
Over-The-Counter Drugs	Handbook of Nonprescription Drugs, Physicians' Desk Reference for Non-Prescription Drugs, DRUGDEX, POISINDEX	IPA, IOWA, MEDLINE
Pharmacokinetics	Applied Pharmacokinetics: Principles of Therapeutic Drug Monitoring, Basic Clinical Pharmacokinetics, AHFS Drug Information, DRUGDEX, Handbook of Clinical Drug Data	IPA, IOWA, MEDLINE
Pharmacology	Goodman and Gilman's Pharmacologic Basis of Therapeutics, AHFS Drug Information, DRUGDEX, Facts and Comparisons	IOWA, IPA, MEDLINE, InPharma
Stability/Compatibility	Guide to Parenteral Admixtures, Handbook of Injectable Drugs, AHFS Drug Information, DRUGDEX	IPA, IOWA, MEDLINE
Toxicology/Poisoning	Clinical Toxicology of Commercial Products, POISINDEX, Poisoning & Toxicology Handbook	Reactions, IPA, IOWA, MEDLINE

appropriately cited in the reference section. Discussion of study limitations established by either the study authors or by drug literature evaluation is also appropriate within this section. The last section is the conclusion. This section should give a brief synopsis of the information provided and should usually include a professional opinion based on the literature cited.

Step VII. Conduct Follow-up and Documentation

This step involves checking with the requestor to make sure his or her question has been sufficiently and completely answered. Of vital importance is to document all the steps taken in this process.

STANDARD REFERENCES

This section provides information on some of the standard references that are used to answer drug information questions. A more extensive review of standard references by categories can be found in the textbook *Drug Information: A Guide for Pharmacists*. Table 8.4 provides some good general tertiary references that can be helpful in answering a wide variety of questions. It is important to note that many of these tertiary references can be found in different formats including hard copy, Web based, CD-ROM based, and PDA based. Table 8.5 outlines some good secondary references that may be available for identifying the primary literature. Table 8.6 provides some guidance to general journals that will often provide good primary literature.

DRUG LITERATURE EVALUATION

Drug literature evaluation is a key component to providing a good-quality answer to a requestor. Being able to separate good data from poor data is essential. Knowing the limitations of any study can help in evaluating the usability of its data. Drug information specialists will often use some standard questions to help in this process. Several references provide guides to evaluating the medical and

---

TABLE 8.4. GENERAL TERTIARY REFERENCES

Facts and Comparisons
Drug Information Handbook
ASHP Drug Information
MICROMEDEX (DRUGDEX, IDENTIDEX, POSIONDEX)

TABLE 8.5. COMMON SECONDARY REFERENCES

SECONDARY SOURCE	BRIEF DESCRIPTION
IOWA	Index by drug and disease and provides full text articles in PDF format
International Pharmaceutical Abstracts (IPA)	Most comprehensive pharmacy database, the best indexing of pharmacy journals from around the world, provides abstracts
MEDLINE	Most comprehensive biomedical database that includes medicine, nursing, pharmacy, and veterinary
InPharma	Shortest lag time between published and indexed articles, good review of drugs from around the world, provides news from the FDA, good for research and development
Reactions	Good source for adverse events, drug interactions, problems with herbal therapy, pregnancy and lactation, and toxicology
Lexis-Nexis	Provides comprehensive biomedical database, provides TV transcripts
Periodical Abstracts	Provides an index of both medical journals and consumer magazines

pharmacy literature. A template of 32 questions has been designed by drug information specialists and can be found in some of these references. The questions in Table 8.7 can be used as a template and are adapted with permission from Malone et al.[2] Table 8.8 has some helpful hints for determining the answers to these questions.

TABLE 8.6. PRIMARY REFERENCES

Annals of Pharmacotherapy
Pharmacotherapy
American Journal of Health-System Pharmacists
Journal of the American Pharmaceutical Association
Journal of the American Medical Association
New England Journal of Medicine
Annals of Internal Medicine

TABLE 8.7. QUESTIONS USED TO GUIDE
THE DRUG LITERATURE EVALUATION PROCESS

1. Is the journal considered reputable? Is the journal appropriate to find an article relating to this particular subject?
2. Do the researchers appear to have the appropriate qualifications for undertaking the study? Was the research performed in an appropriate medical facility?
3. What was the source of financial support for the study?
4. Do the authors give sufficient background information for the study? Did they demonstrate that the study was important and ethical?
5. Are the purpose and the objectives clearly stated and free from bias?
6. Was the study approved by an investigational review board?
7. Does the investigator state the null hypothesis? Is the alternative hypothesis stated?
8. Is the sample size large enough? Is the sample representative of the population?
9. Are the inclusion and exclusion criteria clearly stated, and are they appropriate?
10. Was the study randomized correctly? Even if the study is adequately randomized, are the groups (treatment and control) equivalent?
11. What is the study design? Is it appropriate?
12. Was the study adequately controlled? Were the controls adequate and appropriate?
13. Was the study adequately blinded?
14. Were appropriate doses and regimens used for the disease state under study?
15. Was the length of the study adequate to observe outcomes?
16. If the study is a crossover study, was the washout period adequate?
17. Were operational definitions given?

(continued)

PROFESSIONAL WRITING

Pharmacists and pharmacy students are often required to do professional writing. This may come in different formats, including drug information responses, case presentations, meeting abstracts, research papers, drug monographs, journal clubs, and newsletters.

First steps in professional writing really begin with good preparation. Establish an outline for the paper that is appropriate to the format required for the exercise. Do all research before establishing the outline. Check to make sure that you have primary literature to support the document when appropriate. Table 8.9 provides some helpful hints for writing.

TABLE 8.7. QUESTIONS USED TO GUIDE
THE DRUG LITERATURE EVALUATION PROCESS (*Cont.*)

---

18. Were appropriate statistical tests chosen to assess the data? Were the levels of α and β error chosen before the data were gathered? Were multiple statistical tests applied until a significant result was achieved?
19. Was patient compliance monitored?
20. If multiple observers were collecting data, did the authors describe how variations in measurements were avoided?
21. Did the authors justify the instrumentation used in the study?
22. Were measurements or assessments of effects made at the appropriate times and frequency?
23. Are the data presented in an appropriate, understandable format?
24. Are standard deviations or confidence intervals shown along with mean values?
25. Are there any problems with type I (α) or type II (β) errors?
26. Are there any potential problems with internal validity or external validity? Internal validity types include history, maturation, instrumentation, selection, morbidity, and mortality
27. Are adverse reactions reported in sufficient detail?
28. Are the conclusions supported by the data? Is some factor other than the study treatment responsible for the outcomes?
29. Are the results both statistically and clinically significant?
30. Do the authors discuss study limitations in their conclusions?
31. Were appropriate references used? Are references timely and reputable? Have any of the studies been disproven or updated? Do references cited represent a complete background?
32. Would this article change clinical practice or a recommendation that you would give to a patient or healthcare professional?

The following examples are provided as a guide to professional writing. These examples were done by students and represent a good job at the exercise for the information available at the time of the project.

Drug Information Professional Writing Examples

DRUG INFORMATION QUESTION RESPONSE: RENEE A. POTHAST, PHARM.D., COMPLETED AS PART OF A PHARM.D. ROTATION WHILE A PHARMACY STUDENT AT OHIO NORTHERN UNIVERSITY

Question

Therapy combining an angiotensin-converting enzyme inhibitor with an angiotensin II receptor blocker: is it rational?

TABLE 8.8. HELPFUL HINTS
FOR DRUG LITERATURE EVALUATION

Some helpful hints can also provide some insight to the reader when trying to answer the 32 questions of Table 8.7.

1. A journal is considered reputable if it is peer reviewed.
2. Appropriate qualifications often include some sort of research background or an author on the team who has statistics background. Do the researchers have expertise in the area of study?
3. Often at the end of the article there is information on funding. NIH funding etc. is often considered unbiased. Questions arise if the company marketing the product funds the sponsorship. (This does not necessarily mean it is bad, just a concern.)
4. Sufficient background information would include a good review (timely) of the drug, disease state, or research topic. Was the background concise but comprehensive. Did they indicate why the authors thought this was important or why they needed to know?
5. Purpose is the reason for doing a study, the objectives are how they are going to accomplish the purpose. Very few studies really outline the objectives if they mention the purpose. Some journals now require the authors to state the objective in the abstract.
6. Investigational Review Board (IRB), also known as Institutional Review Board, Human Subjects Committee, etc. They should indicate this over and beyond talking about informed consent.
7. The null hypothesis should be clearly stated as the hypothesis of no difference, with the alternative being the hypothesis of difference. Many times the research question is stated but not in the form of the hypothesis. Ask what you think the null hypothesis would be or should be based on the information given in the article. This formulation of the null hypothesis by the reader will be helpful later to establish type I and type II error as well as trying to obtain information related to external validity.
8. Is the sample large enough, is a good question. The central limit theorem suggests a sample size larger than 30 is necessary to assume normality (normal distribution) and therefore be able to do parametric statistical testing. However, the central limit theorem is not applied here to this question. This question is directed at knowing if the sample is largeenough to statistically prove differences between groups or statistically identify trends in the data. It also is directed at knowing if the sample size is large enough to truly represent the overall population being studied. Good research will identify how they arrived at their sample size. This usually involves a calculation that takes into consideration things like type I and type II error (often you will see power used here instead), standard deviation, and the clinical difference to be detected.
9. Inclusion criteria define who is included in the study, and the exclusion criteria define who is eliminated or not included in the study. Exclusion criteria need to make sense and not be so restrictive that they exclude important

(*continued*)

TABLE 8.8. HELPFUL HINTS
FOR DRUG LITERATURE EVALUATION (*Cont.*)

or good data. Inclusion criteria need to be specific enough that all of the researchers understand who really belongs. Definitions of inclusion criteria are often helpful. For example, the patients must have a fasting blood glucose less than 120 mg/dL.

10. Did they randomize the study? Really randomize, not just say they did. How did they do it? Random number tables or names pulled from a hat are legitimate ways to do this. Did they provide a table or chart comparing the demographic information between groups? Does it look as though the groups are relatively equal, or are they characteristically (demographically) similar? There are other ways to randomize besides simple random samples. These can be legitimate ways to allocate subjects. Research design textbooks will elaborate on these other methods.

11. What is the study design? Several references including the Malone textbook[2] go into more depth about study designs. Common study designs include the clinical trial (experimental design comparing therapies between groups), cohort studies (long-term studies observing disease patterns related to risk factor exposures), case-control studies (comparison of cases who have a condition with controls without the condition to determine if a risk factor could have caused the differences), intention-to-treat (a type of clinical trial that often controls for subjects dropping out of studies prematurely), and meta-analysis (statistical combination of previous studies' data and determining if the conclusions would be different). Does the type of design they chose make sense? Would a different study design have been better to answer the proposed hypothesis?

12. Did they use controls? Did they compare the controls to the treatment subjects (cases)? Often they will provide a demographics table that allows a comparison of control group to treatment group. Do they look similar? Did they run statistical tests that compare the similarity of the two groups. If they did, p-values should be reported; p-values less than 0.05 would indicate that the groups are different, whereas a p-value greater than 0.05 would show the groups to be similar on that characteristic. The next question would be, did they select the groups appropriately? Where did the controls come from? Is that similar to how they selected the treatment group? Some studies will take a treatment group from the community and then select controls from a hospital group. There could be differences between these two groups just based on their selection and not because of treatments provided. Some studies will actually have more than one control matched to each case. This is actually considered to be a good research technique.

13. Was it single-blinded or double-blinded? Single-blind means either the study subject or the investigator is not aware of the treatment, but not both. Usually in a single-blinded study just the subjects or patients are blinded to the therapy they are receiving. In double-blinded studies both the subjects and the researchers or care providers in the study are blinded to the therapy being given. Usually double-blinded is best!

(*continued*)

**TABLE 8.8. HELPFUL HINTS
FOR DRUG LITERATURE EVALUATION (*Cont.*)**

---

14. Doses and regimens? Why or why not? What do general tertiary references such as *Facts and Comparisons* say? Also think about pharmacodynamics and pharmacokinetics when considering this question. The authors may have selected appropriate doses and regimens, but did they consider the half-life of the drug and the length of time it takes to get to steady state? Did the authors consider that a drug pharmacodynamically may take some patients 4 to 6 weeks or longer to see clinical benefit?

15. If they are talking about adequate treatment with a drug for CHF, and they look at only a 2- to 6-week study, is that really long enough? If they are evaluating only short-term results, that would be fine. If they are looking at long-term outcomes, it needs to be longer, for example, 6 months to a year.

16. Crossover studies mean the same subject gets both treatments, one after the other. Note that the washout period should be at least 5 half-lives of the drug to achieve a plasma level of zero, or the washout needs to be long enough that any pharmacodynamic effects of drug therapy are gone. The drug maybe gone from the plasma but may still have tissue concentrations or have affected receptors for a longer period of time. It is also important in a crossover study that each drug or treatment is started at the beginning of the study and then patients are crossed over to the other drug or treatment. For example, if the study involves 40 patients and they are to get both Drug A and Drug B in the study, this would mean that 20 patients would start the study on Drug A and then be crossed over to Drug B while 20 would start on Drug B and then be crossed over to Drug A. If both drugs are started from the beginning, this helps reduce the chance of error that could have happened because of some other effect that was changing the outcome. For example, CHF usually gets worse with time. If you started all of your CHF patients on an ACE inhibitor and then switched them over to a β-blocker, and then the disease got worse, is that because of the β-blocker, or is that the natural progression of the disease? But if you started half of the group on ACE-I and half on β-blockers and then switched each group to the other treatment, and the CHF got worse on the β-blocker treatment regardless of the timing, one could successfully argue that the β-blocker caused this rather than the disease state itself?

17. Operational definition means definitions of the variables, measurements, etc. When they say subjects have glaucoma, what do they mean by that? When they measure a gentamicin level, how are they doing this, and on what machine? How do they define a gentamicin peak level: is that 1 hour after the infusion or a half-hour? How do they define clinical cure? How do they define an exacerbation of a disease state? Think of these questions as though you were part of the research team receiving this document. Could you adequately perform this study based on the definitions they provide?

(continued)

TABLE 8.8. HELPFUL HINTS
FOR DRUG LITERATURE EVALUATION (*Cont.*)

18. Some tests you may have to look up in a statistical book. Did they meet the assumptions for a parametric test? How many groups were they comparing on the outcome variable (two, three, etc)? Did they set α (type I) and β error (type II) before starting the study? Did they do multiple tests until they found the answer they wanted? Was it a fishing trip—were they just looking for an answer of any type?

19. Did they, and how did they, monitor compliance? Was it a good method?

20. This is important. If there were multiple researchers or multiple sites, how did they coordinate the efforts so that they all did the same thing?

21. Instrumentation is the instrument/gauge they used to measure the variables. This could be an actual instrument such as a blood pressure kit or glucose monitor. This could be an instrument such as a survey or questionnaire. If the research used the Visual Analog Scale for pain, which is a scale from 0 to 10 with 10 being the worst pain, this is an instrument.

22. Did they assess measurements when it was appropriate? If not, what would you recommend or the literature recommend?

23. Format is important. Look at the tables and graphs. Are they easy to read? Do they make sense? Do you know what they measured? Do you know the measurement scale? What are they describing? How many of these are hard to read or make no sense? When you get done looking at it, are you not sure if they were giving you the mean with the standard deviation or standard error of the mean?

24. The study should always give standard deviation and not standard error of the mean, in most cases. Standard error of the mean is only appropriate if more than one sample is being studeed. Confidence intervals are a good alternative when they do not give standard deviations or standard deviations are not appropriate.

25. This is tricky. Did they state a null hypothesis (remember that the null hypothesis is the hypothesis of no difference)? If not, can you infer the null hypothesis? Did they accept or reject the null hypothesis at the end of the study? If they accepted the null hypothesis, it is more likely that they made a type II error. If they rejected the null hypothesis, it is more likely that they made a type I error. Realize that a study is vulnerable to both types of errors.

26. External validity deals with the overall generalizability of the study, whereas internal validity deals with the internal methods used to do the study.

26a. External validity has to do with the generalizability of the study. Can you take the results from the study and generalize them to the rest of the population? The key here is to look at whom they studied (really studied) and what type of conclusions they stated based on the data. For example, if I look at mitral value prolapse (mild and moderate forms) in young men (age 18–40), and I am trying to determine if β-blockers help them with improving exercise tolerance, and my conclusion of the study states that

(*continued*)

**TABLE 8.8. HELPFUL HINTS
FOR DRUG LITERATURE EVALUATION (*Cont.*)**

"β-blockers are superior agents in helping improve exercise in mitral value prolapse," there is an external validity problem. From the study, I know that β-blockers are agents that improve exercise tolerance in mild to moderate mitral value prolapse in young men, but I do not know anything about women or serious prolapse problems. You can only make conclusions about what you have studied, and you can only apply your results to your target population. Look for this because it happens often in the medical literature.

26b. Internal validity has to do with the internal structure of the study. This focus is on the materials and methods section of the article. If the internal structure is flawed, then one would question how valid the study would be. For example, some types of internal validity include:

Instrumentation (mentioned above). Is the visual analog scale the best means to measure subjective pain? Is intraocular pressure the best means to measure glaucoma? Is urine output the best means to measure diuretic success in CHF?

History (you may know this as the Hawthorne effect). Did something happen during the study that may have altered the results rather than the intervention or treatment. For example, suppose I established a calcium supplement intervention program for college-age women to improve calcium intake. I designed a good educational program, and I am making the college tour and promoting good calcium intake while in college to prevent later osteoporosis. I then go back and see if the women have changed their behavior and added more calcium to their diets. I have discovered that yes, indeed, they have significantly increased their calcium, and I conclude What a great educational program I have developed! What I did not take into consideration was the Diary Board's latest ad campaign with "Got milk?" In other words, my great program had nothing to do with it, but rather the Milk Board did.

Maturation. This has to do with the subject changing over time. For example, if I gave everyone a copy of the final exam questions as a pretest and then gave the same posttest, I could claim that my superior teaching techniques resulted in an excellent display of knowledge on the final. What is really being displayed is the individual's ability to learn from the pretest. The individual matured. This can happen with disease states as well. For example, a CHF study looking at outcomes must realize that most CHF patients will mature in the disease progression over a 2- to 5-year period of time. Other disease states may improve over time. Some disease states have exacerbations and remissions. How do you know if a drug is preventing exacerbations of multiple sclerosis or if the disease is just in remission as part of its natural course? Did the researchers control for this?

Selection goes back to question 8. How did they select the sample? Was it representative? Did they randomize? Were the controls appropriate?

(*continued*)

TABLE 8.8. HELPFUL HINTS
FOR DRUG LITERATURE EVALUATION (*Cont.*)

Experimentation. Did they pick the right study design? Did they pick a cohort study to look at a rare disease when a case-control would have
been better? Did they have appropriate treatment groups? Did they have
a washout period? Did they cross over treatment groups appropriately?
Attrition refers to dropout rates, morbidity, or even mortality. Did they tell
you who dropped out and why? For example, a study will start off with
150 people, but the data are reported on only 132. Where did the rest
go, and why?

27. Did they tell you about adverse drug reactions (ADRs)? Was it a good explanation, or did it leave something to be desired? Did they tell you the
number of patients who left the study (dropped out) because of ADRs?
28 & 30. This is crucial! They can only conclude about what they studied, and
a good conclusion will discuss limitations to their study. This is considered good research and not admitting disaster.
29. Statistical significance is usually defined as the p-value being less than or
equal to the α (type I) error rate that was set by the researchers a priori. For
example, if the researchers set α at 0.05 and the p-value is reported as
0.013, then the results are statistically significant. Clinical significance,
however, is not dependent on statistical significance. This is related to one's
professional judgment. Do the data suggest a clinical trend but not necessarily have statistical significance?
31. Were the references timely? Did they have a comprehensive list?
32. This one is up to you to defend! How does this change what you recommend? How good was the study in terms of answering questions 1 through
31? Where the results clinically significant?

TABLE 8.9. HELPFUL WRITING HINTS

- Do not plagiarize any part of the paper (put information into your own words)
- Use proper grammar and spelling (read the paper, do not rely on spell check)
- Keep things concise and to the point (do not stray off on tangents)
- Avoid first person (such words as I and we)
- Avoid abbreviations and acronyms (unless described early in the paper)
- Avoid contractions (can't, couldn't, it's)
- Cite any factual information with appropriate referencing
- Reference throughout the paper starting with the first paper cited (do not put
  the references in alphabetical order or chronological order)
- Avoid the internet unless it is specifically appropriate to the document

Introduction

Hypertension and congestive heart failure (CHF) are two cardiovascular conditions common in the American population. In fact, approximately 50 million Americans have hypertension. The incidence increases with age, as one out of every four adults has this condition.[1] Treatment of hypertension is crucial to prevent multiple complications, including coronary heart disease. Control of blood pressure may also decrease the progression of CHF. Medical management of both hypertension and CHF has changed throughout the years. Currently, the effects of the reticular activating system (RAS) have been targeted in designing drug therapy for these conditions.

The RAS is activated in an individual by a variety of states, including sodium restriction and a decline in cardiac output. After the conversion of angiotensinogen to angiotensin I by renin, the angiotensin-converting enzyme (ACE) catalyzes the change of angiotensin I to angiotensin II. It is this peptide hormone, angiotensin II, that mediates the effects of the RAS. Angiotensin receptors can be found in many organs, including the kidneys, heart, blood vessels, brain, and adrenal tissues.[2] Two types of angiotensin II receptor subtypes have been identified. It is believed that activation of the angiotensin II receptor subtype AT_1 instigates the effects commonly associated with the RAS. These are an increase in systolic and diastolic blood pressure via systemic vasoconstriction, the release of adrenal aldosterone, and renal sodium reabsorption. Binding to this receptor also mediates cardiac remodeling through hypertrophy and proliferation. On the other hand, the angiontensin II receptor subtype AT_2 is now believed to exert opposing effects (vasodilation and antiproliferation), but this must still be fully investigated.[3]

The Role of Angiotensin-Converting Enzyme Inhibitors

ACE inhibitors have been found to be very effective when used for hypertension, CHF, and in the post–myocardial infarction (MI) setting. In fact, numerous studies have demonstrated their benefit in these situations, and ACE inhibitors are considered the foundation of combination therapy in CHF patients on the basis of many clinical trials. Enalapril was shown to reduce mortality when used in heart failure patients in the Cooperative North Scandinavian Enalapril Survival Study (CONSENSUS),[4] the Studies of Left Ventricular Dysfunction (SOLVD),[5] and the Veterans Administration Cooperative Vasodilator Heart Failure Trial II (VHeFT II).[6]

The reduction of mortality with ACE inhibitors in post-MI patients has also been demonstrated through clinical trials, including the Survival and Ventricular Enlargement Trial (SAVE)[7] and the Fourth International Study of Infarct Survival (ISIS-4),[8] both of which used captopril. In addition, zofenopril was deemed effective in the Survival of Myocardial Infarction Long-Term Evaluation (SMILE),[9] as was trandolapril in the Trandolapril Cardiac Evaluation (TRACE) study.[10]

The action of ACE inhibitors revolves around the RAS, for they ameliorate some of the effects of angiotensin II by preventing its formation by this pathway. In addition to their effect on the RAS, ACE inhibitors also inhibit the breakdown of bradykinin, enkephalin, and substance P. This most likely contributes to the side effects of cough and angioedema associated with these agents. More recently, the effects on bradykinin are also speculated to contribute to benefits in regard to exercise tolerance encountered by CHF patients on ACE inhibitor therapy.[11] However, this still remains to be fully proven.

Although ACE inhibitors block angiotensin II production by the RAS, long-term suppression of angiotensin II levels are not achieved.[12] One mechanism that is potentially responsible is an increase in angiotensin I levels through the loss of feedback inhibition of renin, overriding the inhibition of ACE.[13] Other mechanisms may be related to alternative pathways of angiotensin II production and activity, including a chymase pathway.[14] Even if the mechanism is not yet clear, it is known that further preventing the detrimental effects of angiotensin II in patients with cardiovascular disease is the goal.

The Role of Angiotensin II Receptor (AT$_1$) Blockers

The newest class of antihypertensive agents, the angiotensin II receptor blockers (ARBs), also exert their beneficial effects by influence on the RAS and are often compared to ACE inhibitors. Clinical data are being gathered to demonstrate the efficacy of ARBs in patients with heart failure and after an MI. The Evaluation of Losartan in the Elderly Study (ELITE) compared the ARB losartan to the ACE inhibitor captopril in CHF patients. Results actually showed a lower mortality rate in patients taking the ARB compared to the ACE inhibitor.[15] However, these findings were not repeated in ELITE II, which did not find the mortality rates to be significantly different between the two agents.[16] Nevertheless, losartan was found to be better tolerated in both studies.[15,16] Additionally, the Study of Patients Intolerant of Converting Enzyme Inhibitors (SPICE) trial found the ARB candesartan cilexetil to reduce mortality in CHF patients who were unable to tolerate an ACE inhibitor.[17]

ARBs are being assessed for use in post-MI patients in the Optimal Therapy in Myocardial Infarction with the Angiotensin II Antagonist Losartan (OPTIMAAL) trial. This randomized trial, currently in progress, is comparing losartan therapy to captopril in high-risk patients $\geq$ 50 years old who have had an acute MI.[18]

ARBs, unlike the ACE inhibitors, exert their effect via binding selectively to the angiotensin II type 1 receptor, AT$_1$. As a result, the hypertensive effects and cardiac remodeling are blocked while angiotensin II is still able to bind to the type 2 receptor, AT$_2$. If binding to the AT$_2$ receptor results in the vasodilation and antiproliferation as currently believed, then there is a theoretical advantage of ARBs over ACE inhibitors. Also, angiotensin II's damaging effects via all pathways are more thoroughly blocked by receptor blocking than by preventing RAS angiotensin II formation as the ACE inhibitors do. Furthermore, the side effect of cough is absent in the ARBs because there is no inhibition of the breakdown of bradykinin.[3,19]

Rationale of Using an ACE Inhibitor and an ARB in Combination

Because of their different means of preventing angiotensin II from binding to its receptor (either by preventing the formation of angiotensin or direct receptor inhibition), ACE inhibitors and ARBs are being evaluated for combined use. In theory, the benefit stems from complete blockage of the angiotensin II by all pathways, resulting in an additive effect of the two agents and the potential advantage of inhibiting the breakdown of bradykinin.[3] When an ACE inhibitor, an ARB, their combination, or placebo was administered to normotensive male volunteers who were mildly sodium depleted, the ACE inhibitor and ARB combination demonstrated a greater reduction in blood pressure, a major additive effect on renin rise signifying a compensatory mechanism, and no effect on plasma aldosterone levels, most likely because aldosterone is regulated through other pathways than solely the RAS.[20]

Clinical Studies Validating the Combined Use for Heart Failure

The effects on afterload were studied by Hamroff et al.[21] in 43 patients with severe CHF who were treated with losartan after being maximally treated with an ACE inhibitor. Following evaluation for 1 month in an outpatient facility, patients were started on losartan 25 mg for the first week, followed by an increase to 50 mg thereafter. All other medications and doses remained constant. Blood pressure, heart rate, serum potassium, sodium, blood urea nitrogen, and creatinine were monitored weekly during the 2 weeks of the study. Repeated-measures analysis and a Bonferroni-adjusted significance level were used to evaluate the data. Results showed a decline in blood pressure as distinguished by a decline in systolic blood pressure from 122 ± 18 mm Hg at baseline to 107 ± 17 mm Hg after the 50-mg dose ($p < 0.0001$). There were no significant changes in electrolytes or renal function during treatment duration. Conclusions included that, as indicated by the decline in blood pressure, therapy with an ARB in these patients further reduces afterload. Limitations consist of a small sample size, short treatment duration, lack of a control group, and an insufficient definition of terms.[21]

    A double-blind, crossover, placebo-controlled study was conducted by Guazzi et al.[11] in 26 stable CHF patients [New York Heart Association (NYHA) class II to III] with a mean age of 58 years. Following randomization, patients received either placebo + placebo, placebo + enalapril (20 mg/day), placebo + losartan (50 mg/day), or enalapril (20 mg/day) + losartan (50 mg/day), or the same drugs in the reverse order, with all treatment periods lasting 8 weeks. Monitoring was completed by quality-of-life questionnaires, neurohormone evaluations, pulmonary function tests, cardiopulmonary exercise testing, chest x-rays, and left ventricular ejection fraction evaluations. Two patients were excluded from the final analysis because of adverse events (hypotension with the enalapril and losartan combination and cough with enalapril). Results included an increase in exercise oxygen uptake and physical performance when the drugs are used in combination, although improved exercise performance was noted with enalapril only. This is thought to be through action on bradykinin. Also, the inhibitory effect of neurohormones was additive, and combination therapy was safe and well tolerated. Quality of life did not significantly change, although the authors believe this to most likely be because the patients were stabilized in digoxin and diuretic therapy prior to study inclusion. Again, a small sample size is a limitation, as were multiple patient variables with the potential to influence the results and a complicated drug regimen.[11]

The Randomized Evaluation of Strategies for Left Ventricular Dysfunction (RESOLVD) pilot study, conducted by the RESOLVD investigators, compared candesartan, enalapril, and their combination over 43 weeks in this multicenter, double-blind, randomized, parallel, placebo-controlled trial. All patients were in the NYHA functional class II, III, or IV for their CHF. The trial included a run-in of three 1-week phases of enalapril 2.5 mg twice daily + placebo, enalapril 2.5 mg twice daily + candesartan 2 mg daily, and enalapril 2.5 mg twice daily + placebo. Randomization followed, and patients received candesartan alone (4.8 or 16 mg daily), candesartan (4 or 8 mg daily) + enalapril (10 mg twice daily), or enalapril (10 mg twice daily). Endpoints were the change in ejection fraction, the 6-minute walk distance, ventricular volumes, and neurohormone levels. Other measurements made included end-systolic volume (ESV), end-diastolic volume (EDV), and quality of life via the Minnesota Living With Heart Failure questionnaire. Statistical analyses occurred by ANOVA, post-hoc Tukey test, and chi-squared test. There were 899 patients in the run-in phase, and 768 were randomized. Patient characteristics were similar between the groups, although fewer patients in the groups containing candesartan were concomitantly receiving β-blockers. Although not statistically significant, there was an increase in ejection fraction in the combined group, compared to enalapril or candesartan alone. Both ESV and EDV increased less with combination therapy. Candesartan alone demonstrated the smallest increase in renin levels but the greatest increase in angiotensin II levels. Aldosterone significantly decreased at 17 weeks with combination therapy ($p < 0.01$), but not at 43 weeks. Blood pressure declined the greatest with the combination therapy throughout the study ($p < 0.05$), as did brain natriuretic peptide ($p < 0.01$). Compared to enalapril, potassium decreased with candesartan ($p < 0.05$) and increased with combination therapy ($p < 0.05$). No significant changes in creatinine, 6-minute walk distance, quality of life, mortality, or hospitalizations was confirmed. The authors concluded that despite limitations of small number unreliability and not being able to predict net clinical effects because of surrogate outcomes, this pilot study did demonstrate the effectiveness and safety of enalapril and candesartan combination therapy to prevent left ventricular remodeling when compared to either agent given alone.[22]

Baruch et al.[12] carried out a randomized, multicenter, double-blind trial in 83 CHF patients in NYHA functional class II, III, or IV. All patients had to have previous ACE inhibitor therapy and, at baseline, were stratified into low- or high-dose ACE inhibitor therapy based on this previous ACE inhibitor dose. Following a 2-week single-blind placebo phase in which the patient's heart failure and compliance were assessed, patients were randomized to receive 4 weeks of therapy with valsartan 80 mg twice daily, valsartan 160 mg twice daily, or placebo. Hemodynamic monitoring and hormone measurements (plasma norepinephrine, aldosterone, atrial natriuretic peptide, and angiotensin II) were completed on day 0 and day 30. On these days, patients received either 10 mg or 20 mg of lisinopril rather than their usual ACE inhibitor to guarantee sustained ACE inhibition. Statistical analysis included Fisher's exact or Cochran-Mantel-Haenszel test to compare baseline characteristics, ANOVA, ANCOVA, and Student's t test. An overall two-sided significance level was upheld at 0.05 by Bonferroni adjustment. Statistical significance was defined for between-treatment comparisons of valsartan versus placebo at $p < 0.025$ and within-treatment analyses of change from baseline at $p < 0.05$. All patients were male because of the number of Veterans Affairs hospitals included. Immediate effects (day 0) showed valsartan to demonstrate statistical significance over placebo in the reduction in pulmonary capillary wedge pressure (PCWP; $p < 0.025$), right arterial pressure ($p < 0.025$), and systolic blood pressure. No significant change in neurohormone levels was appreciated. When the long-term effect (day 28) was evaluated, the fall in pulmonary artery diastolic pressure ($p = 0.013$) and the systolic blood pressure ($p = 0.013$) were significant in the high-dose valsartan group when compared to placebo. Both valsartan doses caused significant declines in the plasma aldosterone level. The medication was well tolerated, with 89% of patients able to complete the trial. Documented side effects did include hypotension, gastrointestinal disturbances, and dizziness. Also, increases in blood urea nitrogen, serum creatinine, and potassium were noted. The authors made the conclusion that angiotensin II levels do persist despite long-term ACE inhibitor therapy.[12]

A double-blind, randomized, large-scale trial, including 5010 patients and carried out in 300 centers in 16 countries, was recently completed by Cohn et al.[23] This trial, the Valsartan Heart Failure Trial (Val-HeFT), investigated the effect valsartan 160 mg twice daily would have on CHF patients (NYHA functional class II, III, or IV) who were already taking the usual therapies for CHF, including ACE inhibitors, β-blockers, diuretics, and digoxin.

Compared to placebo, the valsartan group saw a reduction in all-cause mortality and morbidity by 13.3% ($p = 0.009$) and in hospitalization for CHF by 27.5% ($p < 0.001$). Additionally, therapy with valsartan improved quality of life ($p = 0.005$), NYHA functional class ($p = 0.001$), ejection fraction ($p = 0.001$), and signs and symptoms of heart failure ($p = 0.001$).[23,24]

Swedberg et al.[25] is currently assessing the use of candesartan cilexetil in symptomatic CHF patients in the Candesartan in Heart Failure–Assessment in Mortality and Morbidity (CHARM) trial. This multicenter trial encompasses three parallel, placebo-controlled trials in 6500 patients treated with and without an ACE inhibitor. There is a minimum follow-up period of 2 years, with endpoints including all-cause mortality, effect on MI, hospitalization, and resource utilization.[25]

Clinical Studies Validating the Combined Use for Post-MI

The feasibility, tolerability, and safety of using captopril and losartan was the aim in a randomized, single-blind pilot study by Pasquale et al.[26] Patients admitted for an anterior acute MI, Killip class I to II, who were successfully reperfused within 4 hours after the onset of symptoms and received the target captopril dose of 75 mg/day 3 days postadmission were included. Randomization occurred, and patients received either placebo or losartan titrated up to 25 mg/day. Captopril 75 mg/day was administered to both groups. Blood pressure, heart rate, and electrocardiogram (ECG) were monitored continuously. Neurohormonal levels were monitored at baseline and on days 3 and 10. A hemodynamic study was also completed on all patients 7 to 10 days after admission. Data were analyzed by two-tailed t test, ANOVA, and chi-squared test. The Bonferroni correction was utilized, and statistical significance was set at $p < 0.05$. A total of 42 patents were included in the results. Only the systolic blood pressure was found to be significantly changed with the ARB and ACE inhibitor combination ($p < 0.001$). Even though the ejection fraction was higher in this group than when captopril was given with placebo, the difference was not significant. No side effects were noted. Because of the small sample size, no significant benefits on remodeling, morbidity, or mortality could be found. Also, the single-blind randomization is not ideal, and results cannot be generalized to all post-MI patients because only those who are low risk, thrombolysed, and reperfused were included. Consistent with the objective of the study, the feasibility and safety of this combination encourages further trials in this area.[26]

Pasquale et al. extended the study to include women and a losartan 50 mg/day–only arm and prolonged it for 90 days, when a second ECG was performed. All other aspects remained identical to the first study except for the objective to verify the efficacy of the combined therapy in the early post-MI setting. The losartan-only group acted as a control to gauge the effects of losartan on angiotensin II levels. Ninety-nine patients were randomized, in addition to 23 patients assigned to the losartan-only group.

Data were available for neurohormone and blood pressure assessment from 93 patients. Angiotensin II levels were higher in the losartan-only group on day 10 (this was significantly different from the captopril-only group; $p = 0.006$). Both systolic and diastolic blood pressure was significantly reduced in the captopril + losartan group when compared to the captopril-only group. Patients in the combined group also had a lower ejection fraction than the other two groups, but this did not reach statistical significance. ECG examination at 90 days was completed in 48 patients on captopril only, 47 patients on combined therapy, and 23 patients on losartan only. ESV and ejection fractions were not significantly different between the treatment groups. Nevertheless, there was a statistically significant difference in the ESV within the combination group itself 90 days after treatment ($p = 0.016$) . There were six ischemic events observed in the follow-up (one episode of unstable angina in each group, one episode of reinfarction in the captopril-only and combination groups, and one episode of heart failure in the losartan-only group). It may be deduced from this study that combination therapy is safe and beneficial. However, the same limitations as in the first study apply.[27]

Based on results from the previous two studies, Pasquale et al.[28] designed a similar study to further explore the rationale for ACE inhibitor and ARB combined therapy in other post-MI patients. A randomized, double-blind design was used in patients ≥65 years old who were either not receiving thrombolytic treatment or who had received thrombolytic therapy but had unsuccessful reperfusion. Additionally, a coronary angiography 7 to 10 days postadmission had to demonstrate no patency of the infarct-related artery, and captopril 75 mg/day had to be received by day 3 of admission. Among patients excluded were those with heart failure. On day 3, patients were randomized to receive either captopril 75 mg/day + candesartan 4 mg/day initially but later increased to 8 mg/day based on blood pressure, or captopril 75 mg/day + placebo. Monitoring included blood pressure, heart rate, serum creatinine, serum potassium, Holter monitoring, hemodynamic investigations, and an ECG on days 3 and 10. A two-tailed t test, ANOVA, Bonferroni correction, and chi-squared test were all used to analyze the data; $p < 0.05$ was considered significant. Results are based on 71 patients who met the entry criteria and included a statistically significant lower systolic and diastolic blood pressure in the combined group ($p < 0.001$). The combination group showed a higher, but not significantly so, ejection fraction. Follow-up lasted 1 year with a minimum period of observation of 3 months. ESV values after 90 days were significantly lower in the combination group ($p = 0.03$). During the follow-up, there were two episodes of reinfarction and two episodes of unstable angina in the combination group, compared to one episode of reinfarction and four episodes of unstable angina in the captopril-only group. After 10 days of treatment, an increase in serum potassium >5.5 mmol/L and serum creatinine >2.0 mg/L was experienced by four patients in the combination group and by two patients in the captopril-only group. After a reduction of doses, levels declined and patients continued in the relevant treatment groups. No other significant changes were found. It was concluded that the captopril and candesartan combination is beneficial in elderly, post-MI patients as shown by a greater effect on ESV. Limitations are a small sample size causing ungeneralizability and a failure to show possible benefits on morbidity and mortality and a lack of hemodynamic study completion because of age >75 in 28 patients.[28]

Currently, the Valsartan in Acute Myocardial Infarction (VALIANT) trial is under way to assess the use of valsartan alone or in combination with captopril and the effect on mortality in post-MI patients. Random assignments are made in this trial for patients with CHF symptoms or depressed left ventricular ejection fraction. This is the largest clinical trial using an ACE inhibitor and ARB combination in post-MI patients, is powered at a 90% level to detect a 15% change in mortality, and is projected to run until 2700 deaths have occurred.[29]

Conclusion

The RAS plays a considerable role in the detrimental effects of CHF and MI and can be improved by the use of ACE inhibitors and ARBs. Both of these medications have proven to be safe and effective for patients with CHF and in the post-MI setting. It is only recently that their use together has been practiced medically and substantiated by clinical trials. Additional trials are currently being implemented in these settings to further validate this approach.

References

1. American Heart Association (http://www.americanheart.org/hbp/phys stats. html) 19 March 2001.
2. Hirsch AT, Pinto YM, Schunkert H, Dzau VJ. Potential role of the tissue renin–angiotensin system in the pathophysiology of congestive heart failure. Am J Cardiol 1990;66:22D–32D.
3. Carson PE. Rationale for the use of combination angiotensin-converting enzyme inhibitor/angiotensin II receptor blocker therapy in heart failure. Am Heart J 2000;140(3):361–366.
4. Kjekshus J, Frick H, Swedberg K, Wilhelmsen L. Effects of enalapril on mortality in severe congestive heart failure: results of the Cooperative North Scandinavian Enalapril Survival Study (CONSENSUS). N Engl J Med 1987;316: 1429–1435.
5. Yusuf S, Pitt B, Davis CE, et al. Effect of enalapril on survival in patients with reduced left ventricular ejection fractions and congestive heart failure. N Engl J Med 1991;325:293–302.
6. Cohn JN, Johnson G, Ziesche S, et al. A comparison of enalapril with hydralazine–isosorbide dinitrate in the treatment of chronic congestive heart failure. N Engl J Med 1991;325:303–310.
7. Pfeffer MA, Braunwald E, Moye LA, et al. Effect of captopril on mortality and

   morbidity in patients with left ventricular dysfunction after myocardial infarction. N Engl J Med 1992;327:669–677.

8. ISIS-4 (Fourth International Study of Infarct Survival) Collaborative Group.
   ISIS-4: A randomized factorial trial assessing early oral captopril, oral monon-
   itrate, and intravenous magnesium sulphate in 58,050 patients with suspected acute myocardial infarction. Lancet 1995;345:669–682.

9. Ambrosioni E, Borghi C, Magnani B, for the Survival of Myocardial Infarction Long-
   Term Evaluation (SMILE) study investigators. The effect of the angiotensin-
   converting-enzyme inhibitor zofenopril on mortality and morbidity after anterior
   myocardial infarction. N Engl J Med 1995;332:80–85.

10. Kober L, Torp-Pedersen C, Carlsen JE, et al, for the Trandolapril Cardiac Evaluation (TRACE) study group. A clinical trial of the angiotensin-converting-
   enzyme inhibitor trandolapril in patients with left ventricular dysfunction after
   myocardial infarction. N Engl J Med 1995;333:1670–1676.

11. Guazzi M, Palermo P, Pontone G, et al. Synergistic efficacy of enalapril and losartan on exercise performance and oxygen consumption at peak exercise in congestive heart failure. Am J Cardiol 1999;84:1038–1043.

12. Baruch L, Anand I, Cohen IS, et al, for the Vasodilator Heart Failure Trial (V-
   HeFT) study group. Augmented short- and long-term hemodynamic and hor-
   monal effects of an angiotensin receptor blocker added to angiotensin converting enzyme inhibitor therapy in patients with heart failure. Circulation 1999;
   99:2658–2664.

13. Schunkert H, Ingelfinger JR, Hirsch AT, et al. Feedback regulation of angiotensin
   converting enzyme activity and mRNA levels by angiotensin II. Circ Res 1993;
   72:312–318.

14. Balcells E, Meng QC, Johnson WH, et al. Angiotensin II formation from ACE and
   chymase in human and animal hearts: methods and species considerations. Am
   J Physiol 1997;273:H1769-H1774.

15. Pitt B, Segal R, Martinez FA, G, et al. Randomized trial of losartan versus captopril in patients over 65 with heart failure (Evaluation of Losartan in the Elderly Study, ELITE). Lancet 1997;349:747–752.

16. Pitt B, Poole-Wilson PA, Segal R, et al. Effect of losartan compared with captopril on mortality in patients with symptomatic heart failure: randomized
   trial—the Losartan Heart Failure Survival Study (ELITE II). Lancet 2000;355:
   1582–1587.

17. Granger CB, Ertl G, Kuch J, et al, for the Study of Patients Intolerant of Converting Enzyme Inhibitors (SPICE) Investigators. Randomized trial of candesartan cilexetil in the treatment of patients with congestive heart failure and a
   history of intolerance to angiotensin-converting enzyme inhibitors. Am Heart J
   2000;139:609–617.

18. Dickstein K, Kjekshus J, for the OPTIMAAL study group. Comparison of the effects of losartan and captopril on mortality in patients after acute myocardial infarction: the OPTIMAAL trial design. Am J Cardiol 1999;83:477–481.

19. Gradman AH. Long-term benefits of angiotensin II blockade: is the consensus
   changing? Am J Cardiol 1999;84:16S–21S.

20. Azizi M, Chatellier G, Guyene TT, et al. Additive effects of combined angiotensin-
   converting enzyme inhibition and angiotensin II antagonism on blood pressure
   and renin release in sodium-depleted normotensives. Circulation 1995;92:825–
   834.

21. Hamroff G, Blaufarb I, Mancini D, et al. Angiotensin II-receptor blockade further reduces afterload safely in patients maximally treated with angiotensin-converting enzyme inhibitors for heart failure. J Cardiovasc Pharmacol 1997; 30(4):533–536.

22. McKelvie RS, Yusuf S, Pericak D, et al. Comparison of candesartan, enalapril, and their combination in congestive heart failure. Circulation 1999;100:1056–1064.

23. Cohn JN, Tognoni G, Glazer RD, et al. Rationale and design of the Valsartan Heart Failure Trial: a large multinational trial to assess the effects of valsartan, an angiotensin-receptor blocker, on morbidity and mortality in chronic congestive heart failure [abstract]. J Card Fail 1999;5(2):155–160.

24. Novartis Pharmaceuticals. Novartis issued the following statement in response to the results of the Valsartan Heart Failure Trial (Val-HeFT) announced today at the 73rd Scientific Sessions of the American Heart Association [press release]. (http://www. pharma.us.novartis.com/cgi-bin/pressreleases.pl?Todo=get Story&newsID=95), 15 November 2000.

25. Swedberg K, Pfeffer M, Granger C, et al. Candesartan in heart failure-assessment of reduction in mortality and morbidity (CHARM): rationale and design [abstract]. J Card Fail 1999;5(3):276–282.

26. Pasquale PD, Bucca V, Scalzo S, Paterna S. Safety, tolerability, and neurohormonal changes of the combination captopril plus losartan in the early postinfarction period: a pilot study. Cardiovasc Drugs Ther 1998;12:211–216.

27. Pasquale PD, Bucca V, Scalzo S, et al. Does the addition of losartan improve the beneficial effects of ACE inhibitors in patients with anterior myocardial infarction? A pilot study. Heart 1999;81:606–611.

28. Pasquale PD, Cannizzaro S, Giubilato A, , et al. Effects of the combination of candesartan plus captopril in elderly patients with anterior myocardial infarction. A pilot study. Clin Drug Invest 2000;19(3):173–182.

29. Pfeffer MA. Enhancing cardiac protection after myocardial infarction: rationale for newer clinical trials of angiotensin receptor blockers. Am Heart J 2000; 139:S23–S28.

NEWSLETTER EXAMPLE: BRIAN E. GULBIS, PHARM.D., PREPARED WHILE A PHARMACY STUDENT AT OHIO NORTHERN UNIVERSITY AS PART OF THE PROFESSION OF PHARMACY COURSEWORK

Ubiquinone Use in Cardiovascular Disease

Ubiquinone (coenzyme Q-10, CoQ) is a naturally occurring coenzyme found in aerobic organisms. It was given the name ubiquinone because of its universal, or ubiquitous, occurrence in animal tissues. Since its isolation in 1957, CoQ has been studied throughout Japan, Russia, Europe, and the United States.[1] It is found mostly in the inner mitochondrial membrane, especially in the heart, liver, kidney, and pancreas.[2] CoQ plays an important role in the mitochondrial electron transport chain. NADH and succinate dehydrogenases, and other flavoproteins, donate electrons to CoQ, which transfers them to nonheme iron proteins. The oxidation–reduction reactions that CoQ undergoes during electron transport are an essential part of the proton-pumping mechanism that leads to the generation of ATP in the mitochondria.[3] In addition to its role in the electron transport chain, ubiquinone is also an antioxidant and free radical scavenger, and it is believed to possess membrane-stabilizing properties.[2,4]

Since its discovery, coenzyme Q-10 has been used to aid in the treatment of many cardiovascular diseases, such as congestive heart failure (CHF), cardiac arrhythmias, and hypertension. Although it has not been approved for therapeutic use in the United States, ubiquinone is the primary treatment for cardiovascular disease in approximately 12 million Japanese.[1] Grounds for the use of CoQ in cardiovascular therapy were established in the early 1970s by Folkers et al., who found evidence of decreased levels of coenzyme Q-10 in patients with heart disease.[5] Subsequent studies have shown that there is a correlation between cardiovascular disease and low tissue levels of ubiquinone.[6] However, it is not yet known if the lowered CoQ levels are the cause of or a result of the disease states.

In the early 1990s, a multicenter, randomized, double-blind, placebo-controlled clinical trial was performed by Morisco, Trimarco, and Condorelli to study the effects of coenzyme Q-10 on patients with congestive heart failure. Patients were randomly assigned by a computer-generated allocation schedule that matched age, sex, New York Heart Association class, and treatment used for hemodynamic stabilization. A total of 641 patients were enrolled in the study among 33 centers, with 319 patients placed in the coenzyme Q-10 group and 322 patients in the placebo group. During the study, 16 patients died in the CoQ group, and 21 in the placebo group. Twenty-three patients in the CoQ group dropped out of the study, while 18 patients in the control group dropped out. Neither the number of deaths nor the number of patients who dropped out is statistically significant. There also were no statistically significant differences in the age, sex, weight, cardiovascular drug therapy, or noncardiovascular drug therapy of the two groups. The CoQ group was then given 2 mg/kg per day of coenzyme Q-10 in addition to the cardiovascular drug therapy required to reach hemodynamic stabilization. The other group received a placebo in addition to their regular drug therapy. Patients were then examined after 3, 6, and 12 months of the additional therapy. Evaluation of the efficacy of therapy was based on changes in the functional class of patients in the two groups. There was a statistically significant reduction in the class of the patients in the coenzyme Q-10 group. This means there was an overall improvement in functional status of patients in the CoQ group. There were no significant changes in functional class of patients in the placebo group. In addition, physicians and patients were asked to rate the effects of treatment on a scale of 1 to 3. The mean score given by physicians and patients in the placebo group remained unchanged throughout the study. However, there was a continual increase in the mean score given by physicians and patients in the coenzyme Q-10 group. There was also a statistically smaller incidence of cardiovascular complications, including acute pulmonary edema ($p < 0.001$), cardiac asthma ($p < 0.001$), and arrhythmias ($p < 0.05$) in the CoQ group compared to the placebo group. A final observation showed that about 40% of patients in the placebo group required one or more hospitalizations during the follow-up period, whereas only 20% of the patients in the coenzyme Q-10 group required hospitalization ($p < 0.01$).[7]

In a different multicenter study, by Lampertico and Comis, the efficacy and safety of coenzyme Q-10 as supplementary therapy in patients with heart failure were examined. The study took place in Italy, with 378 physicians participating in the trial. Of those 378 physicians, 201 were cardiologists, and 165 were interns. Physicians were asked to choose no more than five of their patients suffering heart failure who had been stabilized on cardiovascular therapy for at least 3 months to participate in the study. In all, 1715 patients were chosen, with 804 being male and 911 female. Coenzyme Q-10 was added to the traditional cardiovascular therapy at a dose of 50 mg per day in 1423 patients, while 192 patients received CoQ as their only therapy. Treatment was given over a 4-week period. In addition to reporting basic patient data, physicians were asked to evaluate a series of subjective and objective symptoms before treatment began, after 15 days, and after 30 days of therapy. Emphasis was placed on adverse events, and the physician was additionally asked to express an opinion on the efficacy of the therapy. The results of the trial showed a statistically significant subjective and objective improvement in the 1423 patients who received CoQ in addition to their conventional medication. Analysis showed an overall reduction in the intensity of symptoms after 2 and 4 weeks of treatment ($p < 0.01$), and statistically significant differences in systolic and diastolic blood pressure and heart rate were found ($p < 0.01$). Also of note, the incidence of clinical improvement in the group of patients who received only coenzyme Q-10 was the same as the group receiving CoQ in addition to their conventional medication. Incidence of adverse effects decreased from 2.2% after 2 weeks to 0.4% at the end of 4 weeks. Physicians' opinion of treatment efficacy was rated as excellent to good for 71.1% of the patients. A limitation of the study is its focus on people of Italian ethnicity.[2]

Although clinical studies provide scientific data to assess the efficacy of coenzyme Q-10 use, most people do not have the results of these studies readily available to them, nor do they have the ability to effectively analyze these results. Therefore, people turn to other resources for product information. Over the past few years, the Internet has become one of the fastest growing sources of information on anything and everything. People use the Internet to find news on world events, the latest sports scores, and information about new products, including natural products. A query of any major search engine for information on ubiquinone will easily yield over 1000 results. A company called Advance Nutrition has a rather extensive site on coenzyme Q-10. The company describes ubiquinone as "a vital catalyst required for the creation of the energy needed to maintain life."[8] Coenzyme Q-10 functions as a proton and electron carrier that "sparks the mitochondrial energy production which runs all vital body functions."[8] The page claims that the use of their coenzyme Q-10 supplement will "Increase energy levels, increase your VO_2 reading without exercise, lower high blood pressure, detoxify your body, reduce free radicals dramatically, and aid the function of all living cells. . . ."[8] Other sites make similar claims to those of Advance Nutrition. Another company selling ubiquinone supplements, called Natural Warehouse, alleges that use of their CoQ supplement will result in "energy increase, improvement of heart function, prevention and cure of gum disease, a boost to the immune system, and possible life extension."[9]

There is limited scientific evidence to support some of the claims made by these companies. Several clinical trials have shown that ubiquinone supplements probably improve heart function and aid in the treatment of cardiovascular disease. However, there is not yet any conclusive evidence to support the allegations made by these companies. More studies need to be done, and more data need to be collected and analyzed, before the claims of companies such as Advance Nutrition and Natural Warehouse can be either proved or disproved.

Although no dosage guidelines have been established, the administration of 50–150 mg of coenzyme Q-10 daily is considered to have therapeutic benefits. No major adverse effects have been associated with CoQ use at this dosage level.[2] Rare side effects include nausea, epigastric discomfort, loss of appetite, diarrhea, and skin rash. These adverse events have occurred in fewer than 1% of patients taking coenzyme Q-10 supplements.[1,10]

The results of studies have shown that the use of coenzyme Q-10 supplements appears to be effective in the treatment of cardiovascular diseases such as congestive heart failure, cardiac arrhythmias, and hypertension. The safety of CoQ has been established in studies, and no major side effects have been associated with CoQ use. Based on its safety and apparent efficacy, the use of coenzyme Q-10, in combination with conventional medications, can be recommended for the treatment of cardiovascular disease.

References

1. Ubiquinone. Rev Nat Prod 1997;Aug.
2. Lampertico M, Comis S. Italian multicenter study on the efficacy and safety of coenzyme Q10 as adjuvant therapy in heart failure. Clin Invest 1993;71: S129–S133.
3. Marks DB, Marks AD, Smith CM. Basic medical biochemistry: a clinical approach. Baltimore: Williams & Wilkins, 1996:315–316.
4. Ernster L, Dallner G. Biochemical, physiological and medical aspects of ubiquinone function. Biochim Biophys Acta 1995;1271:195–204.
5. Folkers K, Littarru GP, Ho L, Runge TM, Havanonda S, Cooley D. Evidence for a deficiency of coenzyme Q10 in human heart disease. Int Z Vitaminforsch 1970; 40(3):380–390.

6. Mortensen SA. Perspectives on therapy of cardiovascular diseases with coenzyme Q10 (ubiquinone). Clin Invest 1993;71:S116–S123.
7. Morisco C, Trimarco B, Condorelli M. Effect of coenzyme Q10 therapy in patients with congestive heart failure: a long-term multicenter randomized study. Clin Invest 1993;71:S134–S136.
8. Advance Nutrition Co. Enzyme Q10. Advance Nutrition. (http://www.advance nutrition.com/faq.html) Infoseek. 28 Dec 1998.
9. Coenzyme Q10. Nutrition Warehouse. (http://www.nutrition-warehouse.com/ Coenzyme.Q10.html) Infoseek 28 Dec 1998.
10. Anon. Ubidecarenone. DRUGDEX® System. Englewood, CO: MICROMEDEX, Inc., edition expires Feb 1999.

JOURNAL CLUB EXAMPLE: DESTA R. BORLAND, PHARM.D., PREPARED WHILE AN OHIO NORTHERN UNIVERSITY PHARMACY STUDENT AS PART OF AN ASSIGNMENT FOR THE CAPSTONE MODULE

Publication

Abraira C, Colwell JA, Nutall FQ, et al. Veterans Affairs cooperative study on glycemic control and complications in type II diabetes (VA CSDM). Results of the feasibility trial. Veterans Affairs Cooperative Study in Type II Diabetes. Diabetes Care 1995;18(8):1113–1123.

Objective

The objective of the VA CSDM study was to see if a correlation between the incidence of cardiovascular disease and length and severity of hyperglycemia could be established. The study also looked the possible relationship between glucose levels and macrovascular disease in patients with documented non-insulin-dependent diabetes mellitus (NIDDM). The researchers also wished to assess the need for a long-term trial.

Background

The Diabetes Control and Complications Trial (DCCT) published in 1993 examined the long-term macrovascular, microvascular, and neurologic complications that occur in patients with insulin-dependent diabetes mellitus (IDDM), including retinopathy, nephropathy, neuropathy, and cardiovascular disease.[1] The results of this study are not generalizable to patients with NIDDM because of the differences between the two disease states. Because the results of the DCCT could not be applied to patients with NIDDM, researchers felt there was a need for a similar study in these patients.

The use of intensive insulin therapy in patients with type II diabetes in considered to be controversial. Some medical personnel believe that insulin use in NIDDM may increase obesity, hypertension, and dyslipidemia. The only study previously done in this area, the University Group Diabetes Program (UGDP), had failed to establish the benefits of insulin therapy in macrovascular disease in patients with NIDDM.

Methods

The VA CSDM was a multicenter, randomized, prospective feasibility trial conducted in five medical centers over a 2-year period.

Patients

The trial included 153 men 60 ± 6 years of age who had been diagnosed with type II diabetes an average of 7.8 ± 4 years previous to the start of the study.

Inclusion Criteria

The patients included in the trial were adult men between the ages of 40 and 69 years of age who required chronic insulin therapy because other medications had shown clinical failure. A HbA_{1c} of >6.55% and a fasting plasma C-peptide of >0.21 pmol/mL were required at initial screening and verified by the coordinating center. Patients were included if they had a history of preexisting retinopathy or previous cardiovascular disease that was not considered severe or incapacitating with no acute attacks in the past 6 months.

Exclusion Criteria

Patients were excluded if they had a serum creatinine of >141.1 μmol/L (1.6 mg/dL) or an albuminuria >0.5 g/24 h. Other exclusions were patients with clinically evident autonomic neuropathy, current or previous diabetic gangrene, and those with a serious illness, predicted poor compliance, or a diagnosis of NIDDM > 15 years previously.

Outcome Variables

Patients in the study were monitored by a blinded committee of consultants external to the study itself for variables including new myocardial infarction, congestive heart failure, amputation for ischemic gangrene, stroke, angina, coronary artery disease, angioplasty or bypass graft, claudication, transitory ischemic attacks, ischemic ulcers, or cardiovascular mortality. They were also monitored for episodes of severe, moderate, or mild hypoglycemia with symptoms reviewed to decide which category each case fell into. HbA_{1c} and lipid profiles including HDL, LDL, and triglycerides were measured at each quarterly visit and determined by a central lab that had no knowledge of the treatment groups. Fasting plasma C-peptide was measured at entry and after the 2 years had been completed and was determined by a central lab. Also, at each visit, any current or incurrent cases of angina pectoris, smoking, coronary heart disease, transient ischemic attacks, and dyslipidemia were noted. If the patient was being treated for hypertension, the current therapy was documented along with the blood pressure and absence or presence of a foot ulcer, and clinical neuropathy. A central lab, on each 6-month visit determined a urinary albumin excretion level.

An independent Data Monitoring Board periodically evaluated the central laboratories involved in the study. All laboratory accreditations, proficiency-testing programs, and intraassay and interassay coefficients of variation were reviewed to establish that the laboratory was performing properly.

Procedures

Initially, 289 patients were screened for possible inclusion into the study, with only 153 enrolled. Each hospital involved received a standardized operations manual on how to proceed with educating the patients on the dietary plan that should be followed throughout the 2 years that the study would take place. The dietary plan was reinforced at each 3-month ambulatory visit. The health professionals involved were instructed to treat all of the patient's other disease states, such as dyslipidemia, obesity, hypertension, and smoking, according to the American Diabetes Association (ADA) guidelines.

Patients were randomized into either the standard treatment group, which would be treated with one injection of insulin per day and two injections if absolutely necessary, not to exceed two, or the intensively treated group, which was broken into four stepped treatment phases.

Patients in the standard treatment therapy group maintained the same dosing regimen of one injection per day unless they were experiencing diabetic symptoms or reached the HbA_{1c} "alert" level of 12.9% whether or not symptoms were present at the time of testing. These patients were monitored by ambulatory visits every 3 months. At each visit the patients underwent urinary glucose testing, ketonuria testing, and blood glucose testing.

Phase I patients were treated with one bedtime dose of either an intermediate- or long-acting insulin. Phase II patients were given both an evening dose and a daytime dose of glipizide. Phase III patients were administered two injections of insulin daily. Phase IV were dosed multiple insulin injections daily. All patients in the intense treatment group did home blood glucose tests twice daily and once a week at 3 a.m. Patients were stepped through the various phases if they were not meeting their designated target HbA_{1c} level of as close to the normal range as possible (5.1 ± 1%) and a fasting blood glucose of 4.44–6.38 mmol/L (80–115 mg/dL). Patients in this therapy group were also monitored at ambulatory visits at 3-month intervals, and the same tests were performed as with patients in the standard treatment group. These patients also received a monthly visit and weekly phone call for the purpose of monitoring the current doses and making changes in the treatment where necessary. The cardiovascular events and other outcome variables listed above were also monitored at each of the 3-month ambulatory visits.

As previously mentioned, all of the laboratory tests were completed at accredited, centrally located labs. The researchers also split 10% of the specimens and sent half of those specimens to another blinded lab to assess accuracy of the central labs participating.

Statistical Methods

The independent variables of time and treatment were analyzed using a series of chi-squared tests and repeated-measures analysis of variance (ANOVA). Discrete variables and continuous variables were also analyzed using the chi-squared test. All baseline comparisons of the two treatment groups were analyzed using the Student's t test. No p-value or α value was mentioned in the article. The Cox regression analysis was used to determine the relationship between new cardiovascular events and previous cardiovascular disease.[2]

Results/Conclusions

Of the 153 patients involved in the study, 98.6% kept each of their scheduled quarterly visits, and only 4% of those in the intensively treated group were indicated as failing to adhere to the protocol. The average time in the study was 27 months with a range of 18–35 months. Four patients in the intense treatment group failed to complete the study. One left voluntarily at 7 months, one moved without a forwarding address, one fell into an irreversible coma related to a case of septicemia, and one left after being diagnosed with psychotic depression. Results from these four patients, up until their dismissal from the trial, were calculated into the final data. Ninety-six percent of patients in the standard treatment group and 71% of the patients in the intense treatment group were able to follow their treatment protocol throughout the study without interruption.

In the intensively treated group, 85% were in either phase I or phase II, and 15% were in phase III or phase IV at the 1-year marker. By the end of the study most of the patients were receiving two or more daily insulin injections. None of the patients in the standard therapy group were moved to intensified therapy for more than a short period of time. The average insulin dose of patients in the standard treatment group was 23% lower than in the intense treatment group.

Patients in the intense therapy group had fasting glucose levels close to normal range starting at about the 3-month mark and maintained those levels throughout the study. Patients in the standard therapy group were not as close to the normal range, with an average difference between the two groups of 5.46 mmol/L (98.3 mg/dL). The intense therapy group patients were also able to maintain lower HbA_{1c} levels than the patients in the standard therapy group throughout the 2 years of the study. The average difference in HbA_{1c} levels between the two groups was 2.7% starting after the 6-month marker. A small decrease in HbA_{1c} was seen with the addition of glipizide, but the majority of the decrease was seen with the bedtime dose of intermediate- or long-acting insulin. No real change was seen with the twice-daily insulin injections.

At the onset of the study there was no statistical difference in body mass index, patients on therapy for hypertension, hypercholesterolemia, smokers, or those with previous cardiovascular events between the two treatment groups. Throughout the study, there was no statistical difference in body mass index between the two groups. By the end of the 2-year study both groups had experienced a fall in serum triglyceride concentrations with no statistical difference. The fall in LDL levels was also considered not significant for either group. There was a slight increase in patients who required hypercholesterolemia therapy but with no statistical difference. The average blood pressure of the participants did not change throughout. Forty patients experienced 61 new cardiovascular events, but the relationship to each treatment group was not reported. A later article, "Cardiovascular Events and Correlates in the Veterans Affairs Feasibility Trial,"[2] was published in 1997. Sixteen patients (20%) in the standard treatment group and 24 (32%) patients in the intense treatment group experienced new cardiovascular events, but no statistical difference was found in the overall cardiovascular mortality.[2] Five participants in the intensively treated group and two participants in the standard treatment group reported hypoglycemic events. The researchers determined that there was no statistical difference in hypoglycemic events between the two treatment groups.

The major concern of weight gain in NIDDM patients on intense insulin therapy was not seen in this study. It was also determined that patients with type II diabetes could have well-controlled glucose levels without the use of excessively large doses of insulin. A bedtime dose of an intermediate-acting insulin in combination with a daytime glipizide or by itself may be most beneficial in regulating glucose levels. Researchers were also able to establish that "improved glycemic control could be accomplished without differences in adverse events associated with insulin therapy."

Both treatment regimens were considered safe and effective in treating the patients involved. No patients presented with a hyperosmolar state and ketoacidosis throughout the 2-year study. And in the standard treatment group only six patients ever reached the alert HbA_{1c} level of $>12.9\%$.

Reader's Results/Conclusions

The primary objective of the study was met by the large number of cardiovascular events, proving that a further study with a much larger sample size should be conducted to better monitor the effects of insulin therapy on new cardiovascular events and macrovascular disease in patients with diagnosed type II diabetes. The study also showed that it might be possible to treat NIDDM patients with chronic insulin therapy without risk of increasing obesity, hypertension, or dyslipidemia, meaning patients could achieve improved glycemic control without increased risk of adverse events.

The article was written in an understandable fashion and an adequate length. The study was funded by various organizations including many drug manufactures and the DVA Medical Research Service, allowing for lack of bias. The study was approved by an Investigational Review Board and used appropriate references.

Although the article was published in a rather reputable journal and was approved by the institutional review board at each of the participating hospitals, many limitations were evident. The study lacks generalizibility because all of the patients involved were men from within a narrow age range and did not include patients with a >15-year history of NIDDM. The sample size was also relatively small, but because the study was only assessing the need for a larger study, this may have been appropriate. The researchers failed to mention how the patients were randomized into the two treatment groups or how their compliance was monitored throughout the study. The article failed to discuss many aspects of the statistical methods used, including power and α values. The new cardiovascular events of 40 patients were never discussed except to say that they would be mentioned in a later article.

This article should be used as a starting point for further research to be done in the future. By the time this article was published, a proposal for a long-term trial of 1463 patients had already been established to better assess the use of chronic insulin therapy in NIDDM patients.

References

1. The Diabetes Control and Complications Trial. The effect of intensive treatment of diabetes on the development and progression of long-term complications in insulin-dependent diabetes mellitus. N Engl J Med 1993;329(14):977–984.
2. Abraira C, Colwell J, Nutall F, et al. Cardiovascular events and correlates in the Veterans Affairs Diabetes Feasibility Trial. Arch Intern Med 1997;157:181–190.

EXAMPLE OF A DRUG MONOGRAPH: SPARFLOXACIN (ZAGAM®) COMPARISON TO CIPROFLOXACIN (CIPRO®) BY KAREN L. KIER, DRUG INFORMATION CENTER, OHIO NORTHERN UNIVERSITY

Background

Sparfloxacin (Table 8.10) is a new once-daily fluoroquinolone antibiotic by Rhone-Poulenc Rorer that was approved by the FDA on December 19, 1996. This fluoroquinolone has demonstrated activity against a broad spectrum of organisms including gram-positive, gram-negative, and anaerobic bacteria. Sparfloxacin is highly active in vitro against many penicillin-resistant strains of gram-positive pathogens as well as drug-resistant strains of Haemophilus influenzae and Moraxella catarrhalis. It may offer an advantage over other fluoroquinolones by its improved gram-positive cocci coverage and its activity against some anaerobes.[1,12]

TABLE 8.10. COMPARATIVE CHART

	CIPROFLOXACIN[14]	SPARFLOXACIN[1-15]
Description Pharmacology	Fluoroquinolone Synthetic, broad-spectrum bactericidal Interferes with DNA gyrase needed for synthesis of bacterial DNA	Fluoroquinolone Synthetic, broad-spectrum bactericidal Interferes with DNA gyrase needed for synthesis of bacterial DNA
Absorption	Rapidly and well absorbed from GI tract with minimal loss during FPM Food causes delay in absorption [Max serum] = 1–2 h after dosing [Mean] = 12 h. after dosing	92% BA with slow, variable rate of absorption with mean times to peak between 4–5.6 h Food has no effect on absorption Antacids decrease absorption up to 50%
Distribution	Widely distributed Tissue > serum Low CSF concentrations	Achieves high conc. in most tissues 45% bound to plasma proteins
Metabolism	Four metabolites have been found in the urine, together accounting for 15% of an oral dose and having less antimicrobial activity	Undergoes phase II glucuronidation to form conjugate Not metabolized by CYT P450 18.4% excreted renally as metabolite
Elimination	Excreted by renal and nonrenal mechanisms Eliminated through urine and feces	Renal clearance minimal $t\frac{1}{2}$ = 17.6 h

(continued)

TABLE 8.10. COMPARATIVE CHART (*Cont.*)

	CIPROFLOXACIN[14]	SPARFLOXACIN[1-15]

Indications (FDA approved and investigational)	Community-acquired pneumonia
	Lower respiratory infections caused by *E. coli, K. pneumoniae, E. cloacae, P. mirabilits, P. aeruginosa, H. influenzae, H. parainfluenzae, S. pneumoniae.*
	Skin infections caused by *E. coli, K. pneumoniae, E. cloacae, P. mirabilis, P. vulgaris, P. stuartii, M. morganii, C. freundii, S. pyogenes, P. aeruginosa, S. aureus, S. epidermidis*
	Bone/joint infections caused by *E. cloacae, S. marcescens, P. aeruginosa*
	UTI caused by *E. coli, K. pneumoniae, E. cloacae, S. marcescens, P. mirabilis, P. rettgeri, M. morganii, C. diversus, C. freundii, P. aeruginosa, S. epidermidis, E. faecalis*
	Infectious diarrhea
	Typhoid fever
	Sexually transmitted diseases
		Community-acquired pneumonia
		Lower respiratory infections caused by
		    H. influenzae, S. pneumoniae, M. catarrhalis,
		    L. pneumophila, M, pneumoniae, C. psittaci,
		    C. pneumoniae
		Acute bacterial exacerbations of chronic bronchitis
		    caused by *H. influenzae, S. pneumoniae,*
		    M. catarrhalis, C. pneumoniae, H. parainfluenzae,
		    K. pneumoniae, E. cloacae, S. aureus
		Soft tissue infections
		UTI
		Sexually transmitted diseases
		Vancomycin resistance
		Leprosy

(continued)

TABLE 8.10. COMPARATIVE CHART (*Cont.*)

Contraindications	History of hypersensitivity to cipro-floxacin or other quinolone Predisposed to seizures (epilepsy)	History of hypersensitivity to sparfloxacin or other quinolone antibiotics Concomitant treatment with Ia antiarrhythmic agents or predisposed to torsade de pointes (QTc prolongation) Exposure to high levels of UV light Predisposed to seizures (epilepsy)
Warnings	Convulsions, tremors, restlessness, lightheadedness, confusion, hallucinations	Predisposed to epilepsy, liver disease, or kidney disease May make lightheaded or dizzy Skin sensitivity increases; may get rash or sunburn
Precautions	Food decreases absorption Crystalluria, phototoxicity, superinfection, opthalmologic abnormalities Monitor organ functions	Renal failure CNS toxicity Tendon rupture, pain, or inflammation
Carcinogenesis	Mice exposed to UVA light developed a phototoxic response; skin tumor development in 28–52 weeks	Superinfection
Lactation	Excreted in breast milk, but low levels ingested by infant Not recommended (category C)	Not recommended (category C)
Pediatric use	Do not use in children Causes arthropathy and osteochondrosis in immature animals	Do not use in children Causes arthropathy and osteochondrosis in immature animals

(continued)

TABLE 8.10. COMPARATIVE CHART (*Cont.*)

	CIPROFLOXACIN[14]	SPARFLOXACIN[1-15]
Drug interactions	Antacids decrease serum levels Antineoplastic agents may decrease serum levels Azlocillin decreases clearance Cimetidine may interfere with elimination Probenecid decreases renal clearance 50% and increases serum levels 50% Caffeine clearance is reduced Cyclosporin's nephrotoxic effect may be increased Phenytoin serum levels may decrease Anticoagulant effects may be increased Theophylline plasma levels and clearance may increase	Antacids decrease serum levels Disopyramide and amiodarone can cause torsades de pointes and an increase in QTc interval when given concomitantly Theophylline and warfarin levels are *not* affected[11]
Adverse reactions	Nausea, diarrhea, vomiting, and abdominal pain/discomfort HA and restlessness, dizziness Mild, transient rash Increased serum creatinine and BUN concentrations with rare crystalluria Increased conc. of AST and ALT Ruptured tendons, myalgia[8]	Decreased hemoglobin and leukopenia/eosinophilia Cardiac insufficiency, vascular embolism, hypotention, interval prolongation, QTc interval prolongation Insomnia, sleep disorders, agitation, anxiety, delirium Diarrhea, nausea, vomiting, dyspepsia Pseudomembranous colitis Hepatotoxicity Photosensitivity (7.9%) Ruptured tendons, myalgia, arthralgia[8]

(continued)

TABLE 8.10. COMPARATIVE CHART (*Cont.*)

Dosage and administration	Urinary tract: 250–500 mg q 12 h Lower resp. tract, bone and joint, skin: 500–750 mg q 12 h Infectious diarrhea: 500 mg q 12 h Typhoid fever: 500 mg q 12 h Urethral/cervical gonococcal infections: 250 mg single dose	Leprosy: 400 mg LD followed by 200 mg qd × 12 weeks Respiratory tract infection: Bacterial pneumonia, 300 mg qd; over 65 yr. old or acute sinusitis, 400 mg LD 200 mg qd × 10 days; COPD, 200 mg LD followed by 100 mg qd × 7–14 days Soft-tissue infections: 100 mg bid Urethritis: nongonococcal, 300 mg qd 7 or 14 days, 200 mg LD followed by 100 mg qd × 7 days; gonococcal, 300 mg qd × 3 days
Dosage forms	100 mg, 250 mg, 500 mg, 750 mg film-coated tablets; 200 mg and 400 mg inj	200-mg tablets supplied in blister packs of 11 or bottles of 50 tablets
Cost	$82.72 for twenty 500-mg tablets	$87.89 for 11-tablet blister pack

219

What It Is

Sparfloxacin is a difluorinated quinolone antibiotic that is structurally related to ciprofloxacin.[1]

What It Does

Bactericidal activity by inhibition of the enzyme DNA gyrase, which is necessary for the synthesis of DNA by bacteria.

Clinical Trials

An *in vitro* study of activity to human infection isolates showed that sparfloxacin has good activity against anaerobes such as *Peptostreptococci, Clostridium perfingens, Clostridium difficile,* and *Fusobacterium.* Sparfloxacin had significantly better activity against *Bacteroides fragilis* than ciprofloxacin, lomefloxacin, and ofloxacin but was not superior to piperacillin/tazobactam, cefoxitin, imipenem, clindamycin, or metronidazole. This *in vitro* activity may prove to be beneficial in patients with mixed infections that can include anaerobes such as soft tissue infections in patients with diabetes. The limitations of this study included *in vitro* testing, which does not always correlate to *in vivo* response, and the small number of cultures that were performed.[1]

A multicenter, double-blinded, randomized trial comparing sparfloxacin to doxycycline for nongonococal urethritis looked at 725 men. Sparfloxacin was given in a dosing regimen of a 200-mg loading dose on day 1 followed by 100 mg each day for 2 days, and a second group received 100 mg per day for 6 days. This was compared to doxycycline 200 mg once per day for 7 days. For chlamydial infections, rates of relapse or reinfection were similar for both drugs. In addition, the researchers found that 3 days and 7 days of sparfloxacin were also equal in efficacy. Cultures were taken at each office visit by doing an endourethral swab to confirm presence of bacteria. Success of therapy was determined by clinical symptoms and bacteriologic response of the urethral smear. For ureaplasmal urethritis or urethritis of unknown etiology, sparfloxacin had a lower relapse/reinfection rate than doxycycline.[4] A limitation of this study is that the results can be applied only to treating men and not to women. In addition, this study was a multicenter trial that did not control for laboratory or observer differences. This study had limitations in the application of statistical tests. The study used only frequency and descriptive data and did not perform any tests to determine statistically significant results.

A double-blinded, multicenter trial that treated 382 patients for acute purulent sinusitis used sparfloxacin 200 mg once per day for 5 days with a 400-mg loading dose on the first day compared to cefuroxime axetil 250 mg two times per day for 8 days. Patients were classified as success or failure based on clinical symptoms as well as bacterial cultures and radiologic exams. Three hundred seventy-four patients were evaluated in the final results. The success rates as defined by the authors was 82.6% with sparfloxacin and 83.2% with cefuroxime axetil. The most common cultured organisms were H. influenzae and S. pneumoniae. The success rate as well as the side-effect profile were similar between the two drugs.[5] The study limitations included some patients lost to follow-up and not evaluated for the study as well as multiple observers collecting data without mentioning how this variation was to be controlled for by the different researchers. The cultures were analyzed all at one location, which was an appropriate measure to improve internal validity. Another limitation was that not all patients had bacterial cultures or radiologic exams performed. Therefore, success or failure was defined differently for some patients.

A double-blinded, multicenter, randomized trial evaluated 733 patients for acute exacerbation of chronic obstructive pulmonary disease (COPD). The study compared sparfloxacin 100 mg every day with a 200-mg loading dose to amoxicillin 500 mg/clavulanic acid 125 mg three times per day for 7 to 14 days. Patients were evaluated if their FEV_1/FVC ratio was less than 70% and stable. The primary endpoint was improvement in dyspnea and reduction in sputum purulence and volume. Success rates for both treatment groups were equivalent. Sparfloxacin improved dyspnea in 87.4% of patients compared to 88.8% amoxicillin/clavulanic acid. In terms of bacteriologic eradication, sparfloxacin appeared to be superior to amoxicillin/clavulanic acid for Haemophilus influenzae and Moraxella catarrhalis.[6] The study limitations included lack of culture eradication, and not all types of COPD patients were included.

In a prospective, placebo-controlled double-blind study, sparfloxacin 200 mg once daily with a 400-mg loading dose was compared with amoxicillin 1 g three times a day in combination with ofloxacin 200 mg twice a day. This comparison was done in 211 patients admitted to the hospital for community-acquired pneumonia. The efficacy rate was found to be similar between the two groups, with sparfloxacin having a 91.9% rate of success compared to the combination, which showed a lower rate of 81.5%. The adverse effect profile was also found to be similar between the two study drugs.[7] Study limitations included a multicenter trial that did not control for multiple observers. In addition, statistical analysis was limited to frequency data, and statistical significance was not performed. The efficacy rate was considered to be similar via frequency data, but there is a 10% difference in clinical response. This difference could be enough to prove statistical as well as clinical significance.

Comparative Studies

A double-blinded, randomized clinical trial involving 686 patients compared ciprofloxacin to sparfloxacin in complicated urinary tract infections (UTI). This was a multicenter study comparing sparfloxacin 200-mg loading dose followed by 100 mg every day with ciprofloxacin 500 mg twice daily for 10–14 days. Complicated UTI was defined as pyruria and bacteriuria. Evaluations were performed at four different time points during the study. The clinical efficacy of the two products was equivalent at the end of treatment, with sparfloxacin having a clinical cure rate of 87.5% compared to ciprofloxacin's cure rate of 85%. Bacteriologic cure was 72.6% in the sparfloxacin group and 81.4% in the ciprofloxacin group. The side-effect profile was similar in the two groups. However, it was noted that in terms of bacteriologic efficacy ciprofloxacin was superior to sparfloxacin because of persistent pathogens of the Enterobacteriaceae species other than E. coli.[2] Study limitations included the lack of statistical tests to make comparisons to show statistical significance.

A multicenter, double-blinded, randomized clinical trial compared the efficacy of sparfloxacin with ciprofloxacin in acute gonorrhea. The study compared single oral doses of sparfloxacin 200 mg versus ciprofloxacin 250 mg in 238 men with the diagnosis of Neisseria gonorrhoeae. The two drugs were found to be equally effective in the treatment of gonorrhea in men. The primary eradication rate was 99% in the sparfloxacin group and 98% in the ciprofloxacin group. The side effects were similar for both treatment groups.[13] The study was only in the acute environment and does not provide long-term results. The incidence of resistance was not studied. Another limitation was that some patients were lost to follow-up and were dropped from the study analysis.

Recommendation

Ciprofloxacin and sparfloxacin have good gram-negative coverage for most serious infections. The clinical trials support similar rates of eradication and efficacy. The concerns with sparfloxacin are with the drug interactions and the adverse effect of a prolonged QT interval. Because sparfloxacin has these potential problems, the Pharmacy Department recommends to the P&T committee that ciprofloxacin remain as the fluoroquinolone of choice for the institution.

References

1. Nord CE. In vitro activity of quinolones and other antimicrobial agents against anaerobic bacteria. Clin Infect Dis 1996;23(Suppl 1):s15–s18.
2. Naber KG, Di Silverio F, Geddes A, et al. Comparative efficacy of sparfloxacin versus ciprofloxacin in the treatment of complicated urinary tract infection. J Antimicrob Chemother 1996;37(Suppl A):135–144.
3. Rubinstein E. Safety profile of sparfloxacin in the treatment of respiratory tract infections. J Antimicrob Chemother 1996;37(Suppl A):145–160.
4. Phillips I, Dimian, C, Barlow D, et al. A comparative study of two different regimens of sparfloxacin versus doxycycline in the treatment of non-gonococcal urethritis in men. J Antimicrob Chemother 1996;37(Suppl A):123–134.
5. Gehanno P, Berche P, et al. Sparfloxacin versus cefuroxime axetil in the treatment of acute purulent sinusitis. J Antimicrob Chemother 1996;37(Suppl A):93–104.

6. Allegra L, Konietzko N, Leophonte P, et al. Comparative safety and efficacy of sparfloxacin in the treatment of acute exacerbations of chronic obstructive pulmonary disease: a double-blind, randomized, parallel, multicentre study. J Antimicrob Chemother 1996;37(Suppl A):93–104.

7. Portier H, May T, Proust A, et al. Comparative efficacy of sparfloxacin in comparison with amoxicillin plus ofloxacin in the treatment of community-acquired pneumonia. J Antimicrob Chemother 1996;37(Suppl A):83–91.

8. Huston KA. Achilles tendinitis and tendon rupture due to fluoroquinolone antibiotics. N Engl J Med 1994;331:748.

9. Johnson JH, Cooper MA, Andrews JM, et al. Pharmacokinetics and inflammatory fluid penetration of sparfloxacin. Antimicrob Agents Chemother 1992;36: 2444–2446.

10. Ritz M, Lose H, Fabbender M, et al. Multiple-dose pharmacokinetics of sparfloxacin and its influence on fecal flora. Antimicrob Agents Chemother 1994;38:455–459.

11. Takagi K, Yamaki K, Nadai M, et al. Effect of a new quinolone, sparfloxacin, on the pharmacokinetics of theophylline in asthmatic patients. Antimicrob Agents Chemother 1991;35:1137–1141.

12. FDC Pink Sheet. January 6, 1997, 16–17.

13. Moi H, Morel P, Gianotti B, et al. Comparative efficacy and safety of single oral doses of sparfloxacin versus ciprofloxacin in the treatment of acute gonococcal urethritis in men. J Antimicrob Chemother 1996;37(Suppl A):115–122.

14. Anderson PO, Knoben JE. Handbook of Clinical Drug Data, 8th ed. Stamford, CT: Appleton & Lange, 1997.

15. Goa KL, Bryson HM, Markham A. Sparfloxacin. Drugs 1997;53(4):700–725.

EXAMPLE OF PHARMACY & THERAPEUTICS COMMITTEE MONOGRAPH: APRIL M. BAYS, PHARM.D. STUDENT, OHIO NORTHERN UNIVERSITY, AS PART OF A PATIENT CARE ASSESSMENT MODULE ASSIGNMENT: CARVEDILOL (COREG®, SMITHKLINE BEECHAM)

Pharmacology

Carvedilol is a nonselective β-adrenergic blocking agent with α_1-adrenergic blocking activity and no sympathomimetic activity.[1,2] The β-adrenoreceptor blocking activity is present in the $S(-)$ enantiomer, and the α-adrenergic blocking activity is present in both $R(+)$ and $S(-)$ enantiomers at equal potency.[3] The exact mechanism of the antihypertensive effect produced by the β-adrenergic blockade is not known, but it may involve suppression of renin production. The β-adrenergic blocking activity of carvedilol decreases cardiac output, exercise- and/or isoproterenol-induced tachycardia, and reflex orthostatic tachycardia. The α_1-adrenergic blocking activity of carvedilol blunts the pressor effect of phenylephrine, causes vasodilation, and reduces peripheral vascular resistance. Because of the α_1-receptor-blocking activity of carvedilol, blood pressure is lowered more in the standing than the supine position.[2]

The mechanisms by which carvedilol slows the progression of heart failure are not known. Possible mechanisms include up-regulation of the β-adrenergic receptors in the heart, modulation of postreceptor inhibitory G proteins, an effect on left ventricular remodeling, and an improvement in baroreceptor function, which normally can inhibit excess sympathetic outflow.[4]

Carvedilol is rapidly and extensively absorbed following oral administration, with a bioavailability of 25% to 35%, as a result of a significant degree of first-pass metabolism.[1,3] Taking carvedilol with food delays its absorption an additional 1 to 2 hours but does not appear to affect the extent of bioavailability.[3] The volume of distribution at steady-state concentration is approximately 115 L, indicating extensive protein binding (98%), primarily to albumin. Peak plasma concentrations are reached in 1 to 2 hours.[2,5] The drug is extensively metabolized in the liver and primarily excreted by the feces. Small amounts (less than 1%) of unchanged carvedilol are excreted in the urine.[5] The elimination half-life is 7 to 10 hours.[1,5] The primary P450 enzymes responsible for the metabolism of carvedilol are CYP2D6 and CYP2C8.

Indications for Use

Carvedilol is indicated for congestive heart failure and hypertension. In essential hypertension, carvedilol is indicated either alone or in combination with other antihypertensive agents such as thiazide diuretics. Carvedilol, in the treatment of congestive heart failure, is indicated for use in conjunction with digitalis, diuretics, and/or angiotensin-converting enzyme (ACE) inhibitors. It is used to slow the progression of disease as evidenced by cardiovascular death, cardiovascular hospitalization, or the need to adjust other heart failure medications. Carvedilol may be used in patients who are unable to tolerate an ACE inhibitor or in patients who are not receiving digitalis, hydralazine, or nitrate therapy.[1,3,5] Unlabeled uses for carvedilol include angina pectoris and idiopathic cardiomyopathy.

Review of Congestive Heart Failure

Congestive heart failure results when the heart cannot pump blood at a rate comparable to the requirements of metabolizing tissues or can do so only from an elevated filling pressure. As a result, the heart cannot produce enough blood circulation to maintain the body in its normal state. The term "congestive" refers to fluid buildup that occurs with the disease. With less blood leaving your heart, blood returning to your heart gets backed up. As back pressure builds, fluid from your blood can collect in your vital organs, including your lungs and liver. Fluid can also seep into surrounding tissues, causing swelling.[6,7]

Heart attacks, congenital heart disease, heart muscle damage caused by alcohol or viruses, high blood pressure, heart valve abnormalities, and abnormal heart rhythms are the major causes of congestive heart failure. Signs of congestive heart failure include reduced ability to exercise, fatigue, breathing problems, and swelling of the legs.[7,8] The amount of impairment from congestive heart failure ranges from none after appropriate compensation by drugs to the patient being totally bedridden and incapable of normal functioning.[9]

In some cases, congestive heart failure can be corrected by treating an underlying cause, but many times the problem cannot be eliminated. Then, the goal of treatment is to prevent further damage to your heart and help it pump as efficiently as possible. This is usually done through ACE inhibitors, diuretics, digoxin, and β-blockers.

Efficacy

The relatively recent discovery that β-blockers may be used in the treatment of congestive heart failure has lead to many case studies examining the effectiveness of carvedilol. In a double-blinded study by the Australia/New Zealand Heart Failure Research Collaborative Group, 415 patients with chronic stable heart failure were randomly assigned treatment of carvedilol or matching placebo. The primary study outcomes were changes in left-ventricular ejection fraction and treadmill exercise duration. A sample size of 200–225 patients per group was estimated to provide more than 80% power at a statistical significance of 0.05 to detect an absolute change in left ventricular ejection fraction of 2% or more between the groups and a change in treadmill exercise duration of 1 minute or more between groups.

The patients were recruited to the trial from 20 hospitals in Australia and New Zealand. Patients included in the study were those with chronic stable heart failure caused by ischemic heart disease, a left-ventricular ejection fraction of less than 45%, and current New York Heart Association (NYHA) functional class II or III or previous NYHA class II–IV. The mean age of the participants at entry to the study was 67 years, and 80% were men. Principal outcome analysis was by intention to treat. At baseline, 6 months, and 12 months, measurements of left-ventricular ejection fraction and treadmill exercise duration were taken. A double-blinded follow-up continued for an average of 19 months, during which all deaths, hospital admissions, and episodes of worsening heart failure were documented. Results from the study indicate an increase in left ventricular ejection fraction from 28.4% at baseline to 33.5% at 12 months among the patients assigned carvedilol. The placebo group showed little change. However, there was no significant difference between the carvedilol and placebo groups in treadmill exercise duration at 12 months.

The Australia/New Zealand Heart Failure Research Collaborative Group concluded that in patients with chronic stable heart failure caused by ischemic heart disease, the effects of carvedilol on left ventricular function were maintained for at least 1 year from the start of treatment, with no apparent loss of the initial short-term improvement. The increase in left ventricular ejection fraction suggests a sustained improvement in intrinsic myocardial function. Whether there are benefits of β-blocker therapy for these outcomes in other subgroups of patients with heart failure remains uncertain. There have, however, been some reports of benefits in studies of patients with ideopathic cardiomyopathy and in other trials among patients with more severe heart failure.[10]

There are possible concerns with this study. First, the sample size of patients per group was estimated to provide 80% power. Power is the positive spin indicating that when you say the groups are equal, they are in reality equal. A power of 90% tends to be an acceptable standard for most studies. Therefore, the placebo and carvedilol groups may not be as equal as they seem. Additionally, as a result of dropouts and death during the course of the study, the final number of subjects was smaller than the original sample size calculations. This may increase the possibility of a false-negative result. Last, the increase in left-ventricular ejection fraction may not be clinically significant even though it is statistically significant because of the condition of the patient and the response of the patient to the drug.

In a study determining the long-term efficacy of carvedilol in patients with severe chronic heart failure, Krum and colleagues[11] hypothesized that carvedilol produces clinical and hemodynamic improvements in patients who have severe heart failure despite treatment with angiotensin-converting enzyme inhibitors. Patients with chronic heart failure who remained symptomatic were eligible for the study. Heart failure was defined as the presence of dypsnea or fatigue at rest or on exertion for more than 2 months in association with a left ventricular ejection fraction less than or equal to 0.35 as assessed by radionuclide ventriculography. The cause of heart failure was related to numerous different types of cardiac dysfunction. Fifty-six patients with severe chronic heart failure were enrolled in the double-blinded, placebo-controlled study of carvedilol. The 56 patients consisted of 45 men and 11 women (25 to 79 years old). Forty-nine of the 56 patients were randomly assigned to a long-term therapy of carvedilol (33 patients) or placebo (16 patients) while backround therapy remained constant. Patients treated with carvedilol showed an improvement in symptom scores and functional class, whereas these variables did not change in the patients receiving placebo. These clinical benefits were accompanied by an increase in the distance traveled during a 6-minute walk in the carvedilol group. Carvedilol was also associated with a significant improvement in cardiac performance. Patients being treated with carvedilol showed a significant increase in stroke volume index and left-ventricular ejection fraction. Although there was a rise in stroke volume index, the cardiac index did not increase with carvedilol because the heart rate decreased considerably during long treatment with the drug. Last, the plasma epinephrine decreased with the use of carvedilol when compared to the placebo.

For each of the variables being studied, $p < 0.05$, indicating that there was a difference between carvedilol and placebo. In conclusion, this study demonstrated that the β-blockade of carvedilol produces clinical and hemodynamic benefits in patients with severe chronic heart failure in those who can tolerate low doses of the drug. The addition of carvedilol to conventional therapy led to an improvement in symptoms, functional capacity, and submaximal exercise tolerance. This study also demonstrates that carvedilol may be useful in the management of advanced heart failure, regardless of the cause of cardiac dysfunction. The low number of patients enrolled in this study may not have been large enough to detect a statistically significant difference between the treatments. Also, treatment effects may be overestimated with such a small population. Last, the clinical and hemodynamic improvements from carvedilol may not be clinically significant. The improvements may be so insignificant that less expensive treatment options could be used without harming the patient.[11]

Safety

Carvedilol is generally well tolerated at doses up to 50 mg daily. It is contraindicated in patients with NYHA class IV decompensated cardiac failure requiring intravenous inotropic therapy, bronchial asthma or related bronchospastic conditions, second- or third-degree AV block, sick sinus syndrome (unless a permanent pacemaker is in place), cardiogenic shock, and severe brachycardia. The use of carvedilol in patients with clinically manifest hepatic impairment is not recommended. Also, carvedilol is contraindicated in patients with hypersensitivity to the drug.[2,5]

Mild hepatocellular injury confirmed by carvedilol challenge after the discontinuation of treatment has occurred in a few patients, but no deaths from liver failure have been reported. Also, hepatic injury has been reversible. In controlled studies of hypertensive patients, the incidence of liver function abnormalities reported as adverse experiences was 1.1% (13 of 1142) in patients receiving carvedilol and 0.9% (4 of 462) in those receiving placebo. In patients receiving carvedilol with abnormal liver function tests, the drug should be discontinued. Additionally, it should not be given to patients with preexisting liver disease. Carvedilol should also be used cautiously in those with peripheral vascular disease, diabetes, hypoglycemia, thyrotoxicosis, and those undergoing anesthesia and/or major surgery.[4,5]

Most adverse effects reported were of mild to moderate severity. In clinical trials comparing carvedilol monotherapy with placebo, 4.9% of patients treated with less than 50 mg of carvedilol and 5.2% of patients taking placebo discontinued use because of adverse effects. Discontinuation of therapy because of postural hypotension was more common among patients treated with carvedilol (1% versus zero). The overall incidence of adverse effects increased with increasing doses of carvedilol. For individual adverse events this could only be distinguished for dizziness, which increased in frequency from 2% to 5% as the total daily dose increased from 6.25 mg to 50 mg.[3,9] Coreg has been evaluated for safety in congestive heart failure in more than 1900 patients worldwide, of whom 1300 participated in United States clinical trials. Approximately 54% of the total treated population received carvedilol for at least 6 months, and 20% received carvedilol for at least 12 months. The most common side effect among patients was dizziness (32% of the total U.S treated population). Other common side effects of the United States treated population, listed in order of most severe to least severe, are fatigue, upper respiratory tract infection, chest pain, hyperglycemia, diarrhea, bradycardia, hypotension, nausea, and edema. The incidence of adverse reactions does not differ between patients with heart failure who are 65 years of age and older and those who are younger.

Carvedilol has the potential to interact with a number of medications. Because of carvedilol's extensive oxidative liver metabolism, its pharmacokinetics can be profoundly affected by certain drugs that significantly induce or inhibit oxidation. Carvedilol interacts with rifampin, cimetidine, other inhibitors of cytochrome P450 2D6 isoenzyme, digoxin, calcium channel blockers, antidiabetic medications, clonidine, and cyclosporin. Rifampin, an inducer of hepatic metabolism, can reduce plasma concentrations of carvedilol by 70% when carvedilol is coadministered. In contrast, cimetidine may increase plasma concentrations by 30% in patients receiving carvedilol. Other inhibitors of cytochrome P450 2D6 isoenzyme, such as fluoxetine, paroxetine, propafenone, and quinidine, could expect to increase plasma concentrations in patients receiving carvedilol. The concentration of digoxin is increased by 15% when it is used in combination with carvedilol. As a result, digoxin levels should be closely monitored when a combination of these drugs is used. The combination of carvedilol and calcium channel blockers has resulted in rare conduction disturbances. Carvedilol may mask signs and symptoms of hypoglycemia. Clonidine potentiates the blood pressure and heart rate–lowering effects of β-blockers such as carvedilol. When clonidine is used in combination therapy with carvedilol, carvedilol should always be discontinued first. Last, carvedilol increases cyclosporin concentrations.[3,5,8]

When it is taken with food, the rate of absorption is slowed, but the extent of the bioavailability is not affected. Taking with food minimizes the risk of orthostatic hypotension. No food/drug interactions have been noted.

Studies of carvedilol have shown it to have no carcinogenic effect or mutagenicity, and the no-observed-effect dose level for impairment of fertility was 60 mg/kg/day in adult rats. Carvedilol is in pregnancy category C. There are no adequate and well-controlled studies in pregnant women. Carvedilol should be used during pregnancy only if the potential benefit justifies the potential risk to the fetus. It is not known whether this drug is excreted in human milk. Safety and efficacy in patients younger than 18 years of age have not been established. There were no notable differences in efficacy or the incidence of adverse events between elderly and younger patients.[3,5]

Patient monitoring includes blood pressure determinations, blood glucose concentrations, electrocardiogram determinations, heart rate determinations, hepatic function determinations, and renal function determinations.[1] Weight gain of 0.91 to 1.36 kg above their usual "dry" weight should be reported for possible edema. Additionally, at the first sign of liver dysfunction, perform laboratory testing. If the patient has laboratory evidence of liver injury or jaundice, stop therapy and do not restart.[8]

Dose

In congestive heart failure, an initial oral dose of 3.125 mg twice daily is recommended, and if tolerated, the dose may be doubled every 2 weeks up to a maximum dose of 25 to 50 mg twice daily.[1,3,4] Four strengths of carvedilol are available for use: 3.125 mg, 6.25 mg, 12.5 mg, and 25 mg. Tablets are the only available dosage form. Carvedilol should be taken with food to slow the rate of absorption and reduce the risk of postural hypotension.[4] Dosing must be adjusted to meet the individual requirements of each patient on the basis of clinical response. When carvedilol is discontinued, its dosage should be tapered over a 1- to 2-week period, especially in patients with ischemic heart disease. Only small amounts of carvedilol are excreted unchanged in the urine (less than 1% of the dose), and dosing adjustments are not required in patients with renal insufficiency.

Dosage adjustments are not required in chronic hemodialysis patients. However, dose reductions are suggested in patients with hepatic insufficiency. One study by Neugebauer et al. suggests that carvedilol therapy be initiated with approximately 20% of the normal dose in patients with liver cirrhosis. The manufacturer states that carvedilol should not be administered to patients with liver cirrohosis.[1] If the patient's pulse rate drops below 55 beats per minute, the dosage of carvedilol should be reduced. It may also be necessary to adjust the dosages of the patient's other heart failure medications when carvedilol is introduced. At each dosage increase, the patient should be observed for 1 hour for signs of dizziness or lightheadedness. The maximum recommended dosage of carvedilol is 25 mg twice daily in patients weighing less than 85 kg and 50 mg twice daily in patients weighing 85 kg or more.[8]

Cost

The cost for a 1-month supply of carvedilol is $93 average wholesale price. The price per day for carvedilol is $3 average wholesale price.[12] Because carvedilol is the only β-adrenergic blocking agent with α_1-adrenergic blocking activity currently on the market, it is not possible to perform a cost-benefit analysis of carvedilol with any one individual drug having the same pharmacological effect. Carvedilol, however, can be compared by evaluating the conventional method of therapy for congestive heart failure plus carvedilol with the conventional method of therapy alone. The conventional method of therapy includes digoxin, diuretics, and angiotensin-converting enzyme inhibitors.

In a study by Delea et al.,[13] the cost effectiveness of carvedilol for the treatment of congestive heart failure was examined. The conventional therapy consisted of digoxin, furosemide, and enalapril. They examined the conventional method plus carvedilol versus the conventional method alone and found that the cost-effectiveness of carvedilol for congestive heart failure compares favorably to that of other generally accepted medical interventions, even under the assumptions regarding the duration of therapeutic benefit.[13]

Recommendation

Carvedilol appears to be a useful agent in the management of congestive heart failure. Studies have shown that it has a significant impact on the left ventricular ejection fraction, although its benefit in exercise duration remains questionable. Carvedilol is generally well tolerated, and adverse effects appear to be relatively mild to moderate, with dizziness reported as the most common side effect. An unfavorable aspect of carvedilol is its potential to interact negatively with various other medications such as rifampin, cimetidine, inhibitors of cytochrome P450 2D6 isoenzyme, digoxin, calcium channel blockers, antidiabetic medications, clonidine, and cyclosporin. Carvedilol is available only in tablet forms, and dosing ranges from 3.125 mg to 50 mg twice daily.

When one is measuring cost with therapy, patient morbidity must be heavily considered. At a cost of $3 per day average wholesale price (in addition to the conventional therapy), the progression of congestive heart failure can be delayed, resulting in a potentially longer life for the patient.

Considering this information, carvedilol does appear to be a very useful addition to the standard conventional therapy (digoxin, diuretics, and ACE inhibitors) used in the treatment of congestive heart failure and should be available on formulary.

References

1. USPDI Vol I. Drug Information for the Health Care Professional. Englewood, CO: MICROMEDEX, 1999.
2. McEnvoy GK. American Hospital Formulary Service. Bethesda: American Society of Health-System Pharmacists, 2000.
3. Kastrup E. Drug facts and comparisons. St. Louis: Facts and Comparisons, 2000.
4. Frishman W. Carvedilol. Drug Ther 1998;339:1759–1765.
5. Walsh P. Physicians' desk reference. Montvale, NJ: Medical Economics Company, 2000.

6. Hardman JG, Limbird LE, Molinoff PB, Ruddon RW, Gilman AG, eds. Goodman and Gilman's the pharmacological basis of therapeutics, 9th ed. New York: McGraw-Hill, 1996.
7. Senni M, Redfield M. Congestive heart failure in elderly patients. Mayo Clin Proc 1997;72:453–460.
8. Vanderhoff B, Ruppel H, Amsterdam P. Carvedilol: The new role of beta blockers in congestive heart failure. Am Fam Physician 1998;58:1627–1633,1641–1642.
9. Fisher L, Moye L. Carvedilol and the Food and Drug Administration approval process: an introduction. Contr Clin Trials 1999;20:1–15.
10. Australia/New Zealand Heart Failure Research Collaborative Group. Randomized, placebo-controlled trial of carvedilol in patients with congestive heart failure due to ischaemic heart disease. Lancet 1997;349:375–380.
11. Krum H, Sackner-Bernstein J, Goldsmith R. Double-blind, placebo-controlled study of the long-term efficacy of carvedilol in patients with severe chronic heart failure. Circulation 1995;92:1499–1506.
12. Cardinale V. Redbook, 103rd ed. Montvale: Medical Economics Company, 1999.
13. Delea T, Vera-Llonch M, Richner R. Cost effectiveness of carvedilol for heart failure. Am J Cardiol 1999;83:890–896.

SUMMARY

The skills of drug information, drug literature evaluation, and professional communication are essential components of professional pharmacy practice. Information is always a guiding principle in sustaining the professional's knowledge while opening the door for a better-educated patient. One cannot be expected to have all of the answers stored away in one's brain, but one should be able to use one's skills to find the answer.

QUESTIONS

1. What are the seven steps of the modified systematic approach to drug information?
2. What does it mean to get to the "ultimate" question, and why is the category of the question so vital to a good response?
3. What is the difference among primary, secondary, and tertiary literature?
4. What are examples of internal and external validity?
5. What does it mean when an article states that the results were statistically significant?
6. Name five rules for professional writing.

REFERENCES

1. Host TR, Kirkwood CF. Computer-assisted instruction for responding to drug information requests. Paper presented at the 22nd Annual ASHP Midyear Clinical Meeting, December 1997, Atlanta.
2. Malone P, Mosdell KW, Kier KL, Stanovich J. Drug information: a guide for pharmacists, 2nd ed. New York: McGraw-Hill, 2000.

C H A P T E R 9

PHYSICAL ASSESSMENT SKILLS

Cathy Meier

Goals: After reviewing the information in this chapter, you should be able to:

1. Name four skills used during completion of an examination.
2. Describe how to take a pulse.
3. Describe how to place a sphygmomanometer and the technique for taking a blood pressure.
4. List how to proceed through a physical examination.
5. Describe reasons for positive or negative findings for each part of the examination.

INTRODUCTION

Physical assessment or examination has traditionally been reserved for physicians and nurses. Pharmacists are interpreting laboratory data and exam findings to make recommendations but rarely touch a patient. However, as pharmacy progressively becomes a clinical entity, pharmacists are required to hone their examination skills and have greater interaction with patients. This chapter is by no means meant to teach physical exam skills but to provide clues for pharmacists about the importance of the physical exam and key findings.

BASIC TECHNIQUE

Physical examination employs four main skills for effectively assessing a patient. *Inspection* is the practice of examining a patient with the unaided eye, although instruments may be used in certain situations such as during the examination of the eyes or ears. *Palpation* uses the sense of touch to ascertain normal from abnormal findings. *Percussion* involves using a fingertip to "tap" certain body parts to determine whether the compartment is a solid mass or filled with air or fluid. *Auscultation* often requires the use of a stethoscope to listen for normal or abnormal sounds on a patient.[1-6]

A physical exam is often prompted secondarily by a patient's chief complaint of a certain sign or symptom. Any clinician requires certain background

---

**TABLE 9.1. SAMPLE QUESTIONS TO BE
ASKED OF PATIENTS DURING A HISTORY**

- When did this problem start?
- Describe the symptom. If pain, is it stabbing, burning, sharp, etc.?
- Where on your body is this located? Does it move anywhere else?
- Rate your discomfort on a scale from 1 to 10.
- How long during the day does this last? Is there a time that it is worse than others?
- What do you think is the cause of your discomfort?
- Is this problem associated with any other symptoms?
- What makes the symptom worse? What makes it better?

---

information pertaining to that specific complaint. This is referred to as gathering a history on the patient's complaint. For example, a patient may complain of chest pain, morning knee stiffness, or a runny nose. For each of these symptoms, a practioner will be interested in knowing the onset of the symptom, any other accompanying symptoms, activities that worsen the situation, and activities that palliate or relieve the symptom. A prior history of the symptom is important to deciding on treatment as well as the overall timing of the current episode. Patients can be very helpful and descriptive in discussing their complaints. For instance, a patient will, in most cases, be able to describe the severity and/or quality of his discomfort and where the symptom is occurring or radiating. The patient may also give an explanation as to what he feels is causing the problem. A clinician can use the information gained from the patient along with objective testing performed to better make a therapy decision.[1,3,6] Table 9.1 provides sample questions that aid in gaining a reliable history from a patient.

GETTING STARTED

Being examined by a practioner can be a fear-invoking experience for some patients. Adding nurses, pharmacists, and students into the exam arena can cause a patient's anxiety to climb to high levels. When examining a patient or observing someone else examining a patient, you must always remember the patient's rights. The patient has a right to his or her own modesty and comfort. You, as a clinician, need to be alert, thorough, and deliberate. Always record your or someone else's findings accurately and reexamine if needed. Be interested in the patient; act concerned and nonjudgmental, especially if something abnormal is noted. Use language that the patient will understand. Too often healthcare professionals fall into their own medical jargon and do not realize that the patient does not comprehend what they are saying.[1,2] When beginning your assessment, be up front about your identity and your purpose.

For the patient's comfort, it is important to proceed from top to bottom, minimizing the position changes you require. Always respect the patient's requests within reason. Respect the patient and the situation he or she is in. No one wants to be the "intubated COPD-er in room 165, bed B." Patients deserve your respect and to be referred to as the human beings they are.[4]

PRECAUTIONS

When examining and even when observing, it is very important to use Universal Precautions as defined by the CDC for your protection and the patient's. This information can be found on the CDC's web page, http://www.cdc.gov/. Use gloves at all times when coming into contact with bodily fluids. Gowns as well as a mask should be used during certain procedures to protect against airborne debris. Precautions should be undertaken even if you are only observing a procedure. Once you have finished with a procedure or patient contact, immediately wash your hands to prevent the contamination of other patients. Handle all sharps (needles, lancets, scalpels) with care and dispose of them in designated puncture-resistant containers.[7] As a healthcare professional, it is also very important that you receive the necessary vaccinations and remain up to date with your immunization schedule.[1]

VITAL SIGNS

Before beginning the examination, take notice of the patient's temperature, pulse, blood pressure, and respiratory rate, otherwise known as the patient's vital signs. Height and weight are typically included along with the vital signs. Reporting all values is of paramount importance because the lack of an abnormal value is as important as finding an aberrant value.[3]

Temperature. Temperature can be measured using several different methods including oral, axilla, and rectal. In reporting the specific value, it is very important to indicate the place the temperature was taken (Table 9.2). Any reading in excess of 37.8°C (> 100°F) would be considered a fever.[3]

Pulse. When a pulse is taken, three qualities are typically reported: rate, rhythm, and strength. A normal heart rate falls between 60 and 100 beats per minute (bpm). A reading of less than 60 bpm, bradycardia, can be normal in

TABLE 9.2. NORMAL TEMPERATURE VALUES		
Oral	35.8 to 37.3°C	96.4 to 99.1°F
Axilliary	36.3 to 37.8°C	94.9 to 99.6°F
Rectal	36.3 to 37.8°C	94.9 to 99.6°F

certain patients or can be caused by drugs such as β-blockers. Bradycardia can also signal a disease process such as a conduction deficit or hypothyroidism. A rate above 100 bpm, tachycardia, can be secondary to drugs, anxiety, pain, volume depletion, etc. Rhythm is best assessed with ECG devices but can be generally described by palpating a peripheral pulse. Rhythm is typically described as regular, irregularly regular, or irregularly irregular.[3] A regular rhythm is optimal; irregularly regular could signal a rate disturbance such as atrial flutter. In atrial flutter, the pattern of the rhythm, although abnormal, repeats over and over at the same interval. Irregularly-irregular rhythm means that the rhythm is normal in neither interval or pattern. Atrial fibrillation presents in this manner.[1]

Blood pressure. Blood pressure may vary according to race, sex, and age. Normal readings should fall below 140/90. When a patient has more than one reading above 140/90, this is considered abnormal and should be investigated. Most importantly, proper technique is essential in determining an accurate value. Using a cuff that is too small or too large may overestimate the actual reading.[3]

Respiratory Rate. The respiratory rate is usually measured while the patient's pulse is taken. This technique prevents an inaccurate measurement such as can occur when a patient is aware that his breathing is being watched. Normal values fall between 12 and 16 breaths per minute. Fewer than 12 breaths per minute may indicate drug-induced stupor, for example. Above 16 breaths may indicate anxiety, pain, or a number of cardiac or pulmonary disease states. Normal and abnormal patterns of breathing exist, including Cheyne-Stokes (apnea alternating with maximal deep breaths), which can occur in patients with head trauma or CHF. Kussmaul breathing is a pattern of deep, rhythmic breathing often seen in diabetic ketoacidosis. Kussamaul breathing can also signal a hyperventilatory attempt to correct metabolic acidosis.[3]

REVIEW OF SYSTEMS

The examination and report of the examination always follow a particular order. The examiner starts at the head and works down, saving some jobs for last. When recording the information, follow the same progression used during the exam with a general statement describing the person as an introduction. The following system breakdown is to familiarize you with some key findings as they pertain to specific systems and what to look for as you begin examining patients.[3]

General Appearance

This section of the physical exam describes the patient visually. Included in this section are age, race, and gender. General appearance may also mention nutritional status, distress, and a description of general health. An example would be: "This is a 45 YOWF NAD" (This patient is a 45-year-old white female who presents in no acute distress) or "This is a 24 YO WDWNBM." (This is a well-developed, well-nourished black male).[3]

Skin, Hair, Nails

The skin is the largest organ on the body and can be a great clue into a number of disease states. The most common complaint from patients regarding the skin are rashes, lesions, changes in skin color, itching, and changes in hair or nails. It is important to assess a time frame associated with the complaint and any changes the patient has noticed. Ask about any other systemic side effects the patient may be experiencing in conjunction with the skin condition.[1,4] Evaluate the patient's medication regimen for any drugs that may be causing dermatologic problems. Patients receiving vancomycin may experience flushing and redness with itching, nicknamed "redman syndrome" during an infusion. Tetracyclines, sulfonamides, and quinolones can make people more sensitive to the sun, and patients will often present with sunburns. Exposure to the sun while on amiodarone will cause a blue-gray discoloration of the skin.[3,6,8]

It is important but often forgotten during the examination of a skin disorder to inquire about a travel history, occupational exposure, or any close contacts who may have similar problems.[1]

When a patient complains of skin color changes, it is important to note whether the change is generalized or local. Generalized color changes include jaundice from liver failure or cyanosis from hypoxia. Localized color changes may indicate cancerous changes or simple age spots.[1,2]

Patients who complain about hair or nail problems should be evaluated for environmental exposure, especially if the problem is with the hands.[1] Hair loss can accompany certain neoplastic agents, and it is important to reassure the patient that this is to be expected. Alternatively, patients taking minoxidil or cyclosporin may experience an increase in hair growth. Patients who suffer from hyperthyroidism may complain of very thin, silky hair, a key finding in supporting a hyperthyroidism diagnosis.[3,6] For any skin, hair, or nail complaint, investigate a past medical history to find a link or cause to the problem.

Head Eyes Ears Nose Throat

The examination of the head, ears, eyes, nose, and throat (HEENT) will reveal signs and symptoms of a number of disease states. The examination of the head often employs terms such as normocephalic (normal head), microcephalic (small head), or atraumatic (without trauma).[6] Pay attention to these findings while performing your own examination. When examining the head look for changes in hair growth, nits on the scalps, and lumps. Certain diseases can manifest hallmark signs on the head and face. Patients afflicted with Cushing's syndrome often present with puffy faces, known as moon-pie facies, as a result of excess corticosteroid production. Parkinson's disease is well known for its expressionless, mask-like face. Patients with hyperthyroidism often have characteristic bulging eyes called exophthalmos.[3,6] As you proceed with the examination of the head and face, notice the patient's facial expression; is the patient grimacing in pain, anxious? Is the patient making any involuntary movements? Note the skin and check for lesions, color, texture, and hair.

When a practioner examines the eyes, he tests many different aspects including visual fields, ocular movement, and visual acuity. Typically, the eye exam begins with a standard Snellen test or pocket eye card (Fig. 9.1). Visual acuity measures eyesight at an established distance based on population norms. Acuity is expressed as a fraction (20/20). For example, a Snellen result of 20/40 indicates that this patient sees an object at 20 feet that a normal patient would see at 40 feet. The larger the bottom number, the worse the visual acuity.[2] When testing for acuity, the health care professional may also check the intraocular pressure (IOP) to screen for glaucoma. In addition, the practioner should perform an external eye exam. External structures of the eye include the lid, eyebrows and lashes, and the orbits or eye sockets. Patients may complain of redness, itching, and/or pain in any of the external areas to the eye.[1,3,4]

The ophthalmoscope helps visualize the internal structures of the eye, most importantly the retina. It is also important to examine the fundus and the blood vessels of the retina. By visualizing the blood vessels, one can determine eye damage secondary to uncontrolled disease. As an example, uncontrolled hypertension can cause papilledema, A-V nicking, and striate hemorrhages. The ophthalmic exam can also detect forms of retinopathy caused by diseases such as diabetes or hypertension, which becomes present when these diseases remain uncontrolled. It is very important for patients with hypertension or diabetes to have regular eye exams.[1,3,4]

The most common complaints associated with the eyes are loss of vision, pain, diplopia, tearing, dry eyes, discharge, and redness. If the patient is squinting or tearing, find out if the patient is in pain or experiencing burning in the eyes. The patient may complain about itchy, watery eyes; investigate an allergy history.[1] Note any eye movement that is abnormal. A common sign of anticonvulsant therapy is nystagmus, a fine rhythmic oscillation of the eye, seen especially on extreme movement to the left or right.[8]

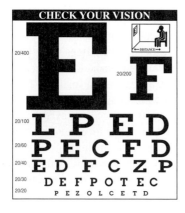

Figure 9.1. Snellen eye chart.

If the patient is experiencing a loss of vision, ascertain whether it was sudden or gradual. If pain is associated with the loss of vision, does light worsen the sensation? Always determine when the last eye exam was to note if a significant change has occurred.[1]

As you move on to the exam of the ear, examine the outer ear for deformities, lumps, and lesions.[1] Check for drainage, pain, and inflammation. If drainage is present, note the color and consistency to assist in diagnosing an infection. Note any hearing aids or devices. Ask questions about earaches, ringing, and dizziness. Ringing in the ears (tinnitus) can be brought on by some medications including aspirin. Also recall that aminoglycosides can damage vestibular and auditory function. Aminoglycosides require strict monitoring and dosing by a pharmacist to prevent these complications.[4]

An ear canal exam, utilizing an otoscope, will visualize the tympanic membrane. Many children present with ear tugging and pain and on examination will have a bulging and red tympanic membrane, suggesting an ear infection called otitis media. Pharmacists can intervene by recommending appropriate antibiotics and medications for symptom control.[1,3]

Many common complaints and reason for visits to a health care professional include nasal congestion and discharge. Patients who have allergies may present with inflamed nostrils, sinus pain, and postnasal drip. Examine both nares (nostrils) to look for these symptoms. Note the color of mucus from the nose. Thick, purulent mucus typically represents infection.[1] Medications can be the cause of a number of common nasal complaints. Warfarin, which is used to prevent the blood from forming unnecessary clots, can cause epistaxis (nose bleeding) if the patient is prescribed more than needed. Overuse of nasal decongestants can cause a condition known as rhinitis medicamentosus.[3]

Check the mouth for sores, tooth and/or gum inflammation, or nodules. Ask if the patient has complaints of dry mouth, hoarseness, or a change in voice, etc.[1] If the patient has mouth sores, review his list of medications. Many chemotherapeutic agents such as methotrexate can cause severe mouth sores called stomatitis. Other medications can cause gingival hyperplasia (gum swelling), including phenytoin and cyclosporin.[8] During the examination have the patient stick out his tongue to examine its symmetry. Look at the area under and around the tongue carefully, as these are common areas for cancerous growth. Note the patient's breath, as the odor can be a clinical clue to certain disease states. Acetone-smelling breath can signal diabetic ketoacidosis, whereas a fishy smell is associated with chronic renal failure. Patients with an infection of the respiratory tract will often have a distinct malodorous breath.[3]

Palpate the neck looking for any unusual lumps, masses, or scars. The patient should be in a relaxed position to facilitate feeling lymph nodes and enlargement. Lymph nodes should not be palpable unless enlarged. Assess the position of the trachea and examine the carotid arteries. Note if the patient is complaining of any pain or stiffness during the exam. If the patient complains of sudden stiffness with headache, refer immediately for emergency care. Neck stiffness with headache can signal meningitis, a medical emergency.[1,3,4]

Respiratory

The respiratory system is made up of the lungs and chest wall working together to support the respiratory needs of the body.[4] The respiratory examination begins by inspecting the chest. Notice the patient's posture, as certain diseases that interfere with posture can also cause difficulty breathing. Watch the patient breathe and appreciate the pattern. Is the patient depending on accessory muscles to breathe somewhat comfortably? Note if breathing is rapid and shallow or slow and irregular. Notice if the patient seems to "favor" one side, called splinting, to protect broken ribs.[6] Patients with chronic obstructive pulmonary disease (COPD) may need to lean forward in order to breathe.[1] COPD patients may also demonstrate clubbed fingers, resulting from years of hypoxia, and may have a thorax that resembles a barrel, referred to as barrel chested. These patients have large, round chests that appear very muscular after years of using all of their thorax muscles to breathe.[4,6] After noting any malformations in appearance, palpate the chest. Note if the patient seems tender in any area. Patients may display crepitus, which feels like packing bubbles when a hand is run over the patient's back. Use percussion to determine the lung composition. Dull sounds usually represent fluid-filled compartments, whereas hyperresonant sounds indicate overinflation.[3,6] Listen to detect any abnormal sounds including wheezing, crackles, or stridor. Note if the patient is coughing and whether it is a dry, hacking cough or a productive "wet" cough. If the patient is coughing up material, record the amount, consistency, and color.[1] Other findings of concern include dyspnea (shortness of breath) and hemoptysis (coughing blood).[2] Find out when the patient last had a PPD test and, if possible, the last chest x-ray. As a pharmacist, it is important to ascertain a smoking history and attempts at smoking cessation. Make sure to check the patient's medication history to make note of any drugs affecting the respiratory system. For example, narcotics can dramatically slow the respiratory rate in an overdose; β-blockers can exacerbate the bronchoconstriction (narrowed airways) seen in asthma, whereas β-agonists improve shortness of breath during an acute asthma exacerbation.[8]

Cardiovascular

The cardiovascular exam employs all four techniques for physical examination, with percussion being used minimally. The examination begins by inspecting the patient to determine the color of skin. Skin can look normal to pale or possibly even blue, denoting lack of oxygen. During inspection, attempt to locate any areas of pulsation.[1] Next palpate the chest for the point of maximal impulse (PMI), located usually at the fifth intercostal space.[4] Murmurs, thrills, and rubs can also be felt on the skin. Murmurs are heard differently than normal heart sounds, as murmurs are longer. Murmurs are caused by turbulent blood flow and can be the result of septal defects, obstructed vessels, dilated vessels, or incompetent valves. When listening to a murmur, it is important to note the time the murmur occurs in the cardiac cycle, the location the murmur is heard at, the "shape" of the mur-

TABLE 9.3. HEART MURMURS	
GRADE	**DESCRIPTION OF MURMUR**
I	Very faint, heard only after listening with stethoscope
II	Quiet, heard immediately after placement of stethoscope
III	Moderately loud
IV	Loud
V	Very loud, possible to hear with stethoscope partly away from chest
VI	Can be heard without the stethoscope

mur, and the quality of the murmur. Murmurs are graded on intensity from I to VI (see Table 9.3).

Thrills are areas palpated on the skin representing areas of turbulence below. Rubs have a "grating" sound, resulting from inflamed tissue rubbing together. Two types of rubs can occur, pericardial and pulmonary. To differentiate between the two, instruct the patient to hold his breath. The pulmonary rub will become silent while holding one's breath, but the pericardial rub will still be audible.[1–3]

Percussion of the cardiac structures will help to identify the left cardiac border, which is near the PMI. Percussion can be used in an attempt to estimate cardiac size.[1]

Auscultation assists in identifying appropriate heart sounds and determining the quality and importance of abnormal sounds. There are four distinct areas for appreciating the various heart sounds. The first area is over the aortic valve, located from the second intercostal space to the apex of the heart. Next, the tricuspid valve is best heard from the lower left sternal border. The mitral valve is best heard around the cardiac apex. Finally, the pulmonic valve is most appreciated in the area of the second and third intercostal space.[2] When listening to the heart, pay attention to the pitch, volume, and duration of heart sounds. Normal heart sounds, S_1 and S_2, are typically referred to as "lub-dub." S_1 represents the closure of the tricuspid and mitral valves. S_2 occurs as the pulmonic and aortic valves close. Two other sounds, S_3 and S_4, can be heard in normal, healthy people but often represent abnormalities.[3,6] In patients older than 30 years of age, S_3 is associated with CHF, and S_4 can result from a noncompliant ventricle. Coronary artery disease is a common cause for a noncompliant ventricle.[6]

If a patient is being assessed for an event of cardiac nature such as a myocardial infarction (heart attack), it is important not only to get objective information including pulse and blood pressure but also obtain a subjective history. Subjective complaints include pain, radiation, and palpitations. Subjectively, patients with CHF may complain of becoming short of breath and requiring more than one pillow to breathe comfortably at night. Patients who are experiencing heart failure may also have systemic signs of disease, manifesting as extremity edema, hepatomegaly, or jugular venous distension.[1,2]

The peripheral vascular exam requires examining the extremities for varicose veins, signs of claudication, or Raynaud's phenomena (digits turn blue on cold exposure). Investigate complaints of calf swelling and tenderness for a possible clot preventing blood flow, known as deep vein thrombosis or DVT, which most likely will require medication to prevent further clotting. Medications such as warfarin or heparin are used in this setting and are referred to as anticoagulants.[3]

For a pharmacist, two important aspects of a good cardiovascular exam include taking an accurate pulse and blood pressure. The radial pulse is the most common site for assessing heart rate. Using the pads of the index and middle fingers, press on the artery until you feel pulsation. Count the number of beats felt over a 15-second time frame. If the pulse is regular in rate and rhythm, multiply the beats by four to find the beats per minute (bpm). If the rhythm is irregular, a cardiac auscultation exam is warranted, as the radial pulse may underestimate the true heart rate. An irregular rhythm can warrant further workup such as an ECG. Determine if the rhythm is regularly irregular, meaning that the rhythm is not a normal pulse rate, but the pattern is consistent, as in atrial *flutter*. Irregularly irregular illustrates a rhythm that is not a normal pulse rate and does not maintain any sort of pattern to the rhythm, as in atrial *fibrillation*.[1,3]

Measuring blood pressure involves use of a sphygmomanometer, a stethoscope, and a cuff. To measure blood pressure, place the cuff around the upper arm and the stethoscope on the artery just below the cuff. It is very important that the cuff is the appropriate size to accurately measure blood pressure. The bag of the cuff should have width that is 40% of the limb circumference, and the length should be 80% of the limb circumference. A cuff that is too short or narrow may give an inaccurately high reading, as does a cuff that is too small for a patient. If you are using a mercury sphygmomanometer, make sure that the column remains vertical, and read the meniscus at eye level. If you are using an aneroid sphygmomanometer, confirm that it has been recalibrated in the recent past. The stethoscope should be placed in the ears with the earpieces facing forward. If the stethoscope has two sides, that is, a bell and a diaphragm, make sure that the side being used is appropriately turned so that sounds will be easily heard[4,9] (Fig. 9.2).

The Joint National Committee released its sixth recommendation on the measurement and treatment of hypertension. Before undergoing a blood pressure measurement, the patient should ideally refrain from smoking and drinking caffeine for 30 minutes. In addition, the patient should rest for 5 minutes before testing, and any tight clothing needs to be loosened. The patient should be sitting flat-footed, and the patient's arm supported. The patient should not cross his or her legs, as this can raise blood pressure. Position the arm so that the artery is at heart level. Support the patient's arm yourself or by using a chair with an armrest. The patient should not support his or her own arm because tensed muscles may raise the blood pressure.

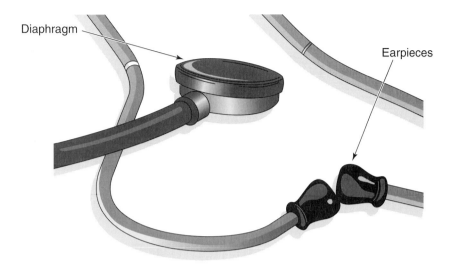

Figure 9.2. Placement of stethoscope.

Begin inflating the cuff while feeling for the radial pulse on the arm. When the radial pulse disappears, add 30 mm Hg to that number and begin deflating the cuff. As the cuff deflates, blood will begin rushing through the artery. When you hear the first pulse, signaling that the blood is flowing again, record that number as the systolic pressure. When the cuff is fully deflated and the pulse disappears again, record that number as the diastolic pressure.[9] Normal readings fall between 100/60 and 140/90, and a single aberrant measure should not be taken as abnormal. Typically, many readings on different days are averaged together to make a diagnosis.[3] Some situations may necessitate measuring the blood pressure in more than one position (i.e., sitting, standing, lying down) or in different limbs. However, repetitive measurement of blood pressure in the same limb can cause venous congestion and lead to inaccurate readings.[4,9]

Breast

Palpation is the most important skill in performing the breast exam. Although a pharmacist may never perform a breast exam, it is important to recognize the unusual. Practitioners will look for lumps, changes in texture and color, and nipple discharge. The most common findings on exam are fibrocystic disease and fibroadenoma. Up to 50% of women have these conditions.[1,4] Inquire when the patient's last mammogram and/or breast exam occurred and note any changes. The American Cancer Society recommends a mammogram annually after the age of 40 with a baseline mammogram done at age 35. If a patient has a family history of breast cancer, annual screening should begin earlier. Women aged 20 to 39 should have a clinical breast exam performed by a physician every 3 years.

RUQ   LUQ

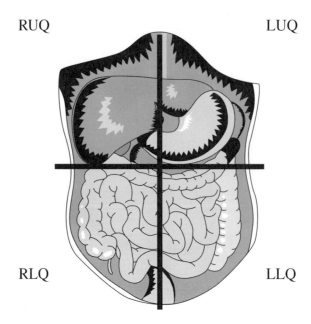

RLQ   LLQ

Figure 9.3. Abdominal quadrants. (From Bates,[2] with permission.)

In addition, the patient should do monthly self-breast examinations.[10] Inquire about the patient's self-exam history and if she has ever felt anything suspicious.

Gastrointestinal

The abdomen is divided into four quadrants to describe the anatomic features (Fig. 9.3). The right upper quadrant (RUQ) contains the liver, gallbladder, pylorus, duodenum, head of the pancreas, right adrenal gland, upper right kidney, hepatic flexure, a portion of the ascending colon, and a portion of the transverse colon. The left upper quadrant (LUQ) houses the left lobe of the liver, spleen, stomach, the body of the pancreas, the left adrenal gland, the upper left kidney, the splenic flexure, and portions of the transverse and descending colons. The lower quadrants contain kidneys, colon, ovaries, fallopian tubes, ureters, spermatic cords, and the uterus and bladder if enlarged. In addition, the appendix can be found in the right lower quadrant (RLQ).[1,3]

There are also nine anatomically descriptive areas on the abdomen used as a "map" to mark various findings (Fig. 9.4). All four aspects of physical exam are employed during examination of the abdomen. It is important to remember as you proceed, however, to auscultate the bowel sounds before percussing or palpating the area, as the latter can influence the sound that will be heard.[6]

Many symptoms associated with the gastrointestinal system are subjective for the patient and can be assessed by questioning. Start by asking about changes

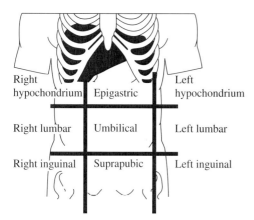

Right hypochondrium	Epigastric	Left hypochondrium
Right lumbar	Umbilical	Left lumbar
Right inguinal	Suprapubic	Left inguinal

Figure 9.4. Anatomic description.

in appetite, nausea, vomiting, or diarrhea. If the patient complains of heartburn, bloating, belching, or reflux symptoms, ask him to quantify the symptoms by using a numbered scale or other device to rate his discomfort. Common concerns for patients include a change in bowel habits or blood in their stool. When blood is present in the stool, you must gain insight into the exact symptomatology. When the blood is bright red, it can be a result of hemorrhoids or lower GI tract malignancy. Dark black, bloody stools, referred to as melena, represent bleeding that is occurring higher in the GI tract. Examine all patients for jaundice, distension, and masses. If jaundice is discovered, investigate the IV history including drugs of abuse, tattoo history, and alcohol consumption, as all can contribute to liver damage.[1] Listen for bowel sounds and the intensity of the sound if present. Bowel sounds should be heard every 5 to 10 seconds as a high-pitched sound. The absence of bowel sounds may represent paralytic ileus, and hyperactive bowel sounds may signal early obstruction. The use of opioid medication can slow bowel sounds considerably and potentially result in obstruction. Record any mention of abdominal pain, colic, and any other significant finding.[4]

Genitourinary

Examination of the genitourinary tract can be an uncomfortable experience for both men and women. It is the examiner's responsibility to remain professional and place the patient at ease to facilitate a thorough exam.

Examining the male genitals involves inspection for abnormalities and palpation for masses and enlargement. Men can present with a number of genitourinary complaints. Common concerns include pain on urination (dysuria), discharge, frequent urination (polyuria), and incontinence.[1] For older men, it is important to ask about hesitancy, dribbling, and strength or size of urine stream, as these questions may assist in diagnosing benign prostatic hypertropy (BPH). Also, men should be questioned about their testicular self-exam history. Inquire whether the patient has swelling, masses, or pain. Most importantly for pharmacists, ensure that the patient is aware that he should do regular exams to prevent any problems in the early stages.[3] Infertility can also impact men, and it is theorized that up to 30% of infertility problems can be linked to the man.[1]

With the evolution of drugs to treat impotence, many men are coming forward to seek help for this condition. Impotence can be described as either erectile or ejaculatory. Causes of impotence can be organic or psychogenic, with the latter accounting for 90% of cases. Diabetes, spinal cord injuries, multiple sclerosis, and direct injury are common organic causes of impotence. Medications to lower blood pressure, especially β-blockers, can cause significant impotence problems and should be investigated when a patient presents with complaints of this nature.[1]

The examination of a woman's genitourinary system involves both an external and internal examination. The outer exam involves noting normal structures and examining for lesions and discharge. The internal examination employs a speculum to visualize the cervix and internal structure and to perform the Pap smear. Women should have regular gynecologic exams every 1 to 3 years, is recommended. It is important to note menstrual history, date of last period, premenstrual symptoms, and quality of menses (heavy versus light, duration, regularity). As a pharmacist, ask about contraception use and satisfaction with this regimen. Ask about any problems with itching, discharge, pain, irregular bleeding, dyspareunia (painful intercourse), and postcoital bleeding. Note any problems the patient has had with fertility and any attempts to correct them.[1,3]

Women present with many of the same urinary complaints as men. Dysuria, polyuria, hematuria, and incontinence are all common complaints from women. Urinary tract infections are more common in women than men and can be easily treated.[1]

A sexual history is very important in both sexes to assess infection risk and need for testing. Although they may be uncomfortable topics, certain areas must be addressed, including number of partners, sexual activity of partners, activities, protection used, frequency, and any problems that may be occurring.[1]

Musculoskeletal

Examining the musculoskeletal system involves inspecting for asymmetry, nodules, masses, and any signs of wasting. When palpating, check for signs of inflammation including warmth, redness, and tenderness. Clinicians will inspect a patient's gait, spine, extremities, neck, and specific joints. Note any abnormalities. For example, rheumatoid arthritis is easily recognized by the deformities on the joints of the hands.[1]

Common complaints attributed to the musculoskeletal system include pain and stiffness, weakness, cramping, back pain, and limited movement. Pharmacists should inquire about methods the patient has used to relieve pain and stiffness, if it helped, and any side effects incurred. Many times, joint difficulties are

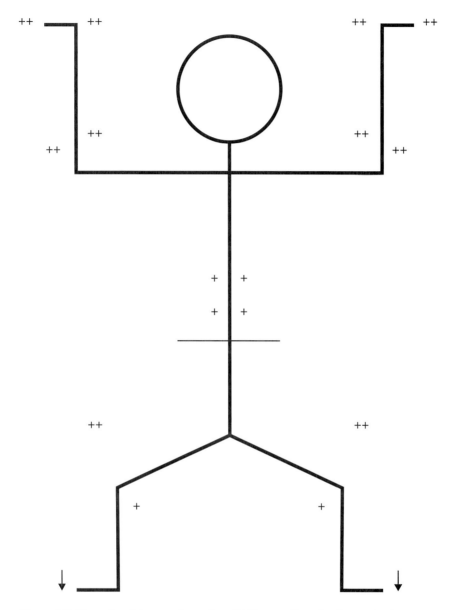

Figure 9.5. Example of deep tendon reflex (DTR) recording. Grading scale: 0 = no response; $+$ = diminished; $++$ = normal; $+++$ = hyperactive; $++++$ = hyperactive, often with clonus.

the result of a previous illness or injury. A good history and physical should contain a thorough investigation of past medical history and evidence of joint- or muscle-damaging incidents.[1]

Neuropsychiatric

A physical exam should involve a complete neurologic exam testing the cranial nerves, deep tendon reflexes (Fig. 9.5), and sensory abilities. Likewise, information may also be gathered as it pertains to seizure history, blackouts, weakness, numbness or tingling, tremors, headaches, or pain. Disturbances in gait, balance, and coordination are also assessed.[1]

The most common neurologic symptom is headache. It is important to discover a pattern or lack thereof to a patient's headaches. Sudden-onset headaches often indicate a serious illness taking place, whereas a constant pain may be indicative of migraines or cluster-type headaches. Other neurologic concerns include loss of consciousness, dizziness, and ataxia. If a patient appears ataxic or complains of feeling "clumsy," carefully check his or her medication profile. A common cause of ataxia is treatment with anticonvulsant drugs.[1]

Part of the neuropsychiatric exam is asking the patient about memory, mood, sleep habits, and overall well-being. The psychiatric exam assesses orientation, consciousness, speech, judgment, memory, and other factors.[4] There are standard tests for memory and orientation available.

Pharmacists can make numerous interventions in the neuropsychiatric exam. Many drugs used in neurologic or psychiatric diseases cause side effects that may only be realized on examination. Examples include nystagmus, gingival hyperplasia, and ataxia and tremor. Patients with COPD taking β-agonists may have a tremor, whereas patients taking a β-blocker may appear sluggish and tired.[8]

PUTTING IT ALL TOGETHER

Always remember before you start the exam to introduce yourself and your purpose. Make the patient as comfortable as possible and begin in an orderly fashion. Minimize the number of position changes and proceed from top to bottom.

Previous sections have described important findings for each of the various organ systems. It is important in the final step to put all the information together in a logical, orderly manner. Most often, an error in examination results not from a lack of knowledge but from a lack of thoroughness and organization. Common errors include failing to detect certain findings, omitting part of an exam, poor technique, misinterpretation of findings, and incorrect recording of information by using improper terms or abbreviations. Illegible handwriting also is a common problem in interpreting an examination.[1]

Using these techniques along with the knowledge gained from systematic description should provide an accurate and thorough physical examination, which will lead to better solving of the patient complaint.

QUESTIONS

1. What is ausculation?
2. What is percussion?
3. What is a normal blood pressure reading?
4. What is one class of medications that causes the finding nystagmus?
5. What is a sphygmomanometer?
6. Why do pharmacists complete a physical examination?

REFERENCES

1. Swartz MH. Textbook of physical diagnosis: history and examination, 3rd ed. Philadelphia: WB Saunders, 1998.
2. Bates B. A guide to physical examination and history taking, 6th ed. Philadelphia: JB Lippicott, 1995.
3. Boh LE. Clinical clerkship manual. Vancouver: Applied Therapeutics, 1993.
4. Tietze KJ. Clinical skills for pharmacists. St Louis: Mosby-Year Book, 1997.
5. Jarvis CM. Perfecting physical assessment: part one. Nursing 1977;7(5):28–37.
6. Lange RL, Calvert JC, Young LY. Physical assessment: a guide for evaluating drug therapy. Vancouver: Applied Therapeutics, 1994.
7. Perspectives in disease prevention and health promotion update: universal precautions for prevention of transmission of human immunodeficiency virus, hepatitis B virus, and other bloodborne pathogens in health-care settings. http://www.cdc.gov/mmwr/preview/mmwrhtml/00000039.htm. September 2000.
8. Lacy CF, Armstrong LL, Lance LL, Goldman MP. Drug information handbook. Hudson: Lexi-Comp, 2000.
9. The sixth report of the Joint National Committee on Prevention, Detection, Evaluation, and Treatment of High Blood Pressure. Bethesda: The National Heart, Lung, and Blood Institute (NHLBI), National Institutes of Health, November, 1997.
10. Breast cancer: detection and symptoms. http://www3.cancer.org/cancerinfo/load_cont.asp?st=ds&ct=5&language=english. September, 2000.

MONITORING DRUG THERAPY

Bruce Parks, Joel R. Pittman, and Kelly Rogers

Goals: After reviewing the information in this chapter, you should be able to:

1. Recognize the role of deductive reasoning in the drug-monitoring process.
2. Know what a patient database is and how it is used to monitor drug therapy.
3. Be able to extract appropriate patient information and integrate it with drug information to formulate a process for monitoring drug therapy.
4. Understand the utility of common calculations used in monitoring drug therapy in a patient, e.g., creatinine clearance, body mass index.
5. Discuss the importance of a chief complaint and history of present illness in monitoring drug therapy.

INTRODUCTION

The purpose of this chapter is to provide some direction primarily for the student who will be beginning his or her first exposure to direct patient care. It will also be helpful for those individuals who already have some experience in this area.

To get the most out of this chapter, prepare yourself to learn to integrate and use your therapeutic and pathophysiology knowledge. Those classroom drug facts along with an understanding of laboratory and diagnostic tests are required to assess and monitor the appropriateness of patient-specific therapeutic regimens. The facts you know must now be used to determine whether the therapeutic regimen is achieving the intended outcome, that is, modification of a disease state to promote cure or mitigation. You must understand the reasons behind treatment failures and what impact this may have on future modifications of the therapy.

Students frequently ask, "What should I read to prepare for your clerkship? A therapeutics text, a pharmacology text, or perhaps specialty journals?" My usual response is none of the above. Your best preparation for this or any other rotation is to read any Sherlock Holmes story. Although this may seem implausible at first, it is actually very sound advice that will stand you in good stead throughout your career. The author of the Sherlock Holmes stories was a physician by training. The methods by which the detective reached his conclusions are illustrative of the type of reasoning taught in medical schools. Sherlock Holmes was a fictional detective in 19th century London who was a proponent of deductive reasoning. This process involves drawing conclusions from general observations. In a clinical venue this is accomplished by combining laboratory and physical data to provide a response to a therapeutic question. For example, it may be observed that a patient with a rising BUN (blood urea nitrogen) and creatinine is being treated with an aminoglycoside antibiotic. With the foregoing information, it could be reasoned that the changes in renal function may be an adverse event produced by the antibiotic. The response is therefore either to make some modification in the dose or frequency of administration of the aminoglycoside or to change to a different class of antibiotic that has the same antibacterial spectrum but does not cause nephrotoxicity.

Monitoring drug therapy is an organized process that provides information necessary to determine whether a patient's therapeutic regimen is achieving the expected outcome or must be changed or adjusted because of a lack of response or undesirable or dangerous adverse drug reactions. Pharmacists must acquire skills in order to interpret certain specific monitoring parameters. These assessment skills combined with pharmacists' knowledge of pharmacokinetics, pharmacotherapeutics, and pharmacoeconomics enhance the ability of the pharmacist to monitor patient outcomes. An understanding of the application and interpretation of laboratory and other diagnostic procedures, such as x-rays, magnetic resonance imaging (MRI), or electrocardiograms (ECG), improves the ability of the pharmacist to assess the patient's condition and provide care. Pharmacists may also be able to enhance patient participation by educating patients on the risks of medication-related problems and how frequent monitoring of key clinical indicators may help reduce those risks.

STEPS FOR MONITORING DRUG THERAPY

When faced with monitoring a patient, the pharmacy student must go through a process of fact finding and collecting data, analyzing the information, drawing conclusions from the information collected, and making recommendations. In order to collect information effectively, the pharmacy student should work to create a patient database (see monitoring form example: Appendix D, Profile 1). Creation of a database helps the student determine what information is pertinent. Using a standardized form helps to organize data in a manner that can be readily retrieved. Information can be obtained from a variety of sources including interviewing the patient, patient's family, or caregiver, patient's chart, past medical records, and/or medication profile. Information can be found as either a hard copy or stored on a computer file in a data bank. From this patient's database, the pharmacy student can make rational decisions about the patient's outcomes, course of treatment, and the medication regimen.

The pharmacy student uses administrative and demographic information as a means of identifying and locating a patient (Fig. 10.1). It will also be used as a means of differentiating patients from each other in case of identical names.

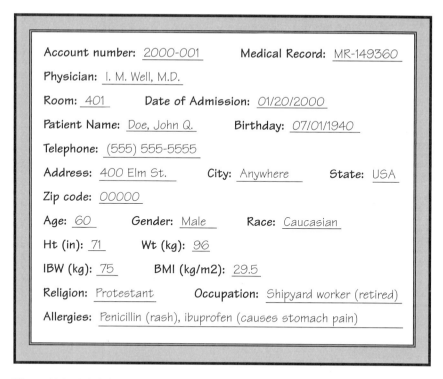

Figure 10.1. Administrative and demographic information.

Account number or medical record number serves as a means of locating infor-
    mation about the patient, such as a patient's older medical record. This is sim-
    ilar to locating a prescription drug profile in the community drug store by us-
    ing a prescription or account number.
Physician or care provider is identified in case the student has questions or rec-
    ommendations about treatment.
Demographic information including items such as name, address, and telephone
    number may be helpful in identifying and contacting the patient.
Age and gender are useful to distinguish male from female patients (for exam-
    ple, for hormone replacement therapy). It is helpful to identify the patient as
    being either pediatric or geriatric. These patients may have altered pharmaco-
    kinetics and pharmacodynamics (Table 10.1).
Religion and occupation may be important in cases where religious beliefs con-
    flict with medical treatment (i.e., Jehovah's Witness patients will not receive
    a blood transfusion). Occupational information may be an important part of
    the patient's history, as it may reveal exposure to toxins (for example, ship-
    builder's exposure to asbestos, painter's exposure to lead, etc.).
Race is relevant because certain medications may not work in specific ethnic
    groups. For example, β-blockers have been shown to be less effective in

TABLE 10.1. AGE-RELATED CHANGES IN DRUG PHARMACOKINETICS

PHARMACOKINETIC PHASE	PHARMACOKINETIC PARAMETER
Gastrointestinal absorption	Unchanged passive diffusion and no change in bioavailabilty for most drugs → Active transport and ↓ bioavailability for some drugs → First-pass effect and ↑ bioavailabilty
Distribution	→ Volume of distribution and ↑ concentration of water-soluble drugs ↑ Volume of distribution and ↑ half-life for fat-soluble drugs ↑ or ↓ Free fraction of highly plasma protein-bound drugs
Hepatic metabolism	→ Clearance and ↑ half-life for some phase I oxidation drugs → Clearance and ↑ half-life of drugs with high extraction ratio
Renal excretion	→ Clearance and ↑ half-life of renally eliminated drugs

254

TABLE 10.2. CALCULATION OF BODY WEIGHT, MASS, AND SURFACE AREA

Ideal Body Weight (IBW)

Male   IBW (kg) = 50 kg + (2.3 kg × height in inches over 60 inches)

Female   IBW (kg) = 45.5 kg + (2.3 kg × height in inches over 60 inches)

Body Mass Index (BMI)

$$BMI\ (kg/m^2) = (weight\ in\ kilograms)/(height\ in\ meters)^2$$

Body Surface Area (BSA) BSA (m^2) =

$$\sqrt{height\ in\ centimeters \times weight\ in\ kilograms\ /3600}$$

African-Americans. Certain ethnic groups have been shown to be poor metabolizers; they are deficient in their ability to oxidize a substrate. Poor metabolizers will not be able to metabolize certain medications well and accumulate medication, resulting in elevated serum concentrations and an increased risk of adverse effects. Extensive metabolizers are persons able to metabolize certain medications rapidly and therefore do not respond to normal doses.

Weight and height permit calculation of ideal body weight (IBW), body mass index (BMI), or body surface area (BSA) (Table 10.2). Ideal Body Weight and Body Surface Area may be important in calculation of the appropriate dose of medication for a patient. Body Mass Index (BMI) is a measurement that estimates a person's body fat. In general, a person is considered obese if he has a BMI of 27 or more.

Allergy information describes both drug and nondrug items that the patient cannot tolerate or that produces a reaction. Allergy can range from minor symptoms such as nasal stuffiness or mild rash to more serious symptoms such as anaphylaxis. It is important for the student to inquire not only about the causes of an allergic reaction but a description of the patient's reaction after exposure to the allergen. You must be able to distinguish between a true allergic reaction and an intolerance or adverse effect to medication. For example, a patient with a true allergy to a medication may break out in a rash, experience swelling, complain of itching of the skin, or describe a difficulty in breathing. This is different from a patient who describes having intolerance to or experiences an adverse effect of medication. In Fig. 10.1, the administrative and demographic information, patient John Doe has listed a true allergy to penicillin. However, the ibuprofen problem is not to be considered a true drug allergy because stomach pain is considered a side effect.

The *chief complaint* is the primary problem that the patient is experiencing. It is usually written in the patient's own words. The student needs to interview the

TABLE 10.3. CHIEF COMPLAINT AND HISTORY OF PRESENT ILLNESS

CC: "My chest is hurting, and it is hard to breathe"

HPI: John Doe is a 60-year-old Caucasian man who presents to the Emergency Department with substernal chest pain that feels as if someone is squeezing his chest. The pain is also radiating down his left arm. The pain began approximately 2 hours ago, while he was raking his yard. Pain was not relieved with rest or nitroglycerin 0.4 mg tablets $\times$ 1, which he swallowed with a glass of water. The patient states, "I always keep these pills with me" and points to a small metal container, which he keeps in his shirt pocket.

patient, family, or caregivers to ask specific questions about the patient's symptoms (Table 10.3).

The *history of present illness* (Table 10.4) describes when the symptoms started, quality, location, concurrent symptoms, what causes the symptoms to worsen, what causes the symptoms to be lessened or relieved, and what the patient has done to relieve the symptoms (including prescription or OTC medication).

The chief complaint and the history of present illness are essential in helping to determine the diagnosis. Appropriate diagnosis aids in selection of appropriate therapy including medication. In addition, problems with the medication therapy may be uncovered. From the information contained in Table 10.3, the student should make a note to counsel the patient on proper use of the nitro-

TABLE 10.4. QUESTIONS CONCERNING PATIENT SYMPTOM(S)

1. Have the symptom(s) occurred before?
2. When did the symptom(s) begin?
3. How long have the symptom(s) been going on?
4. Can you identify where the symptom(s) occur most frequently or have the most pain associated with them?
5. Does anyone else in the household have similar symptom(s) or is there a history of any relatives having these symptom(s)?
6. Does anything cause the symptom(s) to occur or worsen?
7. Does anything cause the symptom(s) to lessen or go away (including medication therapy)?
8. Are there any other associated signs or symptoms (for example, radiating pain, numbness, nausea/vomiting)?

TABLE 10.5. PAST MEDICAL HISTORY

Past Medical History: Hypertension (15 years' duration), Hyperlipidemia (7 years' duration), myocardial infarction (7 years ago)

Surgical History: Cardiac catheterization 7 years ago with percutaneous transluminal coronary angioplasty (PTCA)

glycerin tablets. Counseling includes the proper placement of the medication (sublingual not oral), proper dosing (every 5 minutes until a maximum of three tablets are taken), the need for proper storage, and when to seek emergency treatment.

The *past medical and surgical history* (Table 10.5) lists past and present medical conditions, including any surgeries performed. You must be aware of what concomitant conditions may cause or worsen the patient's acute problem. For example, John Doe has a past history of hypertension, hyperlipidemia, and myocardial infarction that may cause or worsen the chest pain. In addition, you now have a list of diagnoses, and drug regimens and goals of therapy can be formulated. You may increase efficiency by targeting multiple diagnoses with a single drug treatment.

Chronic illnesses may have a *genetic influence* resulting in higher incidences of disease within a family. You should investigate the patient's history or interview the patient, family, or caregiver about any significant past illness or cause of death in any primary family member (Table 10.6). It is important to include the age at which a family member died because it may constitute a risk factor for a disease and therefore be of significance in determining drug therapy. For example, John Doe has an additional risk factor for coronary heart disease because of his father's death at age 54 from an acute myocardial infarction.

The *social history* or *life style* section (Table 10.7) contains information about the patient's living environment, social habits, and financial information, including insurance and prescription drug plan information. This section identifies nondrug treatments that have been tried in the past. Social habits that may improve or worsen the patient's condition such as diet, exercise, use of alcohol,

TABLE 10.6. FAMILY HISTORY

Family History: Father died of acute myocardial infarction at age 54. Mother, age 82, has a history of hypertension, hyperlipidemia, and cardiomyopathy. Patient has two brothers, both with a + history of atherosclerosis and coronary heart disease. One brother with myocardial infarction at age 62.

TABLE 10.7. LIFE STYLE AND SOCIAL HISTORY

Social History:	Patient lives with wife of 36 years. Has two children no longer living at home. Retired from local shipyard, where he was employed as a welder. Patient has insurance and prescription plan through former employer.
Diet:	2-g low sodium, low cholesterol diet
Alcohol use:	three to four 12-ounce beers per day
Tobacco use:	cigarette use 40-pack-year history (1 pack per day × 40 years)
Caffeine use:	eight to 10 cups of coffee per day. Two to three glasses of iced tea with meals
Exercise:	occasional yard work

tobacco, caffeine, illicit drugs, and sexual history may be identified in this section. Remember that drug therapy is only a part of the patient-monitoring process. Pharmacists play a key role in prevention of disease as well as treatment.

The social history and life style section noted in Table 10.7 shows that John Doe is retired; however, he does have health insurance and a prescription drug plan through his old employer. This patient is on a low-sodium and low-cholesterol diet for treatment of his hypertension and hyperlipidemia. Exercise is minimal, with only occasional yard work. In addition, John Doe continues to use alcohol, tobacco, and caffeine in excess amounts. The pharmacy student should counsel this patient on the identified problems. John Doe may have improvement in his illnesses with adherence to a planned schedule of diet, exercise, cessation of smoking, and moderate use of caffeine and alcohol (see Profile 1, Appendix D).

The *physical exam* (Table 10.8) notes any physical findings that serve as objective evidence of a disease or condition.

TABLE 10.8. PHYSICAL EXAM

General:	Moderately obese WM, somewhat anxious, A&O × 3
Heart	RRR, w/o MRG. C/o SOB, denies orthopnea, DOE, or PND, no JVD
Lungs	CTA bilaterally. No rales or rhonchi, c/o nausea associated with CP, denies N/V
CXR	Heart is slightly enlarged. Clear lung fields
ECG	NSR, HR 75, nonspecific ST segment changes in inferior leads
ECHO	—

TABLE 10.9. REASONS FOR USING CLINICAL LABS AS MONITORING TOOLS

1. **Diagnostic:** indicates the presence of disease or health problem. For example, elevated fasting glucose levels may indicate the presence of diabetes.
2. **Baseline:** measurements before initiation of drug therapy. For example, hepatic liver enzyme measurement before starting antihyperlipidemic therapy with HMG-CoA enzyme inhibitors (such as pravastatin).
3. **Monitor:** indicates the progress toward therapeutic goals. For example, decreased total cholesterol and low-density lipoprotein and increased high-density lipoprotein, elevated prothrombin time with warfarin.
4. Adjustment of medication dose indicated by decreased renal or hepatic functioning.
5. Toxic or subtherapeutic concentration of medication.

Clinical laboratory tests along with other monitoring exams, such as the physical exam, x-rays, electrocardiograms (ECG), and magnetic resonance imaging (MRI), are important monitoring indicators (Table 10.9). This information is an important source of objective information. It is important for the pharmacy student to recognize and understand the consequences of abnormal laboratory values in order to make sound decisions concerning medication therapy. In addition, findings from other diagnostic exams, such as x-rays, ECG, and MRI, may indicate a need for medication therapy, track the progress of drug therapy in treating disease, and serve as a monitor for any toxic or adverse effects of medication.

Timing of the laboratory sample may be important; it does make a difference to know when a laboratory sample is drawn. Timing may be critical to the validity of the exam. Laboratory tests are usually drawn fasting or nonfasting. Fasting describes a laboratory sample that is taken from a patient who has not had anything to eat or drink (except water) for at least 9–12 hours. A fasting laboratory sample is usually taken in the morning after a patient awakens. For example, a fasting lipid profile would be more valuable than a nonfasting laboratory sample in determining elevated serum cholesterol. A fasting glucose would be used as a diagnostic tool for diabetes mellitus.

Timing of a laboratory sample is especially critical when sampling drug serum concentrations and may be crucial when a patient is taking a medication with a narrow therapeutic index. A peak level describes a drug serum concentration that is taken after the dose is given and represents the medication's maximum serum concentration. A trough level describes the lowest point of serum concentration of a medication and is taken just before the next dose of medication.

TABLE 10.10. SELECTED THERAPEUTIC RANGES

DRUG	THERAPEUTIC RANGE
Digoxin	0.9–2 ng/mL
Lidocaine	1.5–5 μg/mL
Procainamide/*N*-acetylprocainamide	10–30 μg/mL (total)
Quinidine	2–5 μg/mL
Amikacin	20–30 μg/mL (peak)
	< 5 μg/mL (trough)
Gentamicin, tobramycin, netilmicin	5–10 μg/mL (peak)
	< 2 μg/mL (trough)
Vancomycin	25–35 μg/mL (peak)
	5–10 μg/mL (trough)
Chloramphenicol	10–20 μg/mL
Lithium	0.6–1.4 mEq/L
Carbamazepine	4–12 μg/mL
Ethosuximide	40–100 μg/mL
Phenobarbital	15–40 μg/mL
Phenytoin	10–20 μg/mL
Primidone	5–12 μg/mL
Valproic acid	50–100 μg/mL
Theophylline	10–20 μg/mL
Cyclosporin	150–400 ng/mL (blood)

The use of serum concentrations to monitor drug therapy and make predictions about the absorption, distribution, metabolism, and excretion of a medication is identified as pharmacokinetics. Therapeutic drug monitoring is performed on medications that have a narrow therapeutic index and thus a narrow margin of safety (Table 10.10). Drugs considered to have a narrow therapeutic index must be monitored more frequently than medications that have a wide margin of safety.

Use of specific laboratory tests will also aid in making decisions about proper dosing. Assessment of renal function can be performed using chemistry tests of blood urea nitrogen (BUN) and serum creatinine. Determining the creatinine clearance helps select the proper dosing for medications that are eliminated primarily by renal mechanisms.

Likewise, review of laboratory tests that are specific for hepatic function would indicate a need for dosage adjustment for medications that are primarily eliminated by hepatic mechanisms. Laboratory tests that are specific for hepatic function include lactate dehydrogenase (LDH), aspartate aminotransferase (AST), alanine aminotransferase (ALT), and bilirubin.

TABLE 10.11. ESTIMATED CREATININE CLEARANCE: COCKROFT AND GAULT FORMULA

Estimated creatinine clearance (Cl_{cr}) (mL/min)

$$\text{Male} = \frac{(140 - \text{age}) \times \text{IBW (kg)}}{(72 \times \text{serum creatinine})}$$

Female = estimated creatinine clearance (Cl_{cr}) for male $\times$ 0.85

CASE EXAMPLE: PROFILE 1

John Doe (Appendix D) was admitted to the emergency department with a tentative diagnosis of acute angina. Several laboratory and diagnostic tests aid in clarifying the diagnosis and rule out other potential causes. In this case, acute myocardial infarction is a condition that must be ruled out. In order to help clarify the diagnosis, an electrocardiogram was performed, which showed signs of ischemia but no evidence of myocardial infarction. Laboratory tests that help rule out myocardial infarction included creatine kinase (CK) and its specific isoenzyme CK-MB, lactate dehydrogenase (LDH) and its specific isoenzyme LDH-1, and aspartate aminotransferase (AST). Other clinical markers include serum myoglobin and troponin.

Renal function is estimated using the blood urea nitrogen (BUN) and serum creatinine. In the case example, estimation of the creatinine clearance using the Cockcroft and Gault formula (see Table 10.11) for John Doe would be approximately 76 ml/min. This creatinine clearance value represents adequate renal function and no need for adjustment of any medication that is renally eliminated.

Calculation of the low-density lipoprotein (LDL) fraction using the Friedwald equation (Table 10.12) and laboratory values obtained from the lipid profile reveals a calculated LDL of 174 mg/dL.

According to the guidelines from the third report of the National Cholesterol Education Program, John Doe has multiple risk factors for coronary

TABLE 10.12. LDL CHOLESTEROL CALCULATION

Calculation of LDL choleterol using the Friedwald equation:

$$\text{LDL} = \text{total cholesterol} - \left(\text{HDL} + \frac{\text{TGL}}{5} \right)$$

heart disease. Treatment for hyperlipidemia is necessary because his LDL is ≥ 160 mg/dL. In order to meet his treatment goal for hyperlipidemia, John Doe's LDL goal for treatment with medication needs to be <130 mg/dL. In addition, his HDL is low (<40 mg/dL) and his Triglycerides are 380 mg/dL (Goal is <150 mg/dL).

Vital signs are used to:

1. Help diagnose disease. Abnormal vital signs such as elevated blood pressure, temperature, pulse, respiration rate, or body weight may indicate the presence of disease.
2. Track progression of a patient toward his or her therapeutic goal. Decreased blood pressure, temperature, pulse, or respiratory rate may indicate an improvement in a patient's condition. This may indicate that the patient is responding to the prescribed treatment.

CASE EXAMPLE: PROFILE 1

A review of the patient's vital signs indicates that John Doe has a blood pressure that is slightly elevated. Because this patient has a history of long-standing hypertension, monitoring the blood pressure is in order for you to determine if the current antihypertensive medication regimen is effective. The student may note the elevated blood pressure on a list of potential problems. In establishing a patient-specific monitoring plan, the pharmacy student must make sure that patients are receiving the most rational, appropriate, and cost-effective form of therapy. A review of the patient's medication regimen (Fig. 10.2) is important in establishing any problems that the patient may have.

There are a number of questions that the student should ask about the patient's medication regimen.

1. Is the drug being used for an appropriate diagnosis or indication? Knowing the diagnosis establishes a basis for selection of an appropriate medication. Some medication is used for off-label purposes. You should review scientific literature for evidence of efficacy.
2. Is the dose of the medication appropriate for this specific patient? Take into account patient characteristics such as age, weight, sex, ethnic background, and allergies as well as concurrent disease states and medications used. Is the duration of treatment appropriate?
3. What are the most likely adverse effects caused by this medication? Does the patient exhibit any of these adverse effects?
4. Are there any interactions with other medications or diseases that the patient may have? Is the patient taking each medication at the appropriate time?

Current Medications

Start Date	Medication/Route	Dose/Schedule	Stop Date	Diagnosis
06/15/93	EC Aspirin /po	81 mg daily (7 am)		Post-MI / platelet inhibitor
09/28/96	pravastain/po	20 mg daily (7 am)		Hyperlipidemia
11/02/94	Nitroglycerin transdermal patch	5 mg/24 hr (7 am)		Angina
10/18/90	Atenolol/ po	50 mg daily (7 am)		Hypertension
03/25/94	Amlodipine/ po	5 mg daily (7 am)		Hypertension
06/15/93	Nitroglycerin / sl	0.4 mg prn q 5min for chest pain (max 3 tablets)		Angina
	Acetaminophen/po	500 mg 2 tabs prn		Pain/headache

Time Line – circle actual administration times and record appropriate medications and meals below

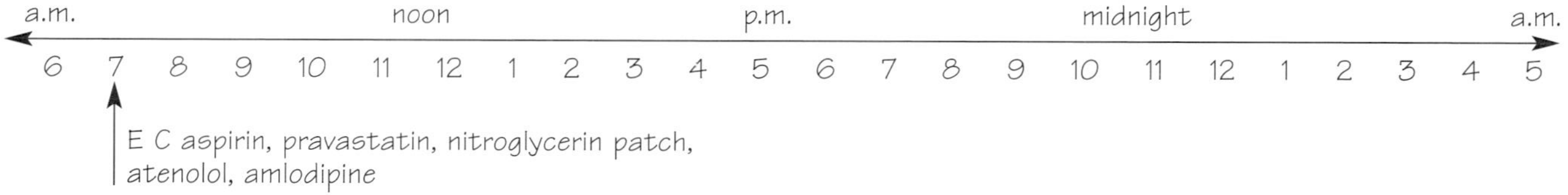

a.m.

6 7 8 9 10 11 12 1 2 3 4 5 6 7 8 9 10 11 12 1 2 3 4 5

noon   p.m.   midnight   a.m.

E C aspirin, pravastatin, nitroglycerin patch, atenolol, amlodipine

Figure 10.2. Medication Profile Review.

263

5. Are there any patient-specific barriers to taking this medication? Is the medication affordable? Are the instructions for use easy to understand? Are there devices that must be used with the medication (syringes, inhalers) about which the patient must be counseled?

6. What proof do you have that the medication is effective? Medication effectiveness can be determined by subjectively asking the patient if their disease has improved, such as pain relief. Objective evidence would include assessment tests or instruments, or improvement of vital signs, diagnostic tests, or laboratory parameters.

Drug interactions and adverse effects present a health risk to patients and a challenge to pharmacists. Patients at high risk for drug interactions and adverse effects include the chronically ill, older, and frail patient, patients with multiple medications, critical-care patients, and patients undergoing high-risk surgery. Adverse effects can be caused by several factors:

1. Characteristic of the medication or drug class, as in gastrointestinal bleeding caused by nonsteroidal antiinflammatory drugs (NSAIDs), hyperglycemia associated with niacin therapy.

2. Characteristic of a toxic effect of a medication. Inhibition of the cytochrome P450 hepatic enzyme system (Table 10.13) will result in increased concentration of medication and a greater risk for toxic adverse effects, as in bradycardia caused by a serum digoxin concentration greater than 2 ng/mL.

3. Decreased concentration of the medication. For example, worsening seizures caused decreased seizure control by a low serum phenytoin concentration.

4. Induction of the cytochrome P450 hepatic enzyme system (Table 10.13), resulting in decreased concentrations of the medications. For example, decreased carbamazepine serum concentration resulting in worsening seizures. Carbamazepine induces its own metabolism in the liver, resulting in lower serum concentrations of the medication.

5. Interference with one medication by another medication. This includes effects such as protein binding, chelation, interference with absorption, interference with elimination, or one medication counteracting another medication.

6. Drugs with similar adverse effects act synergistically to increase the risk of an adverse effect. For example, combined use of a nonsteroidal antiinflammatory agent and aspirin that results in symptoms of gastrointestinal ulceration.

As the number of medications used to treat disease in a patient increases, the risk of drug–drug interactions also increases. Anticipation of adverse effects and educating the patient or caregiver about adverse effects and drug–drug interactions will result in increased awareness and correction or avoidance of any potential problems. Make every effort to counsel the patient and caregivers extensively about the most common side effects and less common side effects that may require alteration of the drug regimen.

TABLE 10.13. CYTOCHROME P450 ENZYME FAMILY AND SELECTED SUBSTRATES
(Taken with permission from Dipiro 4th ed. Table 3-3 p. 29)

CYP1A2	CYP2C9	CYP2C19	CYP2D6	CYP2E1	CYP3A4
Acetaminophen	Diclofenac	Diazepam	Codeine	Ethanol	Alfentanil
Antipyrine	Hexobarbital	Mephenytoin	Debrisoquine	Isoniazid	Alprazolam
Caffeine	Ibuprofen	Omeprazole	Dextromethorphan		Astemizole
Tacrine	Naproxen		Encainide		Carbamazepine
Theophylline	Phenytoin		Fluoxetine		Cisapride
R-Warfarin	Tolbutamide		Haloperidol		Cyclosporine
	S-Warfarin		Loratadine		Diltiazem
			Metoprolol		Erythromycin
			Paroxetine		Felodipine
			Propafenone		Fluconazole
			Risperidone		Itraconazole
			Thioridazine		Ketoconazole
			Venlafaxine		Lidocaine
					Lovastatin
					Midazolam
					Nifedipine
					Qunidine
					Simvastatin
					Tacrolimus
					Terfenadine
					Verapamil

CASE EXAMPLE: PROFILE 1

A review of John Doe's medication profile indicates a need for adjustment of his drug therapy.

Timing of Medication

Changing the dose of pravastatin 20 mg daily from 7 a.m. to bedtime (9 p.m.) will increase the effectiveness of lowering the total cholesterol and low-density lipoprotein (LDL). John Doe should be counseled on intermittent use of the nitroglycerin patch. Application of the nitroglycerin patch for 10 to 12 hours with a nitrate-free interval of 12 to 14 hours will improve this patient's exercise tolerance by decreasing the risk of nitrate tolerance. The enteric-coated aspirin may need to be scheduled at mealtime in order to decrease the risk of abdominal pain.

Adverse Effects

John Doe should be monitored for the following adverse effects:

Enteric-coated aspirin: signs or symptoms of gastrointestinal bleeding or abdominal pain, increased bleeding or bruising.
Pravastatin: gastrointestinal upset, headache, dizziness, muscle pain.
Nitroglycerin transdermal patch: rash, dizziness, hypotension, increased heart rate.
Atenolol: decreased heart rate, hypotension, dizziness, fatigue, constipation, cardiac arrhythmia, edema, heart failure.
Amlodipine: hypotension, flushing, increased heart rate, heart failure, palpitations, chest pain, dizziness, vertigo, unsteady gait, nausea, constipation, loose stools, taste changes.
Acetaminophen: rash, hypersensitivity reactions.

John Doe should be counseled on the most common adverse effects of the medication and ways to prevent these adverse effects.

Proper Use of Medication

Counsel the patient on how to store and use the sublingual nitroglycerin tablets and when to seek medical assistance. Warning the patient to not take more than 4 g of acetaminophen daily will decrease his risk of hepatic injury.

Monitoring Parameters

Monitoring parameters include vital signs, episodes of chest pain, and exercise tolerance.

PUTTING IT ALL TOGETHER

Use of multiple medications requires the integration of individual drug-monitoring plans. This can be achieved by creation of a master flow sheet. A flow sheet specifies a parameter (such as blood pressure) and notes all the medications with the potential for causing a problem.

You should monitor a patient's response to drug therapy continuously by assessing both subjective and objective data. If the patient's response to drug therapy is appropriate, then no alteration of the drug regimen is indicated. Sometimes, a reduction in the dose of medication may be warranted. If the drug regimen does not achieve the desired therapeutic goal or is associated with adverse side effects or toxicities, then an alteration of the therapeutic regimen is indicated (Table 10.14).

Failure of a patient to obtain a therapeutic goal can be related to numerous factors: noncompliance to the drug regimen, inadequate dose of medication, drug–drug interactions, or drug–disease interactions. Each of these aspects needs to be considered. It is important that the pharmacist investigate all pharmacologic and nonpharmacologic reasons why a patient's therapeutic outcome is not achieved.

Decisions to alter the therapeutic regimen are indicated by the response of the patient. Once a new therapeutic plan is decided on, then the process of monitoring drug therapy is started over with new monitoring parameters being set for each patient. Remember that monitoring is based on each individual case. Every patient will have different characteristics and circumstances surrounding him or her. Understanding the process of how to monitor a patient will lessen the chance of missing key information.

Following are a couple of cases for you to use as practice for all of the aforementioned principles.

TABLE 10.14. POSSIBLE OUTCOMES FOR THERAPEUTIC MONITORING

1. Therapeutic regimen provides the expected outcome for the patient. Therapeutic regimen is continued.
2. Therapeutic regimen does not provide the expected clinical outcome.
   a. Dose of current regimen must be increased.
   b. Adjunctive agent is added to current drug regimen.
   c. Current drug regimen is stopped and an alternative agent is started.
3. Therapeutic regimen produces an adverse or unwanted condition. Reduction or discontinuation of current dose or use of an alternative agent should be considered.

PATIENT CASE 1

RN is an 18-m/o WF who presents with a 2-day history of cough and rhinorrhea. Her mother says she "feels warm and has a fever." On examination, she is noted to be fussy and irritable. Vital signs are: T 101°F, RR 24, P 88. Pneumatic otoscopy findings include decreased excursions and a red and inflamed tympanic membrane. She had been treated with amoxicillin for acute otitis media 6 months ago.

Determine the Therapeutic Goal

Cure of the Infection (Acute Otitis Media)

This is the easy part—cure the child, and all else resolves. Because the only way to definitively determine the cause of the infection is to culture a sample from the site of the infection (which in this case would require a myringotomy to obtain middle-ear fluid), the decision about treatment in this case is based on clinical judgment. Although most episodes of acute otitis media are not bacterial, her prior history of AOM would suggest that it would be prudent to treat with antibiotics. The question is, which antibiotic? The Ersatz Pharmaceutical representative was just in the office and left samples of Gorillacillin that treats 75 different organisms. How do you decide between it and amoxicillin?

1. What are the most likely organisms that cause AOM?
2. What are the adverse effects of potential agents?
3. What are the costs (not just acquisition cost)?
4. What dosage forms are available?
5. How often must the drug be given?
6. What patient factors need to be considered?
   a. Are immunizations up to date?
   b. Is the parent likely to give the drug appropriately?
   c. Is there a history of allergy to antibiotics?

Relief of Symptoms (Pain, Fever, Cough)

Cough and fever are natural responses to irritants and infections. Both are innate protective mechanisms designed to help the host get rid of the offending agent. It is probably preferable not to treat these symptoms separately, as they will resolve with cure of the infection. However, from a purely practical standpoint, most parents (or healthcare providers) are not willing to not relieve the cough and fever. What considerations are involved in selecting therapy?

1. Is the cough severe enough that it keeps the child or parents awake?
2. Is the cough dry or productive?
3. Is one antipyretic more effective than another?
4. Are there nonpharmacologic alternatives?

The symptoms produced by AOM are not specific to the disease state. Instead, they are really clinical signs as noted above. The best indicator in this case is the child herself. If the antibiotic therapy is effective, she will return to her normal personality and routine.

What Is the Patient's Response to Therapy?
Evaluate in 24 to 48 hours.

1. Getting better
    a. Make no change in therapy.
    b. Continue full course of therapy—this is dependent on the specific antibiotic chosen, usually 10 days but may be less.
2. No change—reassess
    a. Is it nonadherence?
    b. Inadequate dose?
        i.   Not high enough
        ii. Not administered frequently enough
    c. Natural history of the disease, e.g., it takes a little longer to resolve
    d. Wrong drug or resistance?

Your response depends on what you believe to be the reason for the lack of response. Education of the caregiver (course of AOM, necessity for accurate dosing, frequency of dosing), adjustment of dosage, or change in therapy may be warranted.

3. Getting Worse
    a. Ask the same questions as for no change
    b. Possible concurrent, unrelated illness

The modification of therapy is based on the assessment. The most likely cause of drug failure is nonadherence. This should not be taken to imply child abuse or indifference. It is almost always a consequence of incomplete understanding of the purpose of the treatment and the consequences of not completing the full course of therapy. It could also be the result of a misunderstanding of the proper storage and administration of the drug. In both cases, the pharmacist is in the best position of health care professionals to address these issues. The importance of adequate education of patients and their caregivers cannot be overstressed. It may also be necessary to change therapy by adjusting the dose or frequency of the current drug or changing or adding another drug.

Adverse Effects
Adverse effects associated with antibiotic therapy can be broken into two primary categories. The first and of most concern is an allergic reaction. The most common presentation is an urticarial rash. Fortunately, this is very uncommon and may not require any intervention. However, it is often

difficult to distinguish between nonallergic and allergic rashes, so it may be better to discontinue the antibiotic and change to another chemically unrelated agent, especially since there are many alternatives.

The second and far more likely adverse effects are related to the GI tract and include diarrhea and diaper rash. In many cases they may be self-limited, and no change is necessary, or in the case of diaper rash topical therapy may be sufficient. Diarrhea is an undesirable but not catastrophic consequence and is best left untreated. The administration of a lactobacillus preparation, or eating yogurt with active yeast cultures, although of no proven benefit, is innocuous and provides some comfort to the parents.

How Is the Therapy Modified as a Consequence of the Assessment?

Modification of the therapy as related to lack of efficacy in this case consists of selecting alternative antibiotic therapy. The same principles of selection that apply to the primary therapy should be used here. If adverse effects are a consequence of a possible allergic reaction, antibiotics from a different chemical class for which cross-sensitivity is unlikely should be selected. Modification to decrease or eliminate the GI effects could include giving the drug with food or administering a lactobacillus preparation as previously cited. The use of yogurt addresses both approaches.

PATIENT CASE 2

HL is a 48-yo WM who presents to his primary care physician for a routine check-up and receives a cholesterol screening. He has no significant past medical history and does not smoke or drink. He does not take any routine scheduled medications. His family history is significant for a father who died of a myocardial infarction (MI) at 50. His mother is alive and well at 70, and none of his siblings is known to have heart disease at this time. Pertinent physical findings include a weight of 104 kg, height of 71", BP 130/85, HR 75, RR 12, carotid pulses symmetric bilaterally without bruits, no abdominal pain or bruits, no evidence of xanthomas, xanthelasma, or corneal arcus. His laboratory data reveal normal kidney and liver function. His fasting cholesterol panel shows a total cholesterol of 240 mg/dL, triglycerides 180 mg/dL, high-density lipoprotein (HDL) 30 mg/dL, and calculated low-density lipoprotein (LDL) 174 mg/dL.

What Is Your Initial Assessment of This Patient?

According to the National Cholesterol Education Program Adult Treatment Panel II[1] (NCEP ATII) guidelines, serum cholesterol should be monitored in all adults 20 years of age and older at least once every 5 years. Once hyperlipidemia is identified, a full evaluation of the patient should take place and include a thorough history, physical examination, and baseline laboratory assessments. The initial history and physical exam should include an assessment of any cardiovascular risk factors, family history of premature cardiovascular (CV) disease or lipid disorders, the presence or absence of secondary cause of hyperlipidemia, and the presence or absence of xanthomas, pancreatitis, renal or liver disease, peripheral vascular disease, or cerebral vascular disease. Therefore, your initial assessment of this hyperlipidemic patient is that he has two positive risk factors for coronary artery disease (CAD) which are male > 45 and a family history of premature CAD.

What Is Your Therapeutic Goal for This Patient?

Again, according to the NCEP guidelines, this patient has high blood cholesterol defined as ≥ 240 mg/dL, and his lipoprotein analysis reveals "high-risk LDL cholesterol" defined as ≥ 160 mg/dL. Therefore, a clinical evaluation is warranted. Based on the findings previously stated, this patient is an ideal candidate for diet therapy as well as drug therapy aimed to lower his high cholesterol to a goal LDL of ≤ 130 mg/dL. There have been numerous clinical trials showing the morbidity and mortality benefits of primary prevention with drug therapy in a patient with hypercholesterolemia (WOSCOPS,[2] AFCAPS/TexCAPS,[3] LRC-CPPT,[4] etc.). Therefore, he should be started on a step I diet as recommended by the NCEP ATP II as well as a pharmacologic agent to lower his cholesterol. To choose an appropriate agent, you need to be aware of the effects on the lipid panel and adverse drug effects of each class, as well as each agent within the class. For example, niacin's main effects on lipids are to lower triglycerides, cholesterol, and LDL as well as to raise HDL. However, it should be avoided in patients with diabetes, peptic ulcer disease, or a history of gout. In addition, niacin can pose problems with patient adherence secondary to unwanted side effects such as headache, flushing, or gastrointestinal intolerance. This is not to say niacin should never be used in clinical practice, as it has a very important role in the treatment of hypercholesterolemia, just not necessarily as a first-line agent. The class of drugs most clinicians would choose to treat this patient would be an HMG-CoA reductase inhibitor, or statin. Which statin is chosen should ideally be based on two things: (1) the percentage lowering of LDL required to achieve the goal and (2) the agent and dose to achieve this goal in the most cost effective manner. This patient needs at least a 25% reduction in his LDL, and one should look at the reported lowering of LDL for each dosage form and determine which agent would be the most cost-effective. For example, statin A may lower LDL up to 40% with a starting dose of 10 mg daily and cost the patient $75 for a month's supply. However, statin B may lower LDL only 20% with a starting dose of 20 mg daily and 30% with a dose of 40 mg daily. The 40-mg dose of statin B costs the patient $65 a month. Which statin is the more cost-efficient for this patient? Although statin B 40 mg daily doesn't lower cholesterol as much as statin A 10 mg daily, it is more cost-efficient in our patient who requires only a 25% reduction in his LDL.

The Next Question You Should Ask Yourself Is How Do I Monitor This Patient?

Monitoring parameters are divided into two categories, therapeutic and adverse effect monitoring parameters (MP). Considering therapeutic MPs first, it should seem obvious that the first therapeutic MP for this patient is an LDL ≤ 130 mg/dL. However, do not forget that another important therapeutic MP for our patient is the primary prevention of CAD. An important decision is how often to obtain a lipid panel in a patient being treated for hypercholesterolemia? Usually a lipid panel will be drawn every 6 weeks after initiation of therapy until the goal is achieved. Then, a lipid panel may be reviewed every 6 months thereafter. If a patient is not having the desired therapeutic effects, you may need to adjust his therapy. You may need to increase or decrease the dose or add another agent. After making any changes in a therapeutic regimen, you must continually reassess your patient and determine new therapeutic MPs if necessary.

Adverse MPs may seem more involved. Assuming a statin is chosen to treat this patient'shypercholesterolemia, baseline and follow-up assessments of laboratory parameters are required. Baseline liver function tests (LFTs), mainly alanine transaminase (ALT) and aspartate transaminase (AST), should be done before initiation of therapy with a statin to ensure that the patient has no existing liver dysfunction. Different statin manufacturers may have slightly different recommendations for follow-up assessments of LFTs, but generally, they are obtained at 12 weeks after initiation or dose increase, then every 6 months thereafter. If a patient complains of new-onset or unexplained muscle pain, a creatinine phosphokinase (CPK) should be ordered and assessed to rule out rhabdomyolysis.

If a patient is experiencing an adverse effect, it is always important to determine if it is clinically relevant or not. You may have a patient present with new-onset muscle pain who, on questioning, reveals that he has recently started a new vigorous workout regime. Certainly, it would be prudent to check a CPK to be safe, but it may also be advisable to counsel the patient on exercise moderation and appropriate stretching and cooling-off techniques. Additionally, a patient with an elevated AST is not automatically excluded from receiving a statin. The important question is how much the AST is elevated. Generally, if the LFTs are 1.5–3 times the upper limit of normal, you may want to find the reason for the elevation (recent MI, for example). Determining clinical relevance is something that comes with time and years of practice, but it is an important aspect of clinical practice. If an adverse effect is deemed clinically relevant, you may need to adjust the therapy appropriately by decreasing the dose or changing to a different drug class altogether. Again, after making any changes in a therapeutic regimen, you must continually reassess your patient and determine new adverse MPs if necessary.

If a Patient Is Having No Adverse Effects and Has Reached His Therapeutic Goal, Can You Simply Send Him off and Never See Him Again?

Of course you would never do this. Patient care and monitoring are a continual process and occur for as long as the patient needs a therapeutic intervention, either pharmacologic or nonpharmacologic. For example, in this patient who achieves a goal LDL of ≤ 130 mg/dL and is experiencing no adverse effects, a conceivable monitoring assessment could take place every 6 months. This patient will probably need to be assessed for the rest of his life. Each patient and each clinical scenario is unique and will require different approaches to determining therapeutic goals and monitoring parameters.

QUESTIONS

1. The process of drawing a conclusion from given information and reasoning from the general to the specific is called
   A. Inductive reasoning
   B. Hypothesizing
   C. Regeneration
   D. Deductive reasoning

2. If the primary adverse effect of a drug is bone marrow suppression, which of the following would be the most appropriate laboratory test for monitoring of toxicity?
   A. Liver panel
   B. Complete blood count
   C. Serum glucose
   D. BUN and creatinine

3. A patient has a BUN of 42 mg/dL and a serum creatinine of 2.1 mg/dL. His estimated creatinine clearance is determined to be 19 mL/min. This information would be important for drugs that
   A. are eliminated by the liver
   B. are eliminated by the kidney
   C. are poorly absorbed from the GI tract
   D. have a high first-pass effect

4. A patient taking a nonsteroidal antiinflammatory drug (NSAID) complains of frequent abdominal pain and GI upset. This is an example of
   A. Drug allergy
   B. Drug sensitivity
   C. Drug intolerance
   D. Drug variable

5. Which of the following are appropriate questions concerning the chief complaint and the history of present illness?
   A. How long have the symptoms been occurring?

B. Does anything lessen these symptoms or make them go away?
C. Are there any associated signs or symptoms?
D. All of the above
6. An example of subjective information would be
    A. x-ray report
    B. laboratory test result
    C. physical exam
    D. patient symptoms

REFERENCES

1. Executive Summary of The Third Report of The National Cholesterol Program (NCEP) Expert Panel on Detection, Evaluation, and Treatment of High Blood Cholesterol In Adults (Adult Treatment Panel III) JAMA 2001 May 16;285(19):2486–97.
2. Sheperd J, Cobbe SM, Ford I, et al. Prevention of coronary heart disease with pravastatin in men with hypercholesterolemia. West of Scotland coronary prevention study group. N Engl J Med 1995;333:1301–1307.
3. Downs JR, Clearfield M, Weis S, et al. Primary prevention of acute coronary events with lovastatin in men and women with average cholesterol levels. JAMA 1998;279:1615–1622.
4. The lipid research clinics coronary primary prevention trial results. The relationship of reduction in incidence of coronary heart disease to cholesterol lowering. JAMA 1984;251:365–374.

C H A P T E R 1 1

PRACTICAL PHARMACOKINETICS

Sandra Earle

Goals: After reviewing the information in this chapter, you should be able to:

1. Define dose rate and dose interval and how they influence the average concentration at steady state ($C_{ss,avg}$) and peak-to-trough ratio (P:T).
2. List the factors influencing the bioavailability of an orally administered drug.
3. List the determinants of volume of distribution and determine how changes in volume of distribution may change dosing needs.
4. List the determinants of renal clearance and determine how drugs and disease may alter renal clearance and thus alter $C_{ss,avg}$ and/or P:T of a given drug cleared by the kidney.
5. List the determinants of hepatic clearance and determine how drugs and disease may alter hepatic clearance and thus alter $C_{ss,avg}$ and/or P:T of a given drug cleared by the liver.
6. Given appropriate concentration–time data, calculate k, $t_{1/2}$, C_{max}, C_{min}, and AUC for that drug in that patient.
7. List reasons when therapeutic drug monitoring might be beneficial to the patient's outcome.
8. Discuss the attributes of extended-interval dosing and traditional dosing for aminoglycosides.

INTRODUCTION

The word *pharmacokinetics* strikes fear into the hearts of many students. It should not. Pharmacists must realize that the knowledge of pharmacokinetic principles and the ability to apply that knowledge empowers us to do our job well. We are expected to know how to use drugs effectively and safely. To do this we need to understand how drugs affect the body and also how the body affects the drug. Pharmacokinetics is simply the study of the body's effect on a given drug. Many healthcare practitioners have a good understanding of how drugs work, but only the pharmacist is well educated in pharmacokinetics. Therefore, we must take on the challenge of mastering these principles and their application.

Bioavailability, distribution, and clearance of a drug are important pharmacokinetic parameters to understand. They are introduced early in the chapter and discussed in more detail later. When a drug is introduced to the body, it first must get to the bloodstream in order to reach the systemic receptors. The fraction of given drug that reaches the systemic circulation is the bioavailability (F) of the drug. It will be reported as a percentage or fraction. If a drug's bioavailability is altered, that will affect how much drug is available to work. How the drug distributes in the body is also important to consider. The volume of distribution (V_d) of a drug relates the amount of drug in the body to the measured plasma concentration. Or, how much volume does there have to be to account for the known amount of drug in the body and the concentration measured. The larger the volume of distribution, the higher the amount of tissue binding, and the slower the elimination from the body. Elimination rate constant (k) is dependent on the volume of distribution and the clearance of a drug. Clearance (CL) is defined as the amount of blood that can have all the drug eliminated from it per unit time. Therefore, the units for clearance are volume per time. Clearance is often confused with the amount of drug eliminated per time. How fast a drug can be eliminated from the body is dependent on how efficiently the body can eliminate the drug (CL) and how readily available the drug is to the clearance organ (V_d). If a drug has a large volume, it is not easily available to the clearance organ and will therefore take a longer time to be eliminated even if the efficiency or clearance of the organ of elimination is large. Bioavailability, volume of distribution, and clearance are the parameters that might be affected by drugs, disease, and other interacting entities. With an understanding of these principles, drug and disease interactions can be predicted, and changes can be made in the dosage regimen to accommodate the interaction.

DOSAGE REGIMEN DESIGN

As pharmacists we are often asked to predict and/or react to pharmacokinetic alterations. We cannot easily affect pharmacokinetic parameters such as bioavailability, distribution, or clearance. We can, however, alter the dosing regimen that a patient is getting of a particular drug to control the outcome of any pharmacokinetic alteration. The dosing regimen is made up of two components: dose rate (DR) and dose interval (τ).

Dose rate (DR) is the amount of drug the patient is receiving per time. A constant infusion is an easy example. If a patient is getting a 2 mg/min drip of lidocaine, his dose rate is 2 mg/min. If, however, a patient is getting 1 g of cefotaxime every 8 hours, the dose rate is 125 mg/h or 3 g/day. The dose interval (τ) is how often the patient is receiving the drug. In the above example, the cefotaxime dose interval is every 8 hours. These two components work together to determine the dose. Do not confuse dose with dose rate. For our patient getting 1 g of cefotaxime every 8 hours, if he had renal impairment we would want to decrease his DR and increase his τ. This might mean that the dose remains the same. We might continue to give a dose of 1 g but give it every 12 hours rather than every 8 hours. This would decrease the DR from 3 g/day to 2 g/day while keeping the dose constant.

Average Concentration at Steady State

The two factors targeted when trying to maximize therapeutic efficacy and minimize toxicity are the average concentration at steady state ($C_{ss,avg}$) and the peak-to-trough ratio (P:T) (Fig. 11.1). Think of steady state as an equilibrium. $C_{ss,avg}$ gives us a good picture of the overall average concentration seen during a dosing interval at steady state. It is often the parameter that we are trying to maintain within a given therapeutic range. The determinants of $C_{ss,avg}$ are therefore very important. They include bioavailability (F), dose rate (DR), and clearance (CL) (Eq 11.1).

$$C_{ss,avg} = \frac{F \times DR}{CL}$$ [11.1]

Therefore, if there is a change in CL, F, or DR, there will be an alteration in $C_{ss,avg}$. This may result in a toxic or subtherapeutic concentration. As pharma-

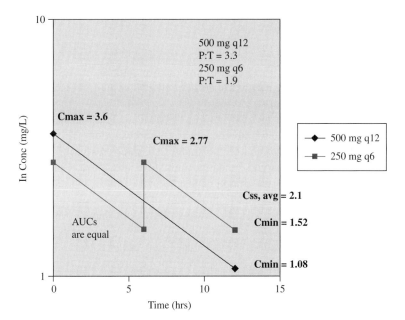

Figure 11.1. Giving the same dose rate with differing τ results in different peak-to-trough ratios but the same AUC and same $C_{ss,avg}$.

cists we can react by altering the DR to accommodate that change. For example, if a patient is on a drug that is cleared by the kidneys and he goes into acute renal failure, the clearance will decrease. The result will be an increase in $C_{ss,avg}$ and possible toxicity. The pharmacist will therefore recommend a decrease in the DR of drug the patient is receiving. This will result in the necessary decrease in the $C_{ss,avg}$. In a second case, if a patient were given an additional drug that decreased the bioavailability of a drug the patient was already on, a decrease in $C_{ss,avg}$ would occur. The pharmacist would respond by suggesting an increase in the DR of the drug the patient was initially taking to increase the $C_{ss,avg}$.

$C_{ss,avg}$ represents total drug, which includes both drug bound to plasma proteins and drug free from plasma proteins. Total drug is what the laboratory typically measures and is what most therapeutic ranges reflect. But only unbound drug can interact at the pharmacologic site, so it alone is the active component. To determine the free/unbound concentration at steady state, the fraction unbound must be known (Eq 11.2).

$$C_{ss,avg,free} = \frac{F \times DR}{CL} \times f_{up} \qquad [11.2]$$

Note that the determinants of $C_{ss,avg}$ and $C_{ss,avg,free}$ are the same other than the addition of the measure of plasma protein binding. (f_{up} is the fraction of drug that is unbound in the plasma.)

Peak-to-Trough Ratio

The peak-to-trough ratio (P:T) is also important in determining a safe, effective dosing regimen. If a drug is not given often enough, it may have an unacceptable P:T. For example, if the drug is given once a day rather than three times daily but the dose rate or total daily dose is the same, the peak concentration will be relatively high, and the trough concentration relatively low. This could result in toxic peak concentrations and subtherapeutic trough concentrations (Fig. 11.1). The smaller the pieces that you divide the daily dose into, the less variation there will be between the peak and trough concentrations. This may be desirable, but it has to be weighed carefully with the ability of patients to comply with difficult dosing regimens. Also, it is not always desirable to have a small P:T. For example, it is advantageous for aminoglycosides to have a large peak-to-trough ratio. High peak concentrations are associated with better bacterial kill, and low trough concentrations may decrease the risk for nephrotoxicity from aminoglycosides. Elimination rate constant (k) and dosing interval (τ) determine the peak-to-trough ratio (P:T) (Eq 11.3).

$$P:T = \frac{1}{e^{-k\tau}} \qquad [11.3]$$

The elimination rate constant (k) is a fractional rate of drug elimination. The units are inverse time. It is a *dependent* variable determined by clearance (CL) and volume of distribution (V_d) (Eq 11.4).

$$k = \frac{CL}{V_d} \qquad [11.4]$$

If there is a change in CL, V_d, or dosing interval (τ), there will be a change in peak-to-trough ratio (P:T). This may result in unacceptably high or low peak concentrations and/or unacceptable trough concentrations. It may be helpful to think about the relationship of elimination rate constant and half-life ($t_{1/2}$). They are inversely proportional (Eq 11.5). Half-life is the time required for the serum concentration to decrease by 50%. Therefore, the determinants of half-life are also volume of distribution (V_d) and clearance (CL) (Eq 11.6). Half-life also is important in determining time to steady state.

$$t_{1/2} = \frac{0.693}{k} \qquad [11.5]$$

$$t_{1/2} = \frac{0.693 \times V_d}{CL} \qquad [11.6]$$

Absolute 100% steady state never occurs, but each half-life cuts the difference in half. Consider this illustration. Pretend the penalty for holding in football is half the distance to the goal. If you had the whole field to go and benefited from this penalty, the first time you would gain 50 yards or half the field. The second time you would gain 25 yards or half of the remaining 50 yards to the goal line. You are now only 25 yards away. The third penalty would put you only 12.5 yards away, etc. If you continue to get that call over and over you would never reach the goal line, right? This idea can be applied to achievement of steady state. After 1, 2, 3, 4, and 5 half-lives, you have achieved 50%, 75%, 87.5%, 93.8%, and 96.9% of steady state, respectively. Thus, it takes 5 half-lives to achieve approximately 97% steady state, so if you are dosing a drug with a $t_{1/2}$ of 10 hours, it would take 50 hours or approximately 2 days to achieve 97% steady state.

It is helpful to realize that with dosing every half-life, the peak-to-trough ratio will be 2. Therefore, the peak concentration will be twice the trough concentration. If dosing is more frequent, there will be less variation between the peak and trough concentrations, and if dosing is more frequent, there will be a greater deviation between peak and trough concentrations (Fig. 11.1). If we go back to the patient on the drug cleared by the kidneys who suddenly goes into acute renal failure, there will be a decrease in CL. The decrease in clearance will result in an increase in the $C_{ss,avg}$ but will also decrease the elimination rate constant (k) and decrease the peak-to-trough ratio (P:T). This may or may not be

clinically acceptable. If this drug were an aminoglycoside, it might be unsatis-
factory. To get the peak-to-trough ratio back to what it was before the onset of
the acute renal failure, you would want to extend the dosing interval. In this case,
you would also need to decrease the dose rate to decrease the $C_{ss,avg}$, as discussed
above. This would happen automatically if you increase the dose interval and
keep the dose the same, as you would be giving less drug per unit time, thus decreasing the dose rate.

   If a decrease in volume of distribution occurred, you would see an increase
in the elimination rate constant (k) and a resulting increase in the peak-to-trough
ratio. Thus, if the dosing regimen remains the same, the peak-to-trough ratio will
increase, possibly causing peak concentrations that result in toxic side effects or
subtherapeutic trough concentrations or both. In this case you would want to decrease the dosing interval to give the drug at more frequent intervals, avoiding
the large peak-to-trough ratio. You would also want to keep the dose rate constant because the $C_{ss,avg}$ has not been changed (no change in CL or F, Eq 11.1).
In this example, for your daily dose to remain constant, your dose per administration would have to decrease.

   In order to determine how we need to alter the dosage regimen, we need to
understand what factors will alter the bioavailability, volume of distribution, and
clearance of drugs.

Bioavailability

For a drug to work it must be made available to the appropriate receptors in the
body. In most cases this means that it must be made available to the systemic
blood flow. The bioavailability defines the fraction of given drug that is able to
reach the systemic blood flow or made available to the receptors. A drug given
intravenously would usually have a bioavailability of 100%. If given via the oral
route, the drug would first have to be absorbed from the gut lumen to the gut
wall; this is the fraction absorbed (f_a). That fraction of drug is then exposed to
possible metabolism in the gut wall. The fraction that escapes gut metabolism
and efflux is symbolized by f_g. Finally, the remaining drug, or $f_a \times f_g$, would then
be transported via the portal vein first to the liver where it may undergo some
metabolism. The fraction that is able to avoid metabolism in the liver is called
the fraction that escapes the first-pass effect (f_{fp}). Therefore, the bioavailable fraction (F) would be the fraction able to be absorbed and then avoid metabolism as
it passes through the gut wall and liver. (Eq 11.7)

$$F = f_a \times f_g \times f_{fp} \qquad\qquad [11.7]$$

Fraction Absorbed

The bioavailability of a drug is determined by many factors including route of administration, dosage form, physiological status of the patient, and the properties

of the drug itself. Following the path of an orally administered drug, the obstacles of getting the drug to the site of action can be identified. First, the drug must be absorbed from the lumen into the gut wall. Most drug absorption in the gut follows the properties of passive diffusion (Fig. 11.2). This means that for a drug to be absorbed, there must be a concentration gradient, and the drug must be in an absorbable form: small enough, relatively lipophilic, and un-ionized. Most absorption occurs in the small intestine because of the great amount of surface area available. Therefore, the rate of absorption is dependent on the drug getting to the site of absorption. Gastric emptying time is often the rate-limiting step in this process. Drug may not have time to be absorbed. This is especially true if there is an increase in gastric motility or if the drug does not have rapid enough dissolution. In this case the drug will be found unchanged in the feces. Another possibility is that the drug may decompose or be adsorbed or complexed in the lumen and thus will be found in the feces in the changed or complexed form.

Fraction Escaping Gut Metabolism

Once the drug makes it out of the lumen into the gut wall, there are both Phase I and Phase II enzymes in the gut wall that may be able to metabolize a portion of the drug (Fig. 11.2). Cytochrome P450 3A enzymes account for more than 70% of the small intestinal cytochrome enzymes (CYP).[1] There are also drug transport systems that can efflux drug from the gut wall back into the gut lumen. The most studied of these drug efflux systems is p-glycoprotein (P-gp), a member of the ABC cassette family of transporters. P-gp has been found in the cells

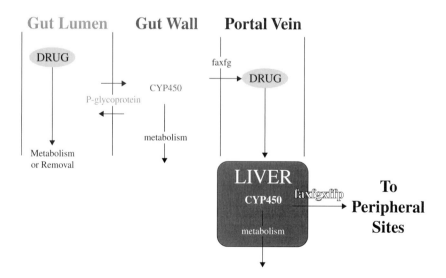

Figure 11.2. Depiction of the trip a drug takes to undergo absorption.

lining the blood–brain barrier, kidney, adrenal glands, and lungs as well as many other tissues. The cells lining the intestinal tract all exhibit P-gp, with the concentrations increasing as you travel down from the esophagus to the colon.[2] The concentrations of CYP in the cells decrease as you travel down the intestinal tract. Many drugs are substrates, inducers, or inhibitors of both the CYP 3A family and P-gp (Tables 11.1–11.3). There is some evidence to suggest P-gp may act as a gatekeeper to regulate the exposure of drug to the CYP enzymes in the gut wall.[3] There are examples of drug–drug and drug–food interactions that can now be explained by this mechanism of gut wall efflux and metabolism. There is great potential for utilizing inducers and inhibitors of these systems to alter the fraction of drug escaping gut metabolism.

Fraction Escaping Hepatic First Pass

Finally, once a drug has been absorbed from the lumen to the gut wall (f_a) and escapes metabolism or efflux from the gut wall (f_g), it is then taken by the portal vein to the liver. The liver is a major organ responsible for the clearance of drugs by metabolism. It is rich with enzymes for both Phase I and Phase II reactions. Drugs extensively metabolized by hepatic enzymes in the liver, called high-extraction drugs, will have a very low bioavailability if given by a first-pass route. (Table 11.4) These drugs must be administered by a non-first-pass route in order to attain sufficient concentrations of parent drug at the receptor site (Table 11.4). An example of this is nitroglycerin; it must be given intravenously, sublingually, or transdermally to be effective. The fraction of drug escaping the first pass for these drugs is primarily dependent on liver blood flow (Q) and liver enzyme activity (CL_{int}) (Eq 11.8).

$$f_{fp} \approx \frac{Q}{CL_{int}} \qquad [11.8]$$

Enterohepatic Cycling

A drug may also undergo biliary elimination and/or enterohepatic cycling. In this case, the drug is absorbed and delivered via the portal vein to the liver; then a portion may be secreted into the bile and stored in the gallbladder. The drug now in the bile will then reenter the intestine. At this point it might be reabsorbed to complete what is called an enterohepatic cycle. There are two other possibilities. The drug might be metabolized in the liver and then secreted into the bile so the metabolite can undergo the enterohepatic cycle. The third possibility is that after the drug reenters the intestine via the bile, it is excreted in the feces. The biliary transport of drugs is similar to renal tubular active secretion and can be competitively inhibited. Drugs that have a high biliary clearance have the following characteristics. They are polar, ionized, and have a molecular weight > 250 g/mol. If a drug is enterohepatically cycling, it is continuously being reintroduced to the systemic circulation.

TABLE 11.1. SELECTED SUBSTRATES OF THE CYP FAMILIES AND P-GLYCOPROTEIN[6,17]

CYP							P-GP
1A2	2C19	2C9	2D6	2E1	3A		
clozapine	amitriptyline	AT2 Blockers:	Antipsych:	acetaminophen	Antihistamines:		Anticancer:
imipramine	diazepam	irbesartan	haloperidol	ethanol	a stemizole		etopside
mexilitine	phenytoin	losartan	risperidone		clorpheniramine		paclitaxel
naproxen	phenobarbital	celecoxib	thioridazine		Benzodiazepine s:		vinblastine
tacrine	PPIs:	fluvastatin	Cardiac:		alprazolam		vincristine
theophylline	omeprazole	glipizide	flecainide		diazepam		Ca channel blockers:
	lasoprazole	NSAIDs:	S-metaprolol		midazolam		diltiazem
	pantoprazole	ibuprofen	mexilitine		triazolam		nicardipine
		naproxen	propafenone		buspirone		verapamil
		piroxicam	timolol		Ca channel blockers:		HIV Protease Inh:
		phenytoin	codeine		amlodipine		ritonavir
		sulfamethoxazole	dextromethorphan		diltiazem		saquinavir
		tamoxifen	ondansetron		felodipine		Hormones
		WARFARIN	tamoxifen		nifedipine		dexamethasone
			TCAs:		nitrendipine		estradiol
			amitriptyline		verapamil		hydrocortisone
			desipramine		CISAPRIDE		Immuno-
			imipramine		HIV Protease Inh:		modulators
			paroxetine		indinavir		cyclosporine
			tramadol		ritonavir		FK506
			venlafaxine		saquinavir		

(continued)

TABLE 11.1. SELECTED SUBSTRATES OF THE CYP FAMILIES AND P-GLYCOPROTEIN[6,17] (Cont.)

	CYP							P-GP
1A2	2C19	2C9	2D6	2E1	3A			
					HMG CoA Reductase Inh:			
					atorvastatin			
					lovastatin			
					simvastatin			
					Immuno-			
					modulators			
					CYCLOSPORINE			
					tacrolimus			
					FK-506			
					Macrolides:			
					clarithromycin			
					erythromycin			
					quinidine			
					quinine			
					sidenafil			
					tamoxifen			
					trazodone			
					vincristine			

TABLE 11.2. SELECTED ENHANCERS OF THE CYP FAMILIES AND P-GLYCOPROTEIN[6,17]

CYP							P-GP
1A2	2C19	2C9	2D6	2E1	3A		
tobacco		rifampin secobarbital		ethanol isoniazid	Antiepileptics: carbamazepine phenobarbital phenytoin rifbutin rifampin St. John's wort troglitazone		Grapefruit juice? Flavonoids kaaepferol quercetin

TABLE 11.3. SELECTED INHIBITORS OF THE CYP FAMILIES AND P-GLYCOPROTEIN[6,17]

	CYP						P-GP
1A2	2C19	2C9	2D6	2E1	3A		
cimetidine Fluoroquinolones: ciprofloxacin levofloxacin fluvoxamine ticlopidine	ketoconazole PPIs: lansoprazole omeprazole SSRIs: fluoxetine fluvoxamine ticlopidine	amiodarone fluconazole isoniazid ticlopidine	Antiarrhythmics: amiodarone quinidine clorpheniramine cimetidine fluoxetine haloperidol paroxetine ritonavir	disulfiram	amiodarone Azole antifungals: itraconazole ketoconazole Antihistamines: astemizole clorpheniramine cimetidine grapefruit juice HIV Protease Inh: Indinavir nelfinavir ritonavir saquinavir Macrolides: clarithromycin erythromycin SSRIs: fluoxetine fluvoxamine		Antiarrhythmics: amiodarone lidocaine quinidine Azole antifungals: itraconazole ketoconazole Ca channel blocker: diltiazem nicardipine nifedipine verapamil Hormones: hydrocortisone progesterone testosterone Immunomodulators cyclosporin FK506 RU486 tamoxifen terfenadine

TABLE 11.4. SELECTED EXAMPLES OF DRUGS UNDERGOING A HIGH FIRST-PASS EFFECT

Amitriptyline	Labetalol
Chlorpromazine	Lidocaine
Cytarabine	Methylphenidate
Desipramine	Metoprolol
Dihydroergotamine	Morphine
Diltiazem	Naloxone
Doxepine	Neostigmine
Doxorubicin	Nicardipine
Encainide	Nicotine
Estradiol	Nifedipine
5-FU	Nitroglycerin
Hydralazine	Pentoxifylline
Imipramine	Propranolol
Isoproterenol	Scopolamine
Isosorbide dintrate	Testosterone
Labetolol	Verapamil

Measuring Bioavailability

To determine the bioavailability of a drug by a given route, a dose is given intravenously and by the route being measured. It is given orally in the example below. The concentration–time curve is characterized for each route, and the area under the curve (AUC) for each route is measured. The bioavailable fraction will be equal to the quotient of the areas if equivalent doses are given (Eq 11.9). If inequivalent doses are given, equation 11.10 is used to correct for the different doses.

$$F = \frac{AUC_{PO}}{AUC_{IV}} \qquad [11.9]$$

$$F = \frac{Dose_{IV} \times AUC_{PO}}{Dose_{PO} \times AUC_{IV}} \qquad [11.10]$$

Determining the f_a, f_g, and f_{fp} components of the total bioavailability is more difficult. It can be done experimentally, but is not routinely done in the clinical arena. The f_{fp} can be calculated from hepatic clearance, if known. Liver blood flow (Q) and the hepatic extraction ratio (E) determine hepatic clearance (CL_H) (Eq 11.11). An average liver blood flow is approximately 90 L/h or 1.5 L/min.

The fraction that escapes the first-pass effect will be the fraction remaining after hepatic extraction (E) (Eq 11.12)

$$CL_H = Q \times E \tag{11.11}$$

$$f_{fp} = 1 - E \tag{11.12}$$

The bioavailability of a drug is important because it is a determinant of the concentration at steady state ($C_{ss,avg}$) (Eq 11.1). It is also important for determining a loading dose if the drug is not given intravenously (Eq 11.13).

$$C_{ss,avg} = \frac{F \times DR}{CL} \tag{11.1}$$

$$LD = \frac{C_{target} \times V_c}{F} \tag{11.13}$$

It is important to recognize all the potential drug–drug, drug–disease, and drug–nutrition interactions that might occur altering the bioavailability of a drug. This may be a problem when changing between products. If there is a change in the dissolution properties, or if the formulation has vehicles that could alter factors involved with f_a or f_g, the bioavailability could be altered. This change in bioavailability might alter the $C_{ss,avg}$ and AUC, thus possibly necessitating a change in dose rate. The FDA does require testing to prove that a generic drug has an equivalent bioavailability to the brand name drug.

Distribution

Once a drug has been made available to the receptors and rest of the body by entering the bloodstream, it distributes, which is the reversible transfer of drug from one place to another. Where a drug distributes is important both therapeutically and from a toxicologic standpoint. The extent of distribution is measured as a volume of distribution.

V_c, V_{ss}, V_z

There are three different volumes used as pharmacokinetic parameters, each having a different purpose. Initially when a drug is given it will distribute into the blood and highly perfused tissues. This is called the central volume of distribution (V_c) and is used to calculate loading doses (Eq 11.14).

$$V_c = \frac{Loading\ Dose}{Initial\ Concentration} \tag{11.14}$$

The volume of distribution at steady state (V_{ss}) represents the volume that the drug occupies when steady state is reached and the drug has been able to come to a distribution equilibrium (Eq 11.15). It represents physiological spaces that describe the determinants of distribution. It is very difficult to measure because it requires measuring drug concentrations in tissues.

$$V_{ss} = \text{Blood volume} + \left(\text{Tissue volume} \times \frac{\text{Unbound fraction in blood}}{\text{Unbound fraction in tissue}} \right) \quad [11.15]$$

The apparent volume of distribution (V_z) is a measurable but calculated volume (Eq 11.16, 11.17). It is determined using the elimination rate constant or the slope of the final elimination phase. It is in most cases very similar to the V_{ss}. Therefore, we routinely assume them to be equal and use the measurable V_z to represent the more physiological V_{ss} and call that the volume of distribution (V_d).

$$V_z = \frac{t_{1/2} \times CL}{0.693} \quad [11.16]$$

$$V_z = \frac{CL}{k} \quad [11.17]$$

The V_c is the smallest volume of distribution, followed by V_z, with V_{ss} being the relatively largest volume. For most drugs V_z is considered to be similar to V_{ss}. When a volume of distribution of a drug (V_d) is referred to, often one is considering the physiological determinants of V_{ss} but measuring the V_z.

The volume of distribution can be thought of as the parameter that relates the amount of drug in the body to the measured plasma concentration. Or, how much volume does there have to be to account for the known amount of drug in the body and the concentration measured. The range of volumes of drugs varies widely from 0.04 to >500 L/kg. One may consider it impossible for a drug to have a volume of distribution of 65 L/kg such as amiodarone. How could this be? It is highly bound to tissues. Consider this analogy.[4] You have discovered oil in your backyard while digging in your garden. You want to calculate how much oil there is to determine if you will drop out of pharmacy school. Using your scientific background, you determine to add a known amount of oil-miscible dye and let it come to equilibrium. You know if you are able to take a sample of the oil once it has come to equilibrium and measure the concentration of dye you will be able to determine the volume of the oil well.

Volume of oil in well (L) = C_{ss} of dye (mg/L) × Known amt of dye added (mg)

By doing this experiment, you determine that you are a multimillionaire and quit pharmacy school. When you pump out the oil well, there is much less than you had calculated. What went wrong? You notice that the rocks in the oil well had bound up much of the dye. If the rocks bound up the dye, then the concentration in the oil was more dilute, making it appear as if the volume was much greater then it physically was. Think of those rocks as tissue binding sites. The larger the volume of distribution, the higher the fraction of drug outside the plasma, which usually means it resides in the tissues.

Determinants of Distribution

A volume of distribution will be dependent on the drug's binding to proteins in the blood and tissues, ability to cross tissue membranes, and partitioning into fat. Delivery of the drug by the blood to the tissues is highly dependent on the perfusion rate of the tissue. The rate of tissue uptake is proportional to how well it is perfused. Recall that a drug must be small enough, unbound, un-ionized, and lipophilic enough to pass through a tissue membrane.

Plasma Protein Binding

Distribution to extravascular tissues can happen only if the drug is not bound to protein in the plasma. Drugs are often bound to proteins in the plasma, most commonly albumin, followed by α_1 acid glycoprotein (AAG), lipoproteins, and corticosteroid-binding protein.

The extent of plasma protein binding varies widely among drugs, ranging from 0.1% to 100% unbound. The fraction that is bound is dependent on the total number of binding sites available or the capacity of the system (N), the association constant (K_a), and the concentration of the drug (C). These determinants are analogous to the capacity (V_{max}), affinity (K_m), and concentration relationship describing hepatic intrinsic clearance. In most cases the concentration is not an important determinant of protein binding for drugs within the therapeutic range. Disopyramide and valproic acid are two exceptions to this statement. They exhibit concentration-dependent plasma protein binding in the therapeutic range.

Drugs and disease can alter the number of binding sites available, thereby changing the fraction unbound of a drug. Also, there can be competition for available binding sites, resulting in an altered fraction unbound of a drug. It is important for pharmacists to be able to recognize and anticipate these interactions.

Binding Proteins

The two most important binding proteins in the plasma are AAG and albumin. Albumin is the most prevalent binding protein in the plasma. It preferentially binds acidic drugs but has a relatively lower binding affinity than AAG. Disease and drugs that can alter albumin concentrations are listed in Table 11.5. α_1 acid glycoprotein (AAG), in contrast, is present in the plasma in low concentrations. But it is an acute-phase reactant and will increase fivefold when in an inflam-

TABLE 11.5. SELECTED EXAMPLES OF CONDITIONS THAT ALTER PLASMA PROTEINS

DECREASE BINDING TO ALBUMIN	INCREASE BINDING TO AAG
Nephrotic syndrome	Crohn's disease
Nephritis	Cancer
Renal failure	Rheumatoid arthritis
Alcoholism	Surgery
Hepatic cirrhosis	Acute myocardial infarction
Burns	Nephrotic syndrome
Pregnancy	Trauma
Surgery	

matory state. Some diseases that increase AAG include those listed in Table 11.5. AAG preferentially binds to basic and neutral compounds. It has a very high affinity for the drugs it binds.

Plasma protein binding interactions are important to anticipate and recognize when a drug is highly protein bound. When a laboratory measures a drug concentration, it is in most cases a total concentration. This includes both bound and unbound drug in the plasma. Only unbound drug is free to interact with the pharmacologic receptors. Therefore, the free concentration is what is important therapeutically. The total concentration will always reflect what is happening with the free concentration as long as there is no change in plasma protein binding. If there is a change in the fraction unbound in the plasma, total concentrations can not be relied on to give a true reflection of what is happening to the active unbound concentration. This is most important with drugs that are highly bound to plasma proteins, with a $f_{up} \leq 0.25$ (Table 11.6). In this case, a small change in the f_{up} will result in a large-magnitude change in the free concentration. Protein-binding interactions are most important in drugs that are highly protein bound.

TABLE 11.6. SELECTED EXAMPLES OF DRUGS HIGHLY BOUND TO PLASMA PROTEINS

Alfentanil	Phenytoin
Amiodarone	Propranolol
Carbamazepine	Quinidine
Ibuprofen	Valproic acid
Nifedipine	Verapamil
Phenobarbital	Warfarin

Tissue Binding

Although plasma protein binding is relatively easily measured, tissue binding is very difficult to determine. Tissue binding can be inferred by measuring the plasma protein binding and volume of distribution (Eq 11.15). Only unbound drug in the plasma (f_{up}) can enter and leave the tissue sites. The relationship between the fraction unbound in the plasma and the fraction unbound in the tissues will determine if the drug is predominately in the tissue or predominately in the plasma. If the drug is more highly bound to plasma proteins than to tissue proteins ($f_{up} < f_{ut}$), it will have a relatively small volume. Even a drug with a strong affinity for its plasma protein binding site can be more highly bound in the tissue ($f_{up} > f_{ut}$). In this case, most of the drug will reside in tissue stores, and therefore, it will have a relatively large volume of distribution. Partitioning into fat is also a tissue-binding site and can result in a depot-like effect increasing the volume of distribution and thus the half-life of a drug in a patient with more fat stores.

Clearance by Hemodialysis

The major determinants of the ability of hemodialysis to remove a drug are getting the drug to the hemodialysis machine and having it available for passive diffusion through the membrane. If a drug has a large volume of distribution, the drug is primarily in the tissues and not in the plasma. The drug must be in the plasma to be delivered to the dialysis machine. If a drug has a sufficiently small volume of distribution, it also must not be highly protein bound to be dialyzed. If it is highly protein bound, the drug–protein complex is too big to diffuse passively through the dialysis membrane and will not be dialyzed. Size itself can be a limiting factor. If a drug is larger than the molecular weight cutoff of the membrane used, it will not be eliminated by hemodialysis. Gwilt and Perrier came up with a quick way to surmise if a drug would be significantly eliminated by hemodialysis[4] (Eq 11.18). If the resulting number was <20, then the drug would not be significantly removed. If it were >80 a significant portion would be removed. If in-between these numbers, it is difficult to tell.

$$\frac{f_{up} \times 100}{V_d(L/kg)} \qquad [11.18]$$

Clearance

Clearance is a measure of the efficiency of drug removal from the body. The two major organs of clearance in the body are the kidneys and the liver. The clearance of a drug by any organ is primarily dependent on the blood flow to that organ (Q) and the efficiency of that organ to eliminate the drug (extraction efficiency, E). The specific factors are different depending on the organ of clearance.

In general, if the kidneys cannot remove a drug in the parent form, it is metabolized to more polar compound by the liver. This allows the metabolite to be removed by the kidneys. To determine which organ of clearance is predominant, the fraction of parent drug excreted unchanged in the urine (f_e) must be determined. For example, if a 100-mg dose of a totally bioavailable drug is given and 80 mg is recovered in the parent form in the urine, the f_e would be 0.8. The remaining 20 mg or 20% of the dose would be cleared by nonrenal routes. These could include the bile, skin, lungs, and/or liver. We usually assume nonrenal clearance to be hepatic clearance. The determinants of both renal and hepatic clearance are discussed.

Renal Clearance

The kidneys rely on three mechanisms to determine renal clearance of drugs. They include glomerular filtration clearance, active secretion, and passive reabsorption. First, drugs are filtered through the glomerulus; then there may be active secretion of the drug from the bloodstream into the proximal tubule; and finally, it can be reabsorbed in the distal tubule by passive diffusion (Fig. 11.3). The determinants of each of these components are discussed below.

Glomerular Filtration Clearance

The glomerulus works as a filter. When a drug arrives at the glomerulus via the renal artery, it will either pass through the filter and into the renal tubule or will not. Whether or not a drug will be filtered is dependent on size of the molecule. If a drug has a very large molecular weight, it will not be filtered. Also, if a drug is bound to a very large protein molecule, it will not be filtered because the protein is too big to be filtered. Recall that a major function of the glomerulus is to keep valuable proteins in the bloodstream and not allow them to be lost via the kidneys. Therefore, if a drug is highly bound to plasma proteins, it will not be filtered. Remember, the clearance of any organ is dependent on the blood flow to the organ and the extraction efficiency of the organ. In this case, the glomerular filtration rate (GFR) is the blood flow, and the extraction efficiency is dictated by the fraction of drug that is free of plasma proteins in the plasma (f_{up}). Therefore, GFR and f_{up} determine glomerular filtration clearance (CL_{gf}) (Eq 11.19).

$$CL_{gf} = GFR \times f_{up} \qquad [11.19]$$

Active Secretion

After a drug is filtered into the tubule it will then travel down to the proximal tubule. As the fluid is traveling down the tubule, there is a vast reabsorption of water. Therefore, tubular fluid becomes more concentrated as it is more distal from the glomerulus. Drugs may be actively secreted from the bloodstream back

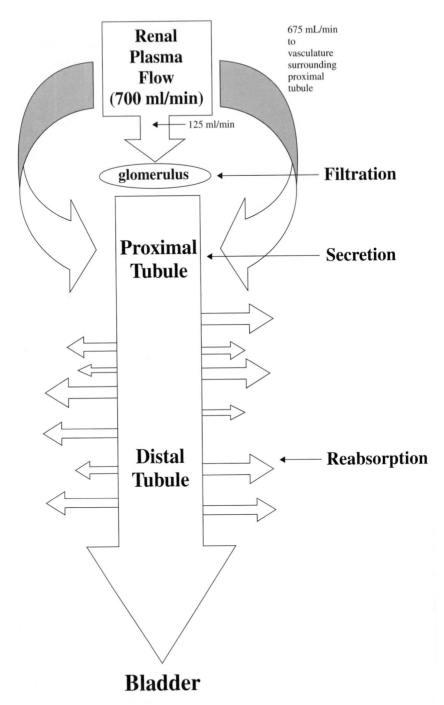

Figure 11.3. Representation of renal clearnace in kidney.

into the renal tubule in the proximal tubule. Because it is an active process, it requires energy and a carrier system. This is a capacity-limited process analogous to hepatic enzymatic metabolism and may be saturated. There are at least two types of carriers known for tubular secretion, one for acids and one for bases. Thus, secreted acids will compete with other secreted acids, and bases will compete with bases for their appropriate carriers. This is an important site for drug–drug interactions. (Recall that biliary clearance is a similar process, with active secretion into the bile containing acid and base carrier systems.)

When two drugs are competing for the same carrier site, the one with the higher affinity for the carrier will be preferentially secreted, leaving the drug with a lesser affinity in the bloodstream. This will result in a decrease in the renal clearance of the drug with a lesser affinity for the carrier, which will produce an increase in $C_{ss,avg}$ and a prolonged half-life. A classic example of this is the probenecid interaction with penicillin. Both of these drugs are competing for the acid secretion carrier sites in the proximal tubule. Probenecid is preferentially secreted because it has a higher affinity for the carrier. Therefore, when probenecid is added to the regimen of a patient taking penicillin, the clearance of penicillin is decreased, resulting in an increased $C_{ss,avg}$ and longer half-life. This is used therapeutically to increase concentrations achieved and allow for less-frequent dosing. Obviously, this type of interaction could result in adversely high concentrations of interacting drugs, so this must be considered when screening for possible drug–drug interactions. Some actively secreted drugs are listed in Table 11.7.

TABLE 11.7. SELECTED EXAMPLES OF DRUGS UNDERGOING ACTIVE TUBULAR SECRETION

ORGANIC ACIDS	ORGANIC BASES
Cephalosporins	Amantadine
Ciprofloxacin	Cimetidine
Clavulanate	Didanosine
Furosemide	Dopamine
Methotrexate	Famciclovir
Penicillins	Meperidine
Probenecid	Morphine
Salicylates	Pseudoephedrine (denantiomer)
Sufonamides	Quinine
Thiazides	Zalcitabine
	Zidovudine

Tubular Reabsorption

Tubular reabsorption, a primarily passive process, occurs in the distal tubule. (Lithium is an exception to this, as it is actively reabsorbed in the proximal tubule.) Passive reabsorption is dependent on the principles of a passive diffusion. Therefore, a drug in the tubule must be relatively lipophilic and uncharged to be reabsorbed. Because it is passive, it is not dependent on a carrier system and cannot be saturated. It is, however, dependent on the concentration gradient. Recall that as fluid moves through the tubule there is a vast reabsorption of water, resulting in more concentrated urine. (Just think what it would be like if our urine output were equal to that of a normal GFR of 125 mL/min!) Therefore, the concentration of drug in the urine will be higher than that of drug in the bloodstream. The drug will passively diffuse from the distal tubular fluid into the less concentrated bloodstream if it is lipophilic enough and uncharged. This would decrease the renal clearance of the drug. Changing the concentration gradient or the fraction of un-ionized drug alters the fraction of drug reabsorbed. Giving an osmotic diuretic such as mannitol alters the concentration gradient. This drug will decrease water reabsorption and therefore minimize the concentration gradient, resulting in less drug being reabsorbed. This would increase renal clearance, decrease $C_{ss,avg}$, and make the half-life shorter. Changing the pH of the tubular fluid alters the ionic character of the drug. For example, a weak acid must be in an acidic environment to be in the primarily un-ionized state. If the pH of the urine is alkalinized, a weak acid will have a smaller fraction of drug in the un-ionized, reabsorbable form, and therefore tubular reabsorption will be decreased. This will result in an increase in renal clearance causing a decreased $C_{ss,avg}$ and a shorter half-life. This is another important area to consider for drug–drug interactions.

Summary

When a drug arrives at the glomerulus, it will be filtered. The fraction of drug that will be filtered is dependent on the protein-binding characteristics. The drug then may be actively secreted or passively reabsorbed in the tubule, increasing or decreasing the renal clearance, respectively. The dominant process is determined by comparing the renal clearance to the filtration clearance (Eq 11.19). If the renal clearance is greater than the filtration clearance, secretion must be the predominant process (Eq 11.20).

$$CL_R > GFR \times f_{up} \qquad [11.20]$$

Passive reabsorption must be the prevailing process if renal clearance is less than the filtered clearance (Eq 11.21).

$$CL_R < GFR \times f_{up} \qquad [11.21]$$

Once the predominant process is identified, drug–drug interactions can be more readily anticipated and acted on.

Hepatic Clearance

Three factors that determine hepatic clearance are liver blood flow (Q), intrinsic clearance (CL_{int}), and fraction unbound in the plasma (f_{up}) (Eq 11.22).

$$CL_H = Q\left(\frac{CL_{int} \times f_{up}}{Q + CL_{int} \times f_{up}}\right) \qquad [11.22]$$

Any organ of clearance is primarily dependent on the blood flow to that organ (Q) and the efficiency of that organ in eliminating the drug (extraction efficiency). Hepatic extraction ratio (E) is dependent on liver blood flow (Q), free intrinsic clearance (CL_{int}), and free fraction in the plasma (f_{up}) (Eq 11.23).

$$E = \frac{CL_{int} \times f_{up}}{Q + CL_{int} \times f_{up}} \qquad [11.23]$$

The extraction ratio (E) and the fraction that escapes the first pass effect in the liver (f_{fp}) are interrelated.

Fraction Escaping Hepatic First Pass

The fraction that escapes the first-pass effect is that fraction that is not extracted by the liver. For example, if 0.8 or 80% of the drug is extracted or metabolized as it passes through the liver, the extraction ratio (E) would be 0.8. In other words, each time that the drug passes through the liver, 80% will be metabolized. This will leave only 0.2 or 20% to escape the first-pass effect and enter the systemic bloodstream. This is symbolized below (Eq 11.24).

$$f_{fp} = 1 - E \qquad [11.24]$$

Thus, the same factors that determine the extraction ratio (E) will determine the fraction that escapes the first pass effect (f_{fp}). A simple algebraic rearrangement and the combination of equations 11.23 and 11.24 demonstrate this relationship (Eq 11.25).

$$f_{fp} = \frac{Q}{Q + CL_{int} \times f_{up}} \qquad [11.25]$$

Liver blood flow (Q), intrinsic clearance (CL_{int}), and free fraction in the plasma (f_{up}) are the three factors that determine hepatic CL (CL_H), hepatic extraction ratio (E), and fraction that escapes the first pass effect (f_{fp}).

TABLE 11.8. SELECTED EXAMPLES OF DRUGS
AND CONDITIONS ALTERING LIVER BLOOD FLOW

Decreased Q (any ↓ in Cardiac Output)	Increase Q (any ↑ in Cardiac Output)
Arrhythmias	Food intake (transient)
β-Blockers	Positive inotropes
Cardiomyopathy	
CHF	
Hepatic cirrhosis	
Shock (transient)	

Liver Blood Flow

Liver blood flow (Q) is the volume of blood entering and exiting the liver per unit time. An average liver blood flow (Q) is about 90 L/h or 1.5 L/min, although disease and drugs can alter it. Table 11.8 lists some of these conditions and drugs.

Free Intrinsic Clearance

The hepatic free intrinsic clearance (CL_{int}) of a drug is the hypothetical measure of the removal of drug by the liver if the drug were not bound to plasma proteins and the delivery to the liver were not limited by liver blood flow. It is easiest to think of free intrinsic clearance as enzyme activity. It can be induced and inhibited by drugs that are enzyme inducers and inhibitors. Three factors determine the free intrinsic clearance (CL_{int}) of a drug: V_{max}, K_m, and concentration (C) (Eq 11.26).

$$CL_{int} = \frac{V_{max}}{K_m + C}$$

[11.26]

Michaelis–Menten

V_{max} is the maximum rate of metabolism. It represents the number of metabolizing enzymes or the capacity of the enzyme system. K_m is the Michaelis constant, which is the concentration at which the rate is half-maximal or $\frac{1}{2}V_{max}$. This is an inverse association constant and gives a measure of the affinity of the drug for the enzyme. The smaller the concentration at which $\frac{1}{2}V_{max}$ is achieved, the greater the affinity of the drug for the enzyme. Finally, the concentration of drug is a determinant of intrinsic clearance. For most drugs the K_m is much greater than the concentrations achieved in the therapeutic range. Mathematically, when there is a sum in the denominator of a fraction and one number is much greater than the other, the smaller number becomes relatively insignificant and can be considered unimportant to the result (Eq 11.26a).

$$CL_{int} = \frac{V_{max}}{K_m + \cancel{C_A}} \approx \frac{V_{max}}{K_m} \qquad [11.26a]$$

If this is done, it is apparent that for most drugs in the therapeutic range, the intrinsic clearance (CL_{int}) will be dependent on V_{max} and K_m only, not concentration. If the concentrations achieved are not much less than the K_m of a drug, concentration becomes a factor determining intrinsic clearance. This will then become nonlinear hepatic clearance. In other words, the intrinsic clearance (CL_{int}), and therefore hepatic clearance (CL_H), will be changing as the concentration changes. This is also called concentration-dependent or Michaelis–Menten kinetics. Phenytoin is a typical example of a drug that has a K_m similar to the concentrations achieved therapeutically. Any drug can exhibit nonlinear clearance if enough is given to permit the concentration to approach the K_m of the drug, as in some overdose situations. Some drugs exhibit nonlinear hepatic clearance in the therapeutic range. Phenytoin is a classic example of this.

Cytochrome P450 System

Drugs and disease can alter intrinsic clearance. The hepatic enzymes metabolize drugs by either Phase I or Phase II reactions. Phase I reactions are nonsynthetic and include oxidation and reduction reactions. Synthetic or Phase II reactions include conjugations, acetylation, and transulfuration. Cytochrome P450 (it maximally absorbs light at 450 nm, which is how it got its name) is an important group of enzymes needed to catalyze most of the oxidation and reduction reactions in the liver. CYP450 can be broken down into several families and subfamilies. Some of the substrates of those families are listed in Table 11.1. These are drugs that are dependent on that family of enzymes for metabolism. They would therefore be vulnerable if there were induction or inhibition of that CYP450 family. Some of the known enhancers and inhibitors of the families are listed in Tables 11.2 and 11.3. An inducing drug will increase the number of enzymes available for metabolism. Therefore, the V_{max} for that enzyme system would increase. The time it takes to induce depends on the half-life of the inducing drug and the enzyme turnover rate, which is 1–6 days.[6] Induction is dose dependent and reversible. Inhibition can occur in several ways. The most common is competitive inhibition. Two drugs may be vying for the same enzyme for metabolism. The drug with the strongest affinity would be preferentially metabolized, thus inhibiting the metabolism of the drug with the lesser affinity. This affinity is called the K_i. This is analogous to the Michaelis constant. The smaller the K_i the stronger the affinity for the enzyme. There can also be noncompetitive inhibition. Time to onset of inhibition is dependent on the half-lives of both the inhibitor and substrate drugs.

Within the families of the CYP there are genetic polymorphisms that have become apparent. Each patient is genetically programmed to have a certain geno-type for each family of CYP. This may result in a slower or faster rate of me-tabolism, depending on the genotype of the patient. Patients with a less common type of slow metabolizing ability for a particular family of CYP enzymes might explain the interpatient variability seen in the pharmacokinetics and adverse events of drugs cleared via these pathways. Drug probes have been studied al-lowing patients to have their phenotypes identified for CYP1A2, 2C19, 2E1, and 3A.[18] This is not done routinely at this time.

Fraction Unbound in Plasma

Unbound fraction in plasma is also an important factor in determining the he-patic clearance of a drug. Factors altering the protein binding of a drug are re-viewed in the Distribution section.

High Hepatic Extraction Drugs

Some drugs undergoing hepatic clearance have a very high extraction ratio and therefore undergo a significant first-pass effect. These drugs can be considered independently from those drugs with a low extraction ratio. Drugs with a high extraction ratio have a very strong attraction for the metabolizing enzyme. There-fore the rate-limiting step for clearance is delivery of the drug to the enzymes or liver blood flow (Q). On the basis of the assumption that liver blood flow is much less than the ability of the liver enzyme to metabolize free drug, some mathe-matical simplifications can be made to establish the important factors determin-ing clearance and bioavailability. Recall the determinants of hepatic clearance (Eq 11.22). When there is a sum in the denominator of a fraction, if one num-ber is much greater than the other, the smaller number becomes unimportant in determining the quotient. By inserting the assumption that $Q << CL_{int} \times f_{up}$, stated above, the factor determining hepatic clearance becomes hepatic blood flow (Q) (Eq 11.27).

$$CL_{H,HighE} = Q \, \frac{CL_{int} \times f_{up}}{\cancel{Q} + CL_{int} \times f_{up}} \approx Q \qquad [11.27]$$

This makes sense considering that the rate-limiting step is hepatic blood flow. It is very important to realize that for a high-extraction drug only an alteration in liver blood flow will change the hepatic clearance. Therefore, only drug and dis-ease interactions that affect Q will cause a change in CL_H.

The factors determining the fraction escaping the first pass effect (f_{fp}) can be determined by applying the above assumption to Eq 11-25 (Eq 11.28).

$$f_{fpHighE} = \frac{Q}{\cancel{Q} + CL_{int} \times f_{up}} \approx \frac{Q}{CL_{int} \times f_{up}} \qquad [11.28]$$

These are high-first-pass drugs, so considering the factors that will affect first pass is important. Note that changes in Q or $CL_{int} \times f_{up}$ may alter the first pass. This f_{up} is the fraction that the liver considers to be free and available for metabolism. High-extraction drugs are usually nonrestrictively cleared. This means the liver "sees" all the drug as being free and available for metabolism. Therefore, a change in f_{up} will probably not alter the f_{fp} appreciably for these drugs (see restrictive and nonrestrictive clearance).

These factors are important because predictions about what drugs and/or disease could alter $C_{ss,avg}$ and peak-to-trough interval can be made if the factors influencing these pharmacokinetic parameters are known. These can be contrasted with the factors determining the clearance and first-pass effect of the drugs with a low hepatic extraction.

Low-Hepatic-Extraction-Ratio Drugs

In contrast to high-extraction drugs, low-extraction drugs have a relatively insignificant attraction for the metabolizing enzyme. The rate-limiting step for the clearance of these drugs is the enzyme activity or intrinsic clearance of unbound drug, not delivery of the drug to the liver. The assumed relationship here is that $Q \gg CL_{int} \times f_{up}$. We can then mathematically simplify Eqs 11.22 and 11.25 to Eq 11.29 and 11.30, respectively.

$$CL_{H,LowE} = Q \frac{CL_{int} \times f_{up}}{Q + \cancel{CL_{int} \times f_{up}}} \approx CL_{int} \times f_{up} \qquad [11.29]$$

$$f_{fpLowE} = \frac{Q}{Q + \cancel{CL_{int} \times f_{up}}} \qquad [11.30]$$

This is very helpful when one is trying to make predictions about drug and disease interactions. Alterations in CL_{int} would be expected to alter CL_H of these drugs. Therefore, when monitoring drugs that are low extraction, it is very important to be aware if they are P450 substrates. If so, they could be subject to drug interactions involving alterations in the P450 system (see Table 11.1). Also, plasma protein binding interactions will cause a change in clearance. It is also useful to remember that the first-pass effect is not a factor for these drugs.

Restrictive and Nonrestrictive Clearance

The hepatic enzymes can only metabolize unbound drugs. Therefore, for most drugs only the free fraction can be metabolized, and the extraction ratio will never be more than the fraction unbound in the plasma ($E < f_{up}$). This is called restrictive clearance. For drugs with a very strong attraction to the hepatic enzyme, the free drug is metabolized very quickly, so quickly it seems as if the enzyme is stripping the drug from the protein. In this case the enzyme appears as if it is able to metabolize both bound and unbound drug. The extraction ratio in this case will be greater than the fraction unbound ($E > f_{up}$). This is called nonrestrictive clearance. Therefore, it can be thought that the hepatic enzyme "sees" both bound and unbound drug as being free and available for metabolism. Restrictively cleared drugs are usually also low-extraction drugs, and nonrestrictively cleared drugs are usually high-extraction drugs.

Predictions

You may be asking yourself, does any of this high versus low extraction, restrictive versus nonrestrictive clearance matter? When we can make the above assumptions it simplifies the things we need to be looking for to determine drug and disease interactions. Recall the two things we are trying to target in most situations, $C_{ss,avg}$ and peak-to-trough ratio. If either or both of these are altered by a change in F, V_d, or CL, we may need to make an alteration in the patient's dosage regimen. Let's examine high- and low-extraction drugs in this way.

Low-Extraction Drugs

A low-extraction drug has a relatively weak attraction for the hepatic enzyme(s) that metabolize it. The rate-limiting step is the intrinsic clearance of the unbound drug. This assumes $Q >> CL_{int} \times f_{up}$. This assumption allows the simplification of the determinants of hepatic clearance ($CL_H \approx CL_{int} \times f_{up}$) and f_{fp} ($f_{fp} \approx 1$) (Eq 11.29, 11.30). Under those assumptions, the determinants of $C_{ss,avg,tot}$ and $C_{ss,avg,free}$ can be determined for this type of drug. (Eq 11.31, 11.32)

$$C_{ss,avg,tot} \approx \frac{(f_a \times f_g \times 1)DR}{CL_{int} \times f_{up}} \qquad [11.31]$$

$$C_{ss,avg,free} \approx \frac{(f_a \times f_g \times 1)DR}{CL_{int} \times \cancel{f}_{up}} \times \cancel{f}_{up} \approx \frac{(f_a \times f_g)DR}{CL_{int}} \qquad [11.32]$$

A change in f_a, f_g, CL_{int}, or f_{up} would alter the total concentration at steady state. But an alteration in $C_{ss,avg,free}$ would be realized only if there were a change in f_a, f_g, or CL_{int}. A change in binding would not alter the free concentration at steady state but would alter the total concentration at steady state. Because total concentration is what is typically measured, the measured concentration would not reflect accurately what was happening with the active free concentration. In this case, it is important to anticipate this problem and react not to the total measured concentration but to what will be occurring with the free drug. If, for example, a drug that is highly bound to plasma proteins (primarily to albumin) and is a low-extraction drug cleared only by the liver is being given to a patient with a poor diet who has a decrease in albumin, the total concentration at steady state will have decreased. The patient is not experiencing any subtherapeutic signs or symptoms, but the physician is concerned because the measured concentration has fallen below the therapeutic range. He wants to increase the dose rate to increase the $C_{ss,avg,tot}$. You, however, caution against this because you know that a decrease in albumin could have increased the free fraction of the drug. This would initially have allowed for more free drug to be available, but when more free drug was available to the hepatic enzymes, clearance increased, and therefore there was no change in free concentration at steady state. In this case, although the total concentration was decreased because of an increase in clearance, the free concentration was not changed at steady state. The dose rate should remain the same. This also reminds us that we should treat the patient in light of the measured concentrations but never treat a measured concentration outside the context of the whole patient.

High-Extraction Drugs

Drugs with a high affinity for their metabolizing enzymes are high-extraction drugs. The rate-limiting step to their clearance is getting the drug to the site of metabolism, which in this case is liver blood flow (Q). Therefore, we assume that $Q \ll CL_{int} \times f_{up}$. This allows for simplification of the determinants of CLH (CLH $\approx$ Q) and f_{fp} ($f_{fp} \approx Q/CL_{int} \times f_u$) (Eqs 11.27 and 11.28). These assumptions are applied to identify the determinants of $C_{ss,avg,tot}$ (Eq 11.33).

$$C_{ss,avg,tot} \approx \frac{\left(f_a \times f_g \times \dfrac{\cancel{Q}}{CL_{int} \times f_{up}}\right)DR}{\cancel{Q}} \approx \frac{(f_a \times f_g)DR}{CL_{int} \times f_{up}} \qquad [11.33]$$

These equations are much more complex than the equations for the low-extraction drugs. This is because high-extraction drugs undergo a significant first-pass effect; therefore, the determinants of f_{fp} become important. In Eq 11.33 the liver blood flow is a determinant of both f_{fp} and CL; they therefore eliminate each other as factors in determining the $C_{ss,avg,tot}$ for a high-extraction drug given orally. Notice that the determinants of $C_{ss,avg,tot}$ for both high-extraction drugs given orally and low extraction drugs are the same. The difference is that $CL_{int} \times f_{up}$ determines clearance for a low-extraction drug but is a factor of f_{fp} for a high-extraction drug given orally.

These drugs are high-first-pass drugs; therefore, we would expect different factors to determine the $C_{ss,avg}$ for drugs given by a non-first-pass route. If a high-extraction drug were given intravenously, the $C_{ss,avg,tot}$ would be dependent on (Eq 11.34)

$$C_{ss,avg,tot} = \frac{DR}{CL} \approx \frac{DR}{Q} \qquad [11.34]$$

Thus, only a change in liver blood flow or dose rate would alter the total concentration of a high-extraction drug given intravenously. The factors determining $C_{ss,avg,free}$ would be (Eq 11.35)

$$C_{ss,avg,free} = \frac{DR}{CL} \times f_{up} \approx \frac{DR}{Q} \times f_{up} \qquad [11.35]$$

Therefore, if a high-extraction drug were given intravenously, and there was a displacement of the drug from its protein binding site, there would be an increase in the $C_{ss,avg,free}$ with no change in the $C_{ss,avg,tot}$. This could result in the measured total concentration being within the therapeutic range but the patient suffering from concentration-related side effects. In this case, the dose rate should be decreased because of the protein binding displacement.

BASIC CALCULATIONS TO DETERMINE INDIVIDUAL PHARMACOKINETIC VARIABLES

Characterization of a Concentration–Time Curve

To determine the initial pharmacokinetic parameters of a given drug, the drug will be administered, and the concentrations of drug in the plasma will be measured over time. If a drug is given as a bolus intravenous injection, bioavailability and rate of administration do not have to be considered. When this is done, the maximum concentration (C_{max}) will be achieved immediately after the drug is given at time zero. The drug will then distribute and be cleared from the body. Because a known amount of drug was introduced into the body, if the C_{max} is measured, the initial volume of distribution (V_c) can be calculated (Eq 11.36). Note this is a variation on Eq 11.14.

$$V_c = \frac{Dose\ (amt)}{C_{max}\ (amt/vol)} \qquad [11.36]$$

To determine the rate of elimination from the body (k), plasma concentrations will be collected and measured at at least two different points in time after administration. From these two time point concentrations, the slope of the line describing the elimination of the drug can be determined (Eq. 11.37):

$$k = \frac{\ln C_2 - \ln C_1}{t_2 - t_1}$$

[11.37]

Notice that this is a simple "rise over run" calculation. Memorization is not necessary if you understand that principle. This number will be negative. That is because it is a negative slope or movement from a higher concentration to a lower one with increasing time. This is a source of confusion. The elimination rate constant is used in equations from this point on as an absolute value. The elimination rate constant is important in determining the fraction of drug eliminated per unit time. The units of this constant are per time (i.e., $second^{-1}$ or $hour^{-1}$). Once the elimination rate constant (k) is calculated, it is quite easy to determine the half-life of the drug ($t_{1/2}$) (Eq 11.5).

$$t_{1/2} = \frac{0.693}{k}$$

[11.5]

Once the elimination rate constant and one other concentration on the concentration–time curve are known, any concentration at any time point can be determined (Eq 11.38).

$$C_2 = C_1 e^{-k(t_2-t_1)}$$

[11.38]

This is just a rearrangement of the above "rise over run" calculation for k (Eq 11.37). If the natural log were taken of each side of this equation, the result would be (Eq 11.39):

$$\ln C_2 = \ln C_1 \times \{-k(t_2 - t_1)\}$$

[11.39]

A simple rearrangement will result in the equation to determine k (Eq 11.37). The realization that C_1 represents the concentration closer to the time of administration and C_2 the concentration further from the administration time or time zero is important. For example, if the C_{max} is known, which, as in our above example, occurred at time zero, Eq 11.38 would look like this:

$$C_2 = C_{max} e^{-k(t_2)}$$

[11.40]

Therefore, the concentration at any time after C_{max} has occurred can be determined by inserting the measured C_{max}, the calculated k, and the time at which you would like to know the concentration. It is helpful to note that the mathematical phrase e^{-kt} represents the fraction remaining at that time t. For example, if the C_{max} was 100 mg/L and 10 hours later the concentration was 30 mg/L, then the fraction remaining (e^{-kt}) at time 10 hours after administration would be 0.3, or 30% remains 10 hours after administration (Eq 11.41).

$$C_2 = C_{max}e^{-kt_2} \qquad\qquad [11.41]$$

$$30 \text{ mg/L} = 100 \text{ mg/L} \times e^{-kt}$$

The log concentration–time curve for a one-compartment model that is linearly cleared is a straight line. It is instructive to think about the equation that describes this drug's behavior in terms of a line. Recall, the equation for a line is $y = mx + b$, where x and y are the parameters on the x and y axes, m is the slope of the line, and b the y-intercept. Equation 11.41 is in that form. By taking the natural log of both sides of the equation and some minor algebraic rearrangements, Eq 11.42 results:

$$\ln C_t = \ln C_{max} - kt$$

$$\ln C_t = (-k)t + \ln C_{max} \qquad\qquad [11.42]$$

where $y = \ln C_t$, $m = -k$, $x = t$, and $b = \ln C_{max}$.

Therefore, the y coordinate will be the natural log of the unknown concentration, and the x coordinate will be the time that the unknown concentration occurs. The slope is the elimination rate, and the y-intercept the natural log of C_{max}. This is a simplified look at a one-compartment model when a drug is given by intravenous bolus.

Multiple Compartments

The simplistic example above is helpful when trying to grasp the basic concepts of a time–concentration curve and the information that can be gathered from it. It is important to realize that drugs are rarely given by IV bolus and rarely if ever have instantaneous distribution. Most often drugs distribute into several groups of tissues at different rates. These are called compartments. Most drugs have at least two compartments; many have more. We do most of our calculations based on the assumption that a drug follows one-compartment pharmacokinetics. This is done for the sake of simplicity. In most cases, assuming one compartment does not result in an unacceptable margin of error.

A two-compartment model is often represented schematically as in Fig. 11.4. In a typical two-compartment model, the first compartment is called the central compartment. It represents the tissues where the drug is presented, and from which the drug is distributed and eliminated. It is physiologically thought of as the blood and highly perfused organs. The second compartment is called the pe-

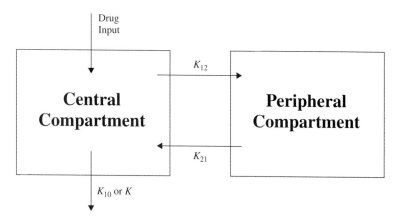

Figure 11.4. A representation of a two-compartment model.

ripheral compartment. This represents the groups of tissue that the drug distributes into more slowly. The drug will also have to move back out of the tissues in the peripheral compartment and return back to the central compartment to be removed. If a concentration–time curve of a two-compartment-model drug were characterized, the line depicting the log concentration versus time would not be straight (Fig 11.5). There would be an initial steeper decline, representing the distribution of the drug. The second phase of the line would be flatter, depicting the slower elimination of the drug. This second phase is called the terminal phase for a two-compartment model. The slope of this terminal phase is what is used

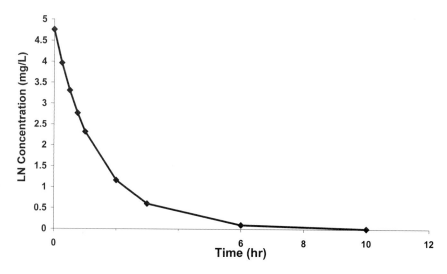

Figure 11.5. Concentration–time curve of two-compartment model.

to determine k and $t_{\frac{1}{2}}$. The biexponential line that is formed by this data can be analyzed to determine a characterization for both compartments, each having a slope (k) and y-intercept (C_{max}) to describe them. When the two compartmental lines are added, the equation to describe the concentration at any time can be determined (Eq 11.43).

$$C_t = C_1 e^{-k_1 t} + C_2 e^{-k_2 t} \qquad [11.43]$$

As more compartments are added, the describing equations and models become increasingly more complex. Most calculations become too cumbersome for humans with a model that assumes more than two compartments.

Area Under the Curve

Area under the curve is a model-independent parameter that is a good measure of drug exposure. The total body clearance can be determined from the dose administered and the area under the time-concentration curve (AUC) (Eq 11.44).

$$CL = \frac{Dose}{AUC} \qquad [11.44]$$

The area under the time–concentration curve can be determined in several ways. The most common is the trapezoidal rule, which is the sum of the areas between each successive concentration–time points (Eq 11.45).

$$AUC_{0-\infty} = \frac{C_1 + C_2}{2}(t_2 - t_1) + \frac{C_2 + C_3}{2}(t_3 - t_2) \cdots + \frac{C_n}{K} \qquad [11.45]$$

As can be seen in the above equation, the areas between successive concentrations are treated as rectangles. The height of each rectangle is the average of the two observed points, and the width of the rectangle is the difference between the two time points. The area between the last observed time point and infinity is a triangle that assumes a log-linear decline. It is based upon the quotient of the last time point observed and the elimination rate constant (K). The sum of these rectangles and the triangle gives a good estimate of the area under the time–concentration curve. The more measured concentrations the better will be the estimate. The AUC is important for determining clearance but can also be used to determine volume of distribution, average concentration at steady state ($C_{ss,avg}$), and bioavailability (Eqs 11.9 and 11.10).

APPLICATION

After reading the above information and doing the problems, you should be able to analyze and make predictions about any new drug that is presented on the market. The first questions might be physiochemical. Is this a chiral compound? Does it have a small therapeutic range? Is it a weak acid or a weak base? How big is it? How lipophilic is it? Is it a P-gp substrate, inducer, or inhibitor? Is it a substrate or known inhibitor or inducer of any of the CYP450 families found in the gut? Is it secreted into bile? Is it highly bound to plasma proteins? If so, which one(s)? What is the volume of distribution?

The next line of questions would address how the drug is cleared. What is its f_e? If it were highly cleared by the kidneys, you would want to determine its protein binding and the predominant process, active secretion versus reabsorption. If a drug were cleared by the liver, you would determine if it were a high- or low-extraction drug and also if it is restrictively or nonrestrictively cleared. You would want to know if it is a substrate or known inhibitor or inducer of any of the CYP450 families. You would also want to know if there were any active metabolites and, if so, how they are cleared. From this information, possible drug and disease interactions can be anticipated and avoided or adjustments made.

Therapeutic Drug Monitoring

Many drugs have large therapeutic ranges, and therefore, therapeutic drug monitoring is not necessary. This does not mean that utilizing and understanding the pharmacokinetic principles learned in the prior discussion cannot be useful to the clinician for these drugs. Table 11.9 lists reasons that drug should have their concentrations monitored. In general, they include drugs whose therapeutic efficacy and/or toxicity cannot be measured by any other means. A few of them are discussed below. The individual parameters of any new or unknown drug can usually be found in the package insert or some other readily available reference.

In general, if a drug is at steady state, it is easy to make needed dose rate adjustments, assuming the drug is cleared linearly and there has been no change in fraction unbound. Recall that the $C_{ss,avg}$ is determined by Eq 11.1.

$$C_{ss,avg} = \frac{F \times DR}{CL} \qquad [11.1]$$

TABLE 11.9. CONDITIONS FAVORING THE USE OF THERAPEUTIC DRUG MONITORING

1. An unpredictable dose–response relationship
2. A correlation between serum concentrations and efficacy/toxicity
3. A lack of a clearly observable clinical endpoint (i.e., blood pressure reduction)
4. A narrow therapeutic range
5. Toxicity or lack of efficacy of drug is dangerous
6. Accurate serum concentration measurement is readily available

In most cases it can be assumed that the CL and F are remaining constant. This is assuming linear clearance and no new drugs or diseases introduced that could alter the F or CL. That being the case, the DR and resulting $C_{ss,avg}$ are proportional. Therefore, a proportion can be set up (Eq 11.46):

$$\frac{DR_1}{C_{ss,avg_1}} = \frac{DR_2}{C_{ss,avg_2}} \qquad [11.46]$$

Therefore, if there is a known $C_{ss,avg}$ that results from a certain given DR, a new DR can be easily calculated for the new target $C_{ss,avg}$.

In some cases $C_{ss,avg}$ is not as helpful as peak and trough concentrations. This is the case for aminoglycosides.

Aminoglycosides and Vancomycin

Most antibiotics have large therapeutic ranges and thus do not warrant, in most cases, therapeutic drug monitoring. Aminoglycosides and vancomycin are two exceptions. They both have narrow therapeutic indices. These are the drugs for which we are very commonly asked to help determine the patient's dosage regimen.

These drugs are cleared exclusively by the kidneys ($f_e = 1$) and are primarily filtered only. They are not highly protein bound and therefore have a clearance that approximates creatinine clearance. They are not chiral compounds and are not subject to genetic polymorphism. They both exhibit multicompartment pharmacokinetics but are treated as if they had one compartment for dosing purposes.

Aminoglycosides

The aminoglycosides (AG) have remained very effective for treating gram-negative aerobic infections for more than 50 years. They are commonly used but are known to be potentially nephro- and ototoxic. The most commonly used drugs in this family are gentamicin and tobramycin. Amikacin is reserved for more resistant organisms, and others are used only topically because of higher rates of nephrotoxiciy. There are data linking efficacy to the C_{max} of AGs and the C_{max} to the MIC (minimum inhibitory concentration needed to inhibit the growth of the bacteria that you are treating) ratio.[7,8] There are also data linking trough concentrations and length of therapy to nephro- and ototoxicity. The nephrotoxicity is probably best characterized by correlating it to exposure time to the drug, which would be measured by the AUC. There are data correlating AUC with toxicity.[9,10]

Traditional Dosing

For many years a traditional individualized approach was taken to dosing with aminoglycosides. This method, popularized by Sawchuck and Zaske,[7] applied one-compartment pharmacokinetics to determine the patient's individual k, C_{max}, C_{min}, and V_d after measuring two or three serum concentrations within a dosing interval. This method advocated targeting a C_{max} of between 4 and 8 mg/L and a C_{min} of < 2 mg/L. The individualized approach targeting these C_{max}s and C_{min}s has been the mainstay of dosing aminoglycosides until recently, when the pharmacodynamic features of the AGs were considered when thinking about dosing strategies.

Extended-Interval Dosing

Aminoglycosides are concentration-dependent killers of aerobic gram-negative bacteria. Therefore, the higher the concentration, the greater the ability of the drug to kill bacteria. They are also able to continue to inhibit the growth of bacteria even after the concentration of AG has fallen below the MIC. This is called the postantibiotic effect (PAE). The PAE allows for an extended dose interval, longer than that predicted based on the MIC of the organism. These two factors taken together make a strong theoretical case for dosing with larger doses less often to enhance efficacy and minimize toxicity. There are several methods published that suggest ways to take advantage of these pharmacodynamic features. The most studied is the Hartford Method.[11] This method has shown to be at least equivalent to traditional methods for both efficacy and toxicities, with a few studies showing a slight advantage to extended-interval dosing for efficacy and nephrotoxicity. A 1998 survey of 249 hospitals nationwide found that approximately 75% report that they are using extended-interval dosing for AG.[12] This approach has been unfortunately named "once-daily dosing." Although using this method does often utilize a q24h schedule, it is not the only dose interval suggested and is increased for those with renal impairment. There are some concerns with how these methods are being implemented and whether there is a true advantage to this method.[13]

Vancomycin

Vancomycin is similar to aminoglycosides in that is cleared by the kidneys and the clearance mirrors creatinine clearance. The pharmacokinetic properties in which it differs from the aminoglycosides are that it has a larger volume of distribution, around 0.4L/kg, and it is about 50% bound to plasma proteins. The pharmacodynamics of this drug are quite different from those of aminoglycosides. It is not dependent on concentration but probably more dependent on the time that the microbe is exposed to the antibiotic. In this case, as opposed to the aminoglycosides, it is important to be sure that the concentration of vancomycin does not fall below effective levels. Therefore, a very small peak-to-trough ratio would be preferred when dosing this drug, whereas a large peak-to-trough ratio is the goal in dosing aminoglycosides.

There has been considerable controversy concerning how useful it is to follow the concentrations of this drug.[14-16] Although measuring a peak concentration seems to be of little value, it is important to ensure that the trough concentration does not fall below the concentration necessary to inhibit growth of the organism.

Traditionally we have assumed a one-compartment model when we calculate individualized pharmacokinetic parameters for patients on vancomycin, but a two- or three-compartment model is probably more accurate. It is hard to justify measuring a peak concentration, but measuring a trough concentration within a half-hour before administration of the next dose to ensure efficacy is probably warranted. If individualization is contemplated, a sample drawn earlier in the dose interval will be necessary.

QUESTIONS

Dosage Regimen Design

1. You read the following quote in a paper that you are evaluating: "There was an increase in the elimination rate constant (K); therefore, there was an increase in clearance." Does this make sense or not?
2. Your patient with epilepsy is well controlled on carbamazepine. He then goes to a mail-order pharmacy, which supplies him with a different brand of carbamazepine that is significantly less bioavailable. What would you expect to see? A(n) increase/decrease/no change in clearance, a(n) increase/decrease/no change in volume, a(n) increase/decrease/no change in $C_{ss,avg}$, and a(n) increase/decrease/no change in half-life.
3. Your patient is well controlled on a drug that is totally cleared by the kidneys. Your patient becomes renally impaired. For this drug, renal impairment decreases the volume of distribution as well as decreasing clearance. Explain how this knowledge will affect your choice of daily dose rate and dose interval.

Renal Clearance

For the given drugs; identify which of the following may explain an increase in $C_{ss,avg}$ and an increase in half-life. Also, in response to these effects, how would you anticipate needing to alter the patient's dosage regimen?

A. Alkalinzation of the urine
B. Acidification of the urine
C. Giving another weak acid; $f_e = 1$; $CL_r > CL_{gf}$
D. Giving another weak base; $f_e = 1$; $CL_r > CL_{gf}$
E. Giving mannitol, which increases urine flow
F. Giving a drug that displaces the drug from plasma protein binding sites
G. None of the above

1. Drug A: $f_e = 1$; weak acid; $CL_r = 14.4$ mL/min; $f_u = 0.85$
2. Drug B: $f_e = 1$; weak acid; $CL_r = 74$ mL/min; $f_u = 0.04$
3. Drug C: $f_e = 1$; weak base; $CL_r = 19.86$ L/hr; $f_u = 0.85$
4. Drug D: $f_e = 1$; neutral; $CL_r = 4$ L/hr; $f_u = 0.9$
5. Drug E: $f_e = 1$; weak acid; $CL_r = 11$ mL/min; $f_u = 0.85$

Hepatic Clearance

You will need to refer to the information in Table 11.10 to answer the questions below. The following are physiological factors that influence pharmacokinetic parameters of clearance, volume. and bioavailable fraction:

A. Fraction absorbed (f_a)
B. Fraction unbound in the plasma (f_u)
C. Fraction unbound in the tissue (f_{ut})
D. Hepatic enzyme activity (CL_{int})
E. Hepatic blood flow (Q)
F. None of the above

Choose as many as apply for the following questions:

1. A change in which of the above would alter phenytoin half-life?
2. A change in which of the above would alter the bioavailability of verapamil?
3. A change in which of the above would alter the total steady-state concentrations of quinidine, given orally?
4. A change in which of the above would alter the free steady-state concentrations of quinidine, given orally?

TABLE 11.10. INFORMATION FOR HEPATIC CLEARANCE REVIEW QUESTIONS

DRUG	f_e	E	f_u	BINDING PROTEINS	METAB CYP ENZYMES
Lidocaine	0.05	0.93	0.25	Alb, AAG	3A4
Propranolol	0.05	0.7	0.1	Alb, AAG	3A4, 2D6
Quinidine	0.18	0.05	0.25	Alb, AAG	3A4
Theophylline	0.1	0.03	0.6	Alb	1A2
Verapamil	0.14	0.75	0.1	Alb, AAG	3A4
Warfarin	0.05	0.005	0.01	Alb	2C9(S)

How would you anticipate needing to change your patient's dosage regimen in the following situations?

5. Addition of cimetidine to the regimen of your patient on a continuous infusion of lidocaine
6. A patient taking quinidine orally post-MI
7. A patient on parenteral propranolol with the onset of CHF
8. Addition of a drug that displaces warfarin from its binding site on albumin
9. Addition of a P4501A2 inhibitor to the regimen of your patient on a continuous infusion of theophylline/aminophylline
10. Removal of a p-glycoprotein inhibitor from the regimen of your patient on oral verapamil (p-glycoprotein substrate)

Basic Calculations

A patient with epilepsy is successfully treated for seizures with Drug A, 400 mg q12h (8 a.m. and 8 p.m.). The usual half-life of the drug is about 12 hours. The patient has been treated for 4 days. The therapeutic range for your lab for Drug A is 5–10 mg/L. Before the patient is discharged, you want to document the serum concentration during a steady-state dosing interval. Four blood samples are drawn:

Time postadministration	Serum concentrations
2 hours	9.5 mg/L
4 hours	8.43 mg/L
6 hours	7.47 mg/L
12 hours	5.21 mg/L

1. Plot the serum concentration–time curve
2. What is the concentration at time = 0?
3. Report k, $t_{1/2}$, and $C_{ss,min}$. Can you determine $C_{ss,max}$?
4. Report AUC and $C_{ss,avg}$.
5. Determine the concentration at 5 hours

Six months later, the same patient returns to the clinic. He reports "breakthrough" seizures in the morning and sometimes in the evening. You obtain a blood sample immediately before his next dose. The serum concentration is 2.8 mg/L
   What might have caused this?
   You measure the following serum concentrations during the dosing interval:

Time postadministration	Serum concentrations
2 hours	13.2 mg/L
4 hours	9.68 mg/L
6 hours	7.10 mg/L
12 hours	2.80 mg/L

A. Plot the serum concentration-time curve
B. Report k, $t_{1/2}$, and $C_{ss,min}$
C. Report AUC and $C_{ss,avg}$
D. Calculate the concentration at 5 hours
D. What do you think has caused this?

REFERENCES

1. Watkins PB, Wrighton SA, Schuetz EG, et al. Identification of glucocorticoid-inducible cytochromes P-450 in the intestinal mucosa of rats and man. J Clin Invest 1987;80:1029–1036.
2. Fojo AT, Ueda K, Slamon DJ, et al. Expression of a multidrug-resistance gene in human tumors and tissues. Proc Natl Acad Sci USA. 1987;84:265–269.
3. Wacher VJ, Silverman JA, Zhang Y, et al. Role of p-glycoprotein and cytochrome P450 3A in limiting oral absorption of peptides and petidomimetics. J Pharm Sci 1998;87:1322–1330.
4. Gwilt PR. Perrier D. Plasma protein binding and distribution characteristics of drugs as indices of their hemodialyzability. Clin Pharmacol Ther 1978;24:154.
5. Adapted from lecture by Janis J. MacKichan, Pharm.D. Ohio State University, Feb., 1985.
6. Michalets EL. Update: clinically significant cytochrome P450 drug interactions. Pharmacotherapy 1998:18;84.
7. Sawchuk RJ, Zaske DE. Pharmacokinetics of dosing regimens which utilize multiple intravenous infusions: gentamicin in burn patients. J Pharmacokinet Biopharm 1976;4:183–195.
8. Kashuba ADM, NafzigerAN, Drusano GL, Bertino JS. Optimizing aminoglycoside therapy for nosocomial pneumonia caused by gram-negative bacteria. Antimicrob Agents Chemother 1999; 43:623–629.
9. Rybak MJ, Abate BJ, Kang SL, et al. Prospective evaluation of the effect of an aminoglycoside dosing regimen on rates of observed nephrotoxicity and ototoxicity. Antimicrob Agents Chemother 1999;43:1549-1555.
10. Kirkpartrick CMJ, Buffull SB, Begg EJ. Once daily aminoglycoside therapy: potential ototoxicity. Antimicrob Agents Chemother 1997;879–880.
11. Nicolau DP, Freeman CD, Belliveau PP, et al. Antimicrob Agents Chemother 1995;39:650–655.
12. Chuck SK, Raber SR, Rodvold KA, et al. National survey of extended-interval aminoglycoside dosing. Clin Infect Dis 2000;30:433–439.
13. Brown GH, Bertino JS, Rotschafer JC. Single daily dosing of aminoglycosides—a community standard? Clin Infect Dis 2000;30:440–441.
14. Edwards DJ, Pancorbo S. Routine monitoring of serum vancomycin concentrations: waiting for proof of its value. Clin Pharm 1987;6:652–654.
15. Freeman CD, Quintiliani R, Nightingale CH. Vancomycin therapeutic drug monitoring: is it necessary? Ann Pharmacother 1993;27:594–598.
16. Saunders NJ. Why monitor peak vancomycin concentrations? Lancet 1994;344:1748–1750.
17. Yu DK. The contribution of P-glycoprotein to pharmacokinetic drug–drug interactions. J Clin Pharmacol 1999;39:1203–1211.
18. Streetman DS. Bertino JS, Nafzinger AN. Phenotyping of drug-metbolizing enzymes in adults: a review of in-vivo cytochrome P450 phenotyping probes. Pharmacogenetics 2000;10:187–216.

MEETING PRECEPTOR'S EXPECTATIONS: ROUNDING, SOAP NOTES, PATIENT EDUCATION

Jacquelyn L. Bainbridge, Ruth C. Taggart, and Janina Z. P. Janes

Goals: After reviewing the information in this chapter, you should be able to:

1. Describe a multidisciplinary team and the role of the pharmacist student.
2. Explain three good practices in writing for documentation.
3. List the elements of the SOAP note and explain how to create such a note. Document patient information in a correct and succinct format.
4. Explain the importance of understanding the patient and his belief system before initiation of medication therapy and how this fits the pharmaceutical care concept.

INTRODUCTION

This chapter is designed to help you prepare for your advanced practice rotations. There is a brief section on what to expect and how to prepare. These expectations are considerably greater than in your early experience or problem-based learning courses. It is time to take those experiences and advance your level of involvement and practice. You have heard through your years of training that pharmacists should practice pharmaceutical care. Pharmaceutical care is defined by Helper and Strand as the responsible provision for drug therapy for the purposes of achieving definite outcomes.[12] It is now time to begin practicing pharmaceutical care.

This entire textbook is about acquiring knowledge and how to use that knowledge to practice in a manner that provides pharmaceutical care to all patients. When providing pharmaceutical care, we focus on the individual patient, advocacy for social services, maximizing realistic therapeutic outcomes, minimizing therapeutic risks, and minimizing cost.[12] The provision of competent pharmaceutical care requires that you have a thorough understanding of the patient, his healthcare beliefs, support systems, and health status. Take what you learn from your preceptors, the facts from your didactic courses, and the pearls in this manual to develop your style of providing pharmaceutical care. It will take time and practice to be comfortable; pharmaceutical care is a philosophy that you must wear. There is not a better time to try it on than now.

CLINICAL ROTATIONS AND PRACTICE EXPECTATIONS

Preparing for Clinical Rotations

Preceptors, professors, and other healthcare professionals have expectations of what you will contribute to a rotation as a pharmacy student. The following suggestions will help you meet those expectations. First, be prepared for anything! The transition from the classroom to the clinical setting can be unsettling if you have not contemplated your new learning environment. Clinical settings are generally structured with numerous rules and regulations that must be followed by the guest practitioner—this means you, the student. Second, review Chapter 1 and be prepared to make a great first impression. Last, consider signing a contract with yourself promising to learn as much as possible during your rotation. Learning is an active process that is your responsibility. Use your time wisely, take advantage of all available resources, and cultivate a positive, enthusiastic attitude.

Preceptors will also expect you to be familiar with multidisciplinary teams, writing SOAP notes, and documenting pharmacy interventions or initiatives. These are key aspects of advanced clinical rotations that require cultivation of professional relationships and integration of didactic knowledge and analytic skills. Practicing SOAP note writing, chart documentation, and immersing yourself in the healthcare team will better prepare you to practice pharmacy in any practice setting.

Multidisciplinary Team Membership and Hospital Rounds

In most teaching institutions you will become a temporary member of a multidisciplinary team. A multidisciplinary team is an aggregate of professionals, sometimes consisting of attending physicians, medical residents and students, pharmacists and students, a nutritionist, ethicist, respiratory therapist, nurse practitioner, physician assistant, and social worker. The multidisciplinary team approach is seen in many hospitals, nursing homes, and private practices. Individual members of the team bring different areas of expertise into the patient care arena. As the pharmacy student you bring knowledge of disease states and the medications available for treatment of the disease, drug mechanisms of action, drug metabolism, duration of action, duration of therapy, and dosing. By offering this unique perspective, the pharmacy student helps avert drug misadventures and ultimately improve patient outcomes.

Patient care rounds are part of clinical rotations in many large teaching hospitals.[1] *Rounding,* in medical terms, means taking the multidisciplinary team to each patient room for discussion of disease and therapies, monitoring patient progress, and to determine patient outcomes. This is sometimes accomplished using only patient charts while the team stays in one place to discuss the patient. Physicians use rounds as an opportunity to evaluate each patient and his or her response to therapeutic intervention. Patient care rounds provide many opportunities for learning.

If you are assigned a rotation site where there are patient care rounds, you should take advantage of the opportunity to participate. When joining a team for rounds, introduce yourself as a pharmacy student, be prepared to ask and answer questions.[1] Participate in all activities, including those you feel "unrelated" to what you think is required of a pharmacist. Attendance at patient rounds enables you to directly observe patients, monitor medications, and practice written and verbal communication skills. It also provides you the chance to practice and test your problem-solving skills as the team works up a patient.

Rounding requires certain etiquette of each team member. Each multidisciplinary team may function a little differently. Table 12.1 lists basic guidelines for participating on rounds.

Find out what the dress code is for the team and dress appropriately. Some disciplines tend to be more relaxed than others. Dress and look like the rest of the members on your team. When wearing a white coat, be sure it is clean and ironed for patient care rounds. Preparation for rounds includes knowing your patients, their medical condition(s), what medications they are taking, and what diagnostic or laboratory tests are ordered or complete.[1] You will need to review the patient's chart an hour or two before the team to gather information. If laboratory results are available, print them or make notes. Other areas to review before rounds include an assessment of the patient's medications for interactions and appropriate dose. Is therapeutic duplication a problem? Are the dose and medication correct for the patient when renal and hepatic function are considered?

TABLE 12.1. RULES OF ETIQUETTE FOR PATIENT CARE ROUNDS

Dress appropriately (see Chapter 1).
Be prepared—carry reference book, notebook, note cards, and pen. Review patient charts *before* rounding starts. Check on all laboratory data.
Listen—don't talk. . . . You may miss important information.
Participate—offer what you know, check on what you do not as soon as possible.
Communicate effectively within standards set by each team.
Respect confidentiality.

Can any medication be switched from IV to PO? Have all suggestions prepared and approved by the preceptor before rounding, or follow the protocol discussed previously with your preceptor in regard to your participation on rounds. Speak up and articulate your knowledge. Many times comments that seem unimportant stimulate discussion and may change the care of a patient. Find out the team protocol or attending physician preference for questions, comments, and general communication on rounds. Listen to everything, ask questions, and follow up with all drug information responses in a timely manner. Maintain confidentiality and keep your patient conversations limited to non-patient-care areas.

Large teaching institution learning environments often differ greatly from those in small cities or smaller communities. Smaller communities may not be able to provide multidisciplinary team experiences as described above. This means that you will have to seek out different ways to learn and individuals to help you. Although it may not seem as exciting or as organized as a team setting, the learning is every bit as valuable.

Writing

For the rest of your pharmacy career you will be required to write in varying styles and formats. It does not matter whether you are writing notes in a chart or a chapter for a textbook; it is important to be clear and concise in your meaning. Always remember your audience and consider their expectations. Make sure you know what it is you want to say. Remember, when writing, if you do not understand the topic yourself, you can not write clearly about it for anyone else. In this chapter we discuss medical writing as it deals with a patient note in a medical chart.

The patient chart is a legal document. It is an effective way to communicate information about a patient to a primary care provider or consulting team. A chart note should be written as though the person reading it does not know the patient. Do not take for granted that others have the same information regarding the patient as you. Chart notes form a record of the patient's condition, response to medication, and procedures for each hospitalization or clinic visit. Chart notes enable the reader to understand what the patient feels, what problems there are, and the impressions of other healthcare professionals. Test results, medications, allergies, vital signs, physical assessment, and consults are all recorded and maintained in charts.

In completing a chart note, there are several "rules" or good practices to guide your writing. First, choose your words carefully so that the meaning of your note is not left open for speculation. Other health care professionals and possibly patient families, lawyers, etc. will read a chart note. It must contain correctly documented information regarding the patient's condition, therapies, and plan. Notes should be written using as few words as possible while still getting the message across to the reader. Table 12.2[2] contains a list of words that you can use to keep the patient chart note clear and concise.

TABLE 12.2. WORDS TO AVOID WHEN WRITING IN THE MEDICAL RECORD[2]

AVOID	WHEN YOU MEAN
In case of	When, if
At the same time as	During
Make an exception for	Except for, or when, exceptions include
At the time	From (specific times, dates, etc.)
Adequate quantity	> 100 cc's (be precise)
In spite of the fact that	Despite
Due to the fact that	Because
At a later date	Later (include a specific date and time if known)
A majority of	Nearly all, most
Accounted for by the fact	Justified by
As a consequence of	The result of
Has the ability of	Can
In order to . . . schedule an appointment	To
In some cases	Occasionally
It is clear that	Obviously
It is apparent	Clearly
It was written by Smith	Smith noted
Take into consideration	Consider
In case that	If

A second good writing practice is to avoid redundancy and bias. Do not repeat yourself within the same note because you feel you need to say the same thing several ways. Do not include personal subjective opinions such as "I find the patient to be distraught and feeling a bit overwhelmed." Be objective; "I found the patient screaming at the top of her voice and threatening to jump out of the window." Do not confuse offering your own subjective opinions with what patients tell you about their feelings. Patient information that is not documented by laboratory results, diagnostic procedures, or physical examination is the chief complaint or subjective information and belongs to that section of your note. Always be careful about including your own biased writing, as it may keep other practitioners from viewing the patient with an open mind.

A third good practice is to avoid using word abbreviations. The meaning of common abbreviations can vary with setting, and their incorrect use may prove embarrassing rather than fashionable. Consider the abbreviation "WNL." It might mean, "within normal limits" or it could mean "we never looked." The term "within normal limits" is subjective and can be interpreted in various ways by other professionals. There is a difference between "DC" and "dc."[3] The first abbreviation means "discharge," and the second means "discontinue." The easiest way to circumvent this problem is to avoid using abbreviations altogether. It is always best to write exactly what you mean when documenting information in charts.

It takes practice to write well, and you should take every opportunity available while on rotations to polish your writing skills. Organizing your writing in a format that is acceptable within the medical community is the next step to writing a good patient chart note.

SOAP Notes

The suggested format for organizing patient notes in medical charts is to use the *SOAP* note. *SOAP* is an acronym that stands for Subjective, Objective, Assessment, and Plan. *S* stands for subjective information that is elicited from interviewing the patient. This section includes information regarding the onset of symptoms, pain intensity, location, duration, and what makes symptoms better or worse. It is imperative to investigate past episodes of similar symptoms and treatment received on prior occasions. You should document the answers to questions:

- How are you feeling today?
- Why are you here today? (This is the chief complaint, presented in quotation marks)
- How have you been feeling? How long has this been going on? Tell me exactly when you feel this started, is it better at some times than others? Is there anything that makes this better or worse?
- Is there a family situation that may be contributing to your health/illness?
- What do you do for work?
- Is there anything else you would like to tell me?

This list is not inclusive. You will need to develop your own style of interview, as discussed in Chapter 3.

O stands for objective findings. This is the section where you document blood pressure, urine output, fever, ability to ambulate, heart sounds, wound size, oxygen saturation, and laboratory values. A complete physical assessment or a problem-focused exam should be included in this section. If you do not perform a physical, then refer to physician notes and document findings particularly relevant to medications.

A stands for assessment. The assessment statement should include the primary and secondary diagnoses and more if applicable. For example, "Problems for this patient include relapsing-remitting multiple sclerosis, exacerbation secondary to urinary tract infection."

P stands for plan. Remember that patient education is always included as part of the plan. The plan is developed based on the subjective and objective information and the final assessment. Developing and writing the plan must be completed with the preceptor's input and approval. Use the cases in the appendix to practice writing your own SOAP note and then review that with your preceptor. Chapters 15 and 16 in this manual have more practice cases.

Treating Patients in the Hospital

For the hospitalized patient, your time frame for achieving a desired outcome is short. Decisions are made quickly because the effectiveness of your plan, or lack of effectiveness, may mean the difference of an extra day(s) stay in the hospital. To accurately evaluate a therapeutic response in any patient, you must know the rationale for the drug treatment, the preferred response, and the time needed to achieve your desired effect.[4] A patient may reach the planned therapeutic goal but the treatment outcome be considered a failure. The treatment may be deemed a failure for two reasons: either the side effects are intolerable to the patient or the outcome was not as expected. In these cases you must have an alternative treatment plan that is ready to implement.

Sometimes when developing a plan, it may seem unnecessary or inefficient to involve the patient because after all you are the health professional and you must know best. Make it a habit early in your career to include patients and family in your planning. It is not unnecessary or inefficient. The patient's capacity for self-care when leaving the hospital is a determining factor when choosing drug therapy and directly linked to issues of patient education and compliance. There is a direct correlation between these issues and the success of drug therapy.[5-7] Patients and families that are active participants in the decision-making process feel that they have some control over the condition.

One way to include the hospitalized patient in planning his care is to present him with treatment options. Consider the patient who is in pain. You say, "We are thinking about changing the way you take your pain medication. Your current medication does not seem to be working as well as it could to control your pain. We would like you to take your pain medication every 4 hours for the next 24 hours to get your pain under control. Once your pain is in control, it is important that you do not let it get out of control. This can be accomplished by asking for your pain medication every 4 to 6 hours as needed. If this therapy does not work, we will discuss changing to another pain medication." This type of dialogue keeps the patient active in his treatment, provides him with options, and lets him know his needs are being considered. Do not forget to allow time for the patient to ask questions once you initiate this kind of discussion. Make the time to educate your patients before they are discharged from the hospital.

Check on your patients regularly while on your hospital rotations. You may have to follow them through moves to several floors. Hospitalized patients can improve or deteriorate rapidly, often in the time it takes you to eat your lunch.

It is important to stay current regarding your pateint's condition, as you may be questioned by a team member for updated information.

Treating Patients in an Ambulatory Care Setting

Treating patients in the hospital setting is very different from treating those who are in ambulatory care settings. Hospital patients are a captive audience. Ambulatory care is defined as "health services rendered to individuals under their own cognizance, any time when they are not in a hospital or other healthcare institutions."[8] Studies have shown that one in three persons engage in self-care for undiagnosed problems or disease states.[8] "The average American experiences one potentially self-treatable health problem every 3 to 4 days."[9] According to self-care studies, at any given time approximately one-third of these patients are taking nonprescribed medications. The clinical correlate of these statistics is that by the time the patient gets to you, they may have already tried several over-the-counter medications, herbal products, and nontraditional medicine techniques.

When patients finally come to clinic, they often have a variety of pharmaceutical agents in their daily regimen. This is even more likely if you live in an area where there is a large demographic of elderly people. The process of "sorting out" prescription medications, over-the-counter medications and alternative medications for interactions can be tedious. When reviewing the patient's current medication list or bottles, be sure to ask why the different medications are being prescribed. Make sure to ask if they are taking the medication, and how. Patients frequently have no idea why they are taking some medications. Always check expiration dates. Many times patients have outdated mediations and continue taking them because they have not been told to stop. Patients commonly have prescriptions for pain medications or antibiotics that are outdated and are kept "just in case." Insist on the disposal of these products and explain the hazards of keeping medications for self treatment. Remember to document all medications: dose, route of administration, dosing schedule, reason for the prescription, when it was started, last laboratory values if indicated, and prescribing physician.

A common mistake made by physicians and pharmacists is forgetting to counsel the patient on the length of treatment with a particular medication, storage requirements, and the danger of taking expired medications. When medications are stored improperly or kept too long, they can lose potency (sublingual nitroglycerin is good for only 6 months once the bottle is open—in more humid climates, 3 months is a better estimate) or become toxic (outdated tetracycline causes Fanconi-like syndrome). Ask patients about medications they have taken in the past for the same problem, duration of therapy, and why it was stopped. As described earlier, patients often see a number of healthcare providers who prescribe medications that interact. Every patient visit should begin with a medication review and be documented in the patient record.

Treating the patient in the ambulatory setting requires that you quickly get the information, develop a plan, and educate the patient. Keep in mind your patient most likely wanted to leave a half-hour ago, and you have 10 more patients waiting to see you before the end of the day. Developing the skills to see the patients quickly and efficiently and obtain all their information takes practice. You should be able to do it all by the end of your rotation if you are persistent in your efforts to achieve.

Patient Education

In both inpatient and outpatient settings, you will be required to provide patient education or counseling on their medications. The importance of this cannot be overemphasized. The best drug available can be prescribed for a patient, and the therapy will fail if the patient is not properly educated on how to take the medication, cannot afford to buy the medication, does not want to take the medication, or has limited self-care abilities. Patient education failure and self-care limitations are often misconstrued as patient noncompliance.[8] The fault is often not that of the patient but that of the healthcare practitioner.

Treatment failure and compliance issues are often avoidable. The patient education you provide must take into consideration the patient's cognitive abilities, literacy, beliefs, language barriers, financial situation, and support system. The frequency of the dosing schedule impacts patient compliance. Cramer et al. report that compliance rates for once-daily dosing is 87%, 81% for twice-daily dosing, 77% for three-times-a-day, and only 39% for four-times-a-day dosing.[10] Cognitive impairment may make the patient appear to be noncompliant, especially if the medication regimen is confusing and has multiple dosing or dosing adjustments that the patient must make.[8] In cases where the patient is noncompliant, compensatory aides such as pillboxes, written instructions for the patient or caregiver, and numbering of bottles are some ideas that can prevent drug misadventures.

Patients are often confused when a brand name such as Percocet 5/325® appears on the prescription and they receive oxycodone 5 mg /acetaminophen 325 mg from the pharmacy. Part of the patient education should include placing both the brand and generic name on all medication labels and patient education sheets. This helps to avoid confusion and duplication of therapy.

Patients must be educated regarding correct dose, time of dosing, and foods or drugs that may interfere with the efficacy of the new drug.[5] You should explain the difference between common and frequently experienced nonharmful side effects and dangerous ones that must be reported immediately. Include in your discussion when the side effects are most likely to occur, interventions available to minimize discomfort and physical harm, and when and where to reach a healthcare professional if needed.[4] Ask the patient to repeat this information back to you and ensure there are no further questions. Understanding the dosage amount and scheduling is crucial for patients. This is true for all drug therapy but is often confusing when PRN dosing is part of the regimen. For example, patients with diabetes using a sliding-scale insulin dosage must understand that the amount of insulin they take may change if blood glucose is outside of set acceptable parameters. The sliding-scale directions should be in writing with specifics on when to check glucose levels and how to treat elevated or low glucose serum values. Explain diet and food interactions to the patient and provide them with an information sheet that can be taken home. Make sure the patient understands the goals of therapy before leaving your office.[5]

Pharmacists often find it worthwhile to compose patient information sheets on commonly used drugs; this information is now provided by most community pharmacies. Teaching sheets give the patient and the pharmacist a chance to discuss the information provided. Written information reinforces pertinent advice and serves as a concrete reminder. Practitioners who provide written instructions can tailor the instructions to be patient specific. Tailoring written instructions requires knowledge of the patient as a person and an understanding of the patient's beliefs, life style, social and family support systems, and any barriers to compliance. Patients find written instructions from their practitioner or pharmacist more personal than the generic instructions and precautions that are provided by outpatient and ambulatory pharmacies.[11] Copies of these education sheets should be placed in the patient's medical record. This is an easy and effective way to document patient teaching and often required by law. Table 12.3 is an example of a tailored patient information sheet.

Practicing as a Professional Pharmacist

The time that you spend on your rotations is the time you need to practice becoming a professional. It seems to be an easy task to be a pharmacist. After all, you have been watching for years, and you are sure you can do it with both eyes shut and arms tied behind your back. You need to practice, just as if you are taking music lessons or learning to ski or painting. Many duties of being a pharmacist may come naturally to you. Others, such as becoming a good listener, writer, and team member, all require that you watch and then practice what you see others doing. Incorporating the facts into everyday functioning requires that you stop and problem solve and that you know what questions to ask. You can do this only by repetition and observation.

Professionalism is not learned from a text. Rather, it is learned through socialization and mentorship that begins early in the educational process.[12] You may have already learned or observed behaviors, in pharmacies or from your teachers, that you feel will define your own attitudes of professionalism. You will continue to learn appropriate professional practices as you progress on to your advanced practical experience rotations. Seek out the mentors who can help you grow as a professional in attitude and behavior.

You should anticipate that the preceptors will provide you with realistic expectations of professional practice customs.[12] Your preceptor should help you blend classroom learning and real-life clinical experiences that will test your professional judgment and values. Rules that are taught in the classroom may not

TABLE 12.3. PATIENT INFORMATION SHEET

NEURONTIN®[14]/GABAPENTIN

You have been given a prescription for Neurontin®. Neurontin® is a medication commonly used for seizures. It has been prescribed for you to decrease spasms, stiffness, abnormal eye movements, or pain. You will be receiving much lower doses than seizure patients receive. Possible side effects include drowsiness, anxiety, unsteady walk, blurry vision, dry mouth, constipation, dizziness, and hiccups. To minimize side effects, and to maximize benefit from the drug, you will start out taking very low doses and gradually increase, as outlined below. Although some people experience the desired effects within the first few days, most require careful dosing increases.

Take 300 mg of Neurontin® as described below. Remember that if your symptoms subside before you reach the full dosing schedule prescribed, there is no need to increase the dose. If the side effects such as drowsiness are troublesome, wait 2 to 3 more days before increasing your dose.

1. Space the doses fairly evenly throughout the day. For example, a schedule of 7 a.m., 2 p.m., and 9 p.m. works well for many people.
2. Take with food to decrease the possibility of nausea.
3. If you take antacids, take the Neurontin® 1 hour before or 2 hours after the antacids.
4. Be sure to tell your healthcare professional if you are taking Tagamet® (cimetidine).
5. Avoid hazardous activities if you experience drowsiness or dizziness.
6. Increase fluids (at least 2 quarts a day) and fiber in your diet to lessen the possibility of constipation.
7. Do not abruptly discontinue this medication.

Day	Morning	Afternoon	Evening
September 1–3			1 300-mg capsule
September 4–6	1 300-mg capsule		1 300-mg capsule
September 7–9	1 300-mg capsule	1 300-mg capsule	1 300-mg capsule
September 10–12	1 300-mg capsule	1 300-mg capsule	2 300-mg capsules
September 13–15	2 300-mg capsules	1 300-mg capsule	2 300-mg capsules
September 16–18	2 300-mg capsules	2 300-mg capsules	2 300-mg capsules
September 19–21	2 300-mg capsules	2 300-mg capsules	3 300-mg capsules
September 22–24	3 300-mg capsules	2 300-mg capsules	3 300-mg capsules
September 25–27	3 300-mg capsules	3 300-mg capsules	3 300-mg capsules

Please call the office with any problems, concerns, or questions. We may increase or decrease your dose based on our symptoms and any side effects. Office telephone # _____ After hours # _____

327

be followed or practical in real-life clinical situations, thus testing the limits of your professional attitudes and behavior. The more practice you seek, the better you will become at making these decisions on your own.

It takes time to develop a professional image. Your positive and professional approach to the practice improves your credibility with physicians, nurses, and other healthcare providers who will be participants in your clinical education.[13] A professional image enhances the confidence others have in you and confidence in yourself. A caring manner, assurance of your clinical knowledge, integrity, and a positive attitude will make your clinical rotations a successful experience.[13]

QUESTIONS

1. Why is student professionalism an important concept?
2. Why is it important for the student to communicate effectively in the medical record?
3. What information about the patient and his health status is required before any drug recommendations are made?
4. What factors might inhibit patient compliance?
5. List members of a multidisciplinary medical team.

REFERENCES

1. Boh LE, Hanson KK. Clerkship goals and objectives. In: Boh LE, ed. Clinical clerkship manual. Vancouver, WA: Applied Therapeutics, 1997;1–16.
2. Day RA. How to write & publish a scientific paper, 5th ed, Appendix 4. Phoenix: Oryx Press, 1998;238–243
3. Taber's cyclopedic medical dictionary,. 17th ed. Philadelphia: FA Davis, 1993;2352–2355.
4. Boyko WL, Yorkowski PJ, Ivey MF, Armistead JA, Roberts BL. Pharmacist influence on economic and morbidity outcomes in a tertiary care teaching hospital. Am J Health-Syst Pharmacy 1997;54:1591–1595.
5. Lehne RA, Moore L, Crosby L, Hamilton D. Pharmacology for nursing care. Philadelphia: WB Saunders, 1994:9–22.
6. Kern DE. Patient compliance with medical advice. In: Barker LR, Burton JR, Zieve PD, eds. Principles of ambulatory medicine, 4th ed. Baltimore: Williams & Wilkins, 1994:49.
7. Kern DE, Roberts JC. Preventive medicine and ambulatory practice. In: Barker LR, Burton JR, Zieve PD, eds. Principles of ambulatory medicine, 4th ed. Baltimore: Williams & Wilkins, 1994:25–26.
8. Barker LR, Roberts JC. Distinctive characteristics of ambulatory medicine. In: Barker LR, Burton JR, Zieve PD, eds. Principles of ambulatory medicine, 4th ed. Baltimore: Williams & Wilkins, 1994:3–19.
9. Limon L, Cimmino A, Lakamp J, eds. Nonprescription products: patient assessment handbook. Washington, DC: American Pharmaceutical Association, 1997:16–24.
10. Cramer JA, Mattson RH, Prevey ML, Scheyer RD, Ouellette VL. How often is medication taken as prescribed? A novel assessment technique. JAMA. 1989;261:3273–3277.
11. Kern DE. Patient compliance with medical advice. In: Barker LR, Burton JR, Zieve PD, eds. Principles of ambulatory medicine, 4th ed. Baltimore: Williams & Wilkins; 1994:49.
12. Hill WT. White paper on pharmacy student professionalism. J Am Pharmaceut Assoc 2000;40:1.
13. Hazebrook LS. Standards of professional conduct. In: Boh LE, ed. Clinical clerkship manual. Vancouver, WA: Applied Therapeutics, 1997:1–9.
14. Lacy CF, Armstrong LL, Goldman MP, Lance LL, eds. Drug information handbook, 8th ed. Hudson, OH: Lexi-Comp, 2000–2001:538–539.

BIBLIOGRAPHY

Helper DC, Strand LM. Opportunities and responsibilities in pharmaceutical care. Am J Hosp Pharm 1990;47:533–543.

Pierpaoli PG. What is a professional? Hosp Pharm Times. 1992;May:9–10.

Schneider PJ. Recommendations for pharmacists from the institute of medicine. Continuing education series in pharmacy and managed care. 2000;May/June(7):5–8.

Schoenbach VJ, Wagner EH, Beery WL. Health-risk appraisal: Review of evidence of effectiveness. Health Serv Res 1987;22:4.

Chase PA, Bainbridge J. Care plan for documenting pharmacist activities. Am J Hosp Pharm. 1993; 50:1885–1888.

Schwartz CE, Cole BF, Gelber RD. Measuring patient-centered outcomes in neurologic disease: Extending the Q-TWIST method. Arch Neurol 1995;52(8):754–762.

Katzung BG. Special aspects of geriatric pharmacology. In: Katzung BG, ed. Basic & Clinical Pharmacology, 7th ed. Stamford, CT: Appleton & Lange, 1998:989–991.

Rawlins MD, Thompson JW. Mechanisms of adverse drug reactions. In: Davies DM, ed. Textbook of adverse drug reactions, 4th ed. Oxford: Oxford University Press, 1991:18–45.

MEDWATCH Conference June 10, 1994. Clinical therapeutics and the recognition of drug-induced disease. A continuing education article. Washington, DC: Provided as a service by the staff college, Food and Drug Administration, Center for Drug Evaluation and Research. June 1995:1–4.

Manasse HR Jr. Medication use in an imperfect world: Drug misadventuring as an issue of public policy, Part 1. Am J Hosp Pharm. 1989;46:929–944.

Bates DW, Cullen DJ, Laird N, et al. Incidence of adverse drug events and potential adverse drug events. JAMA 1995;274:29–34.

ASHP Report: ASHP guidelines for preventing medication errors in hospitals. Am J Hosp Pharm 1993;50:305–314.

Bandura A. Self-efficacy; toward a unifying theory of behavior change. Psychol Bull 1997;84:191.

Shaw GB. Heartbreak house. The complete plays of George Bernard Shaw. London: Odhams, 1937:789.

Jones WHS. Hippocrates, Vol I. London: Loeb Classical Library, Harvard University Press, 1923.

Jones RA, Lopez LM, Beall DG. Cost-effective implementation of clinical pharmacy services in an ambulatory care clinic. Hosp Pharm 1991;26(9):778–782.

Huth EJ. Writing and publishing in medicine, 3rd ed. Baltimore: Williams & Wilkins, 1999:143.

CHARTING NEW PATHWAYS: AN INTRODUCTION TO MANAGED-CARE PHARMACY EXPERIENTIAL LEARNING ROTATION

Darlene M. Mednick, Tracy S. Hunter,
and Cristina E. Bello

Goals: After reviewing the information in this chapter, you should be able to:

1. Discuss the historical origins of managed health care and pharmacy benefit management.
2. Define commonly used managed care terms.
3. Explain factors influencing the cost of medications.
4. Present tools and approaches that managed care pharmacists can use to improve patient outcomes and provide cost effective care.
5. Describe the place of pharmacoeconomic research in the practice of managed care pharmacy.
6. Describe the career opportunities for practice in the managed care setting.
7. Outline steps to take to prepare for a managed care rotation or residency.

INTRODUCTION

According to Edward F. X. Hughes, Ph.D., a conceptual leader in the field, managed care is the application of standard business practices to the delivery of health care in the tradition of the American free enterprise system.[1] Another working definition of managed care is that it is the provision of health care with a corresponding concern for appropriate resource utilization. However, the simple phrase "managed health care" is often used to describe many new approaches to the organization and delivery of health services. As a result, this label stirs emotional responses from both reformers, who view it as an opportunity for improving the delivery of American health care, and from health care providers, who sometimes perceive it as a threat to their professional autonomy.

Two primary driving forces have shaped the world of American managed care as we know it today. The first is the professional imperative toward ensuring proper care, sometimes referred to as the "quality issue." The second is the drive to make money by improving bottom-line savings through cost-effective measures. Although seemingly divergent, these issues are both essential and inseparable in a capitalist economy. Sound economic practices are necessary because every organization needs a healthy bottom line in order to cover operating expenses. Correspondingly, the provision of health care has a significant social purpose, which dictates that professionals strive toward improving health outcomes. Doing so with a minimum of waste is both desirable and necessary to successfully perform that task.

Large managed-care organizations (or MCOs) introduced modern business management techniques into an area of our economy where these techniques had not historically been applied—the health care sector. As in any business setting, management assumes the responsibility of making decisions regarding the appropriate mix of the factors necessary to produce a product. In this case, the product is the health care of a defined population. Other standard business tasks that healthcare managers routinely perform are to negotiate prices for factors of production; strive to achieve the best quality product for the least cost; and systematically measure and continuously improve the outcomes of their product. These and other efficiencies are the basic methods that managed-care organizations employ in order to meet their mandated goals.

The purpose of this chapter is to prepare you as pharmacy students for your managed-care clerkship. It provides a brief survey of managed care in the United States, the historical context for the growth and development of pharmacy benefits managers (PBMs), as well as a discussion of definitions of some commonly used terms in order to help prepare you to best apply and develop your clinical and administrative skills in the managed-healthcare environment.

Managed-care clerkships are a unique learning experience in that they combine both the clinical and practical knowledge obtained in the pharmacy curriculum with the dynamics of the real-world business environment. For that reason, a typical managed-care clerkship experience is difficult to predict. No single job description adequately describes a managed-care pharmacist. In this environment pharmacists perform a variety of services and functions in assorted practice settings ranging from health plans, insurers, employers, and physician groups to acting as pharmacy benefits managers or as healthcare benefits consultants. Managed-care pharmacists are crucial to the design, development, and implementation of all aspects vital to the managed-care industry. However, the essential tools employed—those of persuasion, analytic evaluation, and clinical decision making as well as creative thinking—are necessary in all settings. To fully appreciate your role and better function in this area, you will need to rely heavily on these skills as well as an understanding of the history and philosophy affecting the evolution of health care in this nation.

MANAGED CARE IN THE UNITED STATES

The concept of managed care in this country dates back to the 1920s with the development of the first prepaid health plans. The launch of the Kaiser Health Plan during World War II is generally regarded as the first clinic-based system of managed care with a recognizable modern organizational structure.

After the war, various American employers began offering health plans to workers with a variety of benefits, ranging up to 100% coverage. Prescription medicines were eventually included in the standard healthcare benefit package. Labeled a Pharmacy Benefit, this coverage is defined as the payment for medications provided under terms of a contract with an insurer or payer.

As health care in general became more specialized and expensive, Medicare was implemented in the 1960s as a federal form of prepaid health coverage. In an effort to control increasing costs for medical services and expand access to health care, the Health Maintenance Organization (HMO) Act was introduced in 1973. This allowed HMO companies to offer their stock publicly and resulted in an influx of capital that soon catapulted them ahead of fee-for-service and indemnity health insurance plans. Today, with over three-quarters of the workforce in the United States "managed" by HMOs, Preferred Provider Organizations (PPOs), and other MCOs, these organizations have become important players in the healthcare delivery system.[2]

The 1980s witnessed the inception of healthcare management as an industry. HMOs were profitable business ventures with over 29 million patients enrolled.[3] Enrollment in HMOs climbed steadily to 56 million by 1995.[4] The 1990s also saw the consolidation of managed-care plans into large national corporations and the formation of groups such as the National Committee on Quality Assurance (NCQA) in an attempt to standardize and apply metrics to safeguard the quality of health care provided under managed care.

Despite changes in healthcare policy and the popularity of HMOs, healthcare costs continued to rise in the United States. Costs increased from 6% of the Gross Domestic Product (GDP) in 1965 to 14% in 1996.[5] It is predicted by the Health Care Financing Administration that healthcare costs will continue to escalate and that it will soon equal approximately 16.6% of the GDP or approximately 2 trillion dollars.[6] The need for cost-effective management and allocation of health resources will continue to be a major fact of life in the healthcare environment in the new millennium.

EVOLUTION OF PHARMACY BENEFITS MANAGERS

Because healthcare costs have increased exponentially, with prescription drug costs becoming the fastest growing component (more than other parts of total medical expenses including inpatient hospital costs), effectively managing the pharmacy benefit has become increasingly important. Further, the challenge of managing the pharmacy benefit is complicated by overall increasing use of prescription drugs, selecting newer more expensive products, clinical regimens that encourage the earlier use of maintenance drugs, and by the fact that the FDA has granted more new drug approvals than ever before.

In order to ensure that payers were able to continue providing a pharmacy benefit, healthcare policy makers began to rely on managed-care strategies and sound business principles to deal with the dilemma of providing quality care while controlling costs. Payers (employers, retiree groups, government, etc.) that were struggling to offer a pharmacy benefit increasingly began turn to MCOs and Pharmacy Benefits Managers (PBMs) to administer the benefit and control escalating costs. The term "Pharmacy Benefits Manager" may refer to a person, but the label typically applies to a firm that delivers, monitors, and manages the prescription drug portion of health insurance plans on behalf of plan sponsors (such as a self-insured employer, insurance company, or HMO) and that engages in, or directs, the practice of pharmacy.

Several factors have contributed to the success of PBMs. In the early years of managed care (1965–1980), when prescription drugs did not represent the high percentage of total healthcare dollars that they do today, most pharmacy benefits were administered exclusively by major medical plans. As HMOs and preferred provider organizations (PPOs) continued to expand, health plans began to look outside of their organization for specialized expertise. Nascent PBM firms rose to fill that emerging need to provide cost savings and at the same time ensure appropriate utilization in a way that would ultimately improve the health care of members or beneficiaries. Payers looked to PBMs to manage access to the prescription benefit, educate healthcare providers on optimal prescribing practices, provide quality-driven clinical management, and process manufacturer discounts and rebates. In other words, they provide special guidance for maximizing the benefits of prescription medications while controlling costs.

Today, employers, insurers, HMOs, PPOs, and government all utilize PBMs to assist in the administrative and clinical management of the prescription drug benefit. The introduction of online electronic claims processing coupled with the implementation of *copays* (a cost-sharing arrangement where the enrollee pays a specified flat amount for a specific service) and *cost sharing* (payment method where a person pays some of the health costs in order to receive medical care) has further heralded the increasing reliance on PBMs.

Currently, payers have been less able to rely on rebate dollars (price reductions paid by manufacturers for volume utilization and increasing market share) and are faced with capitation (a specified amount paid periodically to a health provider for a group of specified health services, regardless of quantity rendered) and risk-sharing contracts. PBMs have been able to meet these challenges with formulary management, outcomes-based therapy, and health management (also known as disease-state management or DSM).

DRIVERS OF PHARMACY COSTS

As noted above, the rising costs associated with pharmaceuticals can be assigned to many causes. Superficial analysis often credits the graying of America or points to pricing and marketing practices of the pharmaceutical industry and the recovery of costs of new product development as the primary culprits. In reality, a number of other complex factors interact and significantly contribute to the rising cost of pharmaceuticals. They include:

Demographic shifts within the US population
Dramatic growth in the treatment of chronic illness
Medications previously used to treat disease (e.g., cholesterol) are now being used to reduce risk factorsEnhanced consumer demand (primarily from direct-to-consumer advertising, educational programs, and higher expectations of success on the part of patients)
Escalation in the adoption of new products (product mix)
Price inflation
The costs of drug misadventures and inappropriate usage.[7]

The aging Baby Boomer generation is now and will continue to be a primary driver of pharmacy cost for many years. This very large population is now becoming older and experiencing more illness. Along with this trend toward aging comes a new attitude toward drug utilization. It is not unusual for this population to take medications in an attempt to reduce risk factors for certain diseases. Further, unlike previous generations, Boomers are not opposed to taking prescription medications for long periods of time. Thus, in this group, maintenance drugs may begin earlier, often as early as age 40 rather than the typical 65 years of age.

Other factors driving the increasing pharmacy cost paradigm derive from recent innovations in biotechnology and the emergence of new drugs. Remarkable and revolutionary medications have been developed for people who need them, but the expenses involved in development and testing unfortunately add to growing healthcare costs. Furthermore, hundreds of "biotech" products are currently in the pipeline, and those costs will ultimately have to be absorbed at some point.

Contemporary medical guidelines calling for earlier or more aggressive treatment of certain diseases also impact the economics of the pharmacy benefit. For many diseases, the latest treatment guidelines call for new combination regimens of three or four medications. Some guidelines encourage using higher doses of existing medications for extended periods of time than were previously administered. Additionally, patients are becoming more diligent about taking their medication as prescribed, a result of new drugs with fewer side effects or more convenient dosage forms, higher consumer awareness, and the education efforts of health providers geared toward compliance.

Direct-to-consumer (DTC) advertising also impacts pharmacy costs by increasing consumer demand for pharmaceuticals in general and especially for the advertised product. In 1999 alone, $1.8 billion was spent on DTC advertising geared toward creating consumer awareness.[8] In an age of informed consumers bombarded with information through television, newspapers, and the Internet, the result of increased awareness is increased demand and usage. Health plans often must cover the increased demand even though the actual benefit of added drug usage spurred on by DTC advertising is controversial and often questioned by experts. Some medications marketed through DTC advertising offer no measurable benefit to the patients through better outcomes and improved quality of life (QOL). Many argue that these products do not benefit the payers directly, by lowering total medical costs for a health plan, or indirectly, through decreases in work absenteeism and increases in productivity.

Although these and many other factors based on a health plan's demographics may influence economics to varying degrees, they offer pharmacists working in conjunction with other healthcare professionals an opportunity to develop and administer effective programs and services that will ultimately improve quality and manage costs. Finding that perfect balance will continue to be a crucial concern in the coming years and a chance for pharmacists to have a positive impact on society.

FINDING THE SOLUTION

There are many tools and techniques available to employers and health plans for managing their prescription drug benefit. Pharmacy benefits managers generally present and administer a menu of programs that can be adopted as appropriate for the objectives of a given group or healthcare plan. In general, prescription drug management techniques fall into two primary categories, plan design and benefit management. Plan design focuses on economic issues, defining access to and allocation of the payer's drug dollars through coverage decisions, preference of retail and home delivery distribution channels, selection of drugs, and quality management initiatives. Healthcare utilization is significantly influenced by enrollment and payment demographics such as the age, gender, and family size of the enrollees. Changes in utilization are affected by groups with a mix of single employees and employees with dependents as well as by women of childbearing age who experience a higher-than-average incidence of obstetric utilization. Members over 60 years of age have a higher rate of utilization in diagnostic categories such as neoplasm and circulatory system disorders. The introduction of new medical procedures and equipment can increase the cost of delivering medical care, as do physicians practicing defensive medicine and the rising cost of medical malpractice insurance.

Benefit management primarily focuses on clinical issues, evaluating safety, appropriate use of drugs, as well as the implementation and oversight of accepted clinical treatment guidelines. Government mandates and election of nonstandard benefits influence the cost of health coverage. Factors such as life-style choices (for example, smoking and alcohol consumption, sexual practices, or drug abuse), economic adversity, environmental hazards, job stress, or natural disasters influencing the member's health status can also affect the cost of the benefit.

Both plan design and benefit management should be considered in searching for a total solution to manage utilization, costs, and quality. Each component is crucial to success. For instance, even the most aggressive use of benefit management techniques cannot overcome a poorly conceived plan design with very low copayments and/or overly generous benefits or lack of oversight.

The following is a brief overview of various plan designs and benefit management methods used by managed-care organizations. They are only a part of the "tools of the trade" necessary to be mastered by managed care pharmacists to manage the pharmacy benefit.

Cost Sharing

Cost sharing defines the apportionment of costs between payer and the patient/member. Under this payment method, the patient/member pays some of the health costs in order to receive medical care. Often incentives are included to encourage cost-effective practices. For example, copayments may be classified as single or multiple-tier copays or flat dollar or percentage (coinsurance). Lower cost-sharing levels are used as incentives to encourage patients to accept and use generic drugs, preferred or formulary drugs, and/or home delivery distribution channels for obtaining prescriptions.

Inclusions and Exclusions

Inclusions and exclusions are terms that define coverage rules or limit certain drug categories that will or will not be covered under a plan. Standard exclusions to the prescription benefit often are experimental drugs or medication used for cosmetic purposes such as Renova® for wrinkles. The payer may also select other exclusions that are plan-specific and widely varied. For example, the topic of the exclusion of oral contraceptives by certain employers has been of recent interest in the national media.

Retail Pharmacy Networks

Retail pharmacy networks concentrate purchasing power and secure discounts by limiting the number of pharmacies where members can be reimbursed for drug expenses. The network can be classified as either broad or narrow. Performance-based networks provide incentives to pharmacies for dispensing generic and formulary drugs and achieving utilization-review standards of excellence. Financial penalties for failure to meet minimum standards can also be imposed as a method of ensuring optimal performance.

Home Delivery Pharmacy Service

Direct home delivery via the mail or other methods of distribution is a cost-effective channel for maintenance drugs. This plan design selection is associated with higher generic substitution and formulary compliance rates and lower overhead costs. In recent times, online pharmacies have engaged in providing this service.

Generic Drug Incentives

Generic drugs (those not protected by trademark) cost about one-third of their brand-name equivalents and represent an important cost savings for health plans. Financial incentives in the form of lowered copayments for generic substitutions or higher copayments for brand-name drugs are considered important tools toward effectively managing costs while maintaining quality of care.

Formulary Management

A formulary is a listing of preferred medications selected for quality and cost-effectiveness. Formulary management allows for selection and review of the list of drugs available for reimbursement. With the formulary, the manager has the ability to move market share of a product and thus negotiate lower prices and larger rebates from pharmaceutical manufacturers. The types of formularies include:

Open formulary: members pay the same copay for preferred and nonpreferred drugs.

Incentive formulary: provides incentives to use generics and preferred drugs through lower copayments.

Closed formulary: coverage of nonpreferred drugs only if there is no viable preferred drug alternative.

Utilization Review, Utilization Management, and Drug Utilization Review

Utilization review (UR) is the evaluation of the necessity, appropriateness, and efficiency of the use of services, procedures, and medications in the healthcare environment. It is a method of tracking, reviewing, and rendering opinions regarding care provided to patients and a key component in utilization management (UM). In a hospital, this includes review of the appropriateness of admissions, services ordered and provided, length of a stay, and discharge practices, on both concurrent and retrospective bases. Utilization review primarily involves the review of patient records and patient bills but may also include telephone conversations with providers. It typically involves the use of protocols, benchmarks, or data that managers then use to compare specific cases to an aggregate set of cases. Measurement of utilization of all medical services in combination is usually presented in terms of dollar expenditures. Use is expressed in rates per unit of population at risk for a study period such as the number of admissions to the hospital per 1000 persons over age 65 per year or the number of visits to a physician per person per year for an annual physical. UR is one of the primary tools utilized by MCOs and health plans to manage or control overutilization, reduce costs, and manage care. Managed-care organizations will sometimes refuse to reimburse or pay for services that do not meet their own sets of UR standards.

Another tool used in utilization management is the drug utilization review (DUR), also sometimes called drug use evaluation (DUE). This is an analysis of an insured population's drug utilization with the goal of determining how to reduce the cost of usage. Reviews often result in recommendations to practitioners, including generic substitutions, use of formularies, use of copayments for prescriptions, and educational interventions. In some cases, practitioners are penalized or rewarded depending on their drug prescription-related costs and utilization. Some critics claim that these incentives can adversely affect doctor decisions, but others see this as a solution to overprescribing.

Concurrent Review Programs

A concurrent review program is the evaluation of the necessity, appropriateness, and efficiency of a procedure or drug utilization during the same time frame that the care is provided. This often takes place in the pharmacy with an electronic point-of-service (POS) claims-processing system. With this information, managers can apply guidelines and rules during the dispensing process to identify and act on opportunities for quality improvement and savings.

Retrospective Utilization Review Programs

Retrospective programs are systems for analyzing medical necessity and appropriateness of services rendered by a review that is conducted after the service has been provided to a patient. The review focuses on determining the appropriateness, necessity, quality, and reasonableness of healthcare services provided or medications that were dispensed. Although seen as less desirable than concurrent review, retrospective programs apply guidelines to identify prescribing and dispensing patterns and intervene through reporting, profiling, and education and offer another opportunity for quality and cost improvements.[9]

Performance Indicators

The expenses related to prescription medications are carefully monitored by managed-care pharmacists on a plan-wide basis rather than an individual patient basis. To facilitate the analysis, the cost of the benefit is typically reported in terms of per member per month (PMPM) format or per member per year (PMPY) format for payments and utilization. In reviewing these statistics, the term *member* is defined as each individual eligible for coverage and properly enrolled under a contract.

Payments are reported in aggregate dollars to facilitate comparisons. For example, all the costs associated with medical institutions are reported on an inpatient and outpatient basis and by total facilities (both added together). In addition, professional payments are figured as the total dollars paid for professional services received by the member. A grand total of all medically related expenses is then calculated.

Payments per person are calculated as in equations 13.1 and 13.2.

$$\text{Payment per employee} = \frac{\text{Grand total of payments}}{\text{Employees (average number)}} \qquad [13.1]$$

$$\text{Payment per member} = \frac{\text{Grand total of payments}}{\text{Members (average number)}} \qquad [13.2]$$

To analyze the expenses of the plan or group, the total paid for the group's prescription drug products is calculated. Aggregate calculations allow the benefit managers to track costs and utilization and compare their experience with similar groups. Two key indicators for pharmacy costs are calculated by equations 13.3 and 13.4.

$$\frac{\text{Prescription drug payments/}}{\text{Prescription}} = \frac{\text{Total dollars spent on medications}}{\text{Number of scripts}} \qquad [13.3]$$

$$\text{Prescriptions per 1000 members} = \frac{(\text{Scripts} \times 1000 \times \text{AF})}{\text{Number of members (average)}} \qquad [13.4]$$

where AF = 12 divided by the number of months in the study period.

One of the most commonly used key indicators for monitoring and reporting drug utilization is the PMPM (per member per month) formula for drug costs. This rough figure is tracked monthly and is shown in equation 13.5:

$$\frac{\text{Prescription drug payments}}{\text{Members (average)} \times \text{months in study period}} \qquad [13.5]$$

Other performance indicators that are closely monitored are generic/brand fill rates, generic utilization rates, average ingredient costs, and formulary compliance rates. The generic/brand fill rates and generic utilization rates both represent the generic utilization within the plan and are used to track and refine plan prescribing patterns. Average ingredient costs are reported for plans, regions, and even nationally. For instance, it was recently reported that the average wholesale ingredient costs rose 16.2% nationally in the year 2000.[10] National cost data can be an important tool to put a plan's performance into perspective. If costs rose 10% nationally but the local plan experienced a 20% rise, then a study of the reasons for the discrepancy would be necessary.

Practice Summaries (Physician Profiling)

Creating practice summaries is a method of aggregating data in formats that display patterns of healthcare services (such as prescribing patterns) over a defined period of time. The practice summary reports that are generated are sometimes referred to as physician report cards or a physican profile. These reports can be used to identify and encourage change in prescribers with the greatest potential opportunity for quality improvement and savings.

Health Management (Disease State Management, DSM)

Health management is a comprehensive program that identifies a population of patients with or at risk for a disease and provides a framework for delivering care based on evidence-based medicine. Health management helps patients and prescribers control, alleviate, or prevent illness, resulting in improved outcomes in the areas of quality, cost, health status, and patient satisfaction.

Point-of-Care (POC) Connectivity

POC connectivity improves efficiency, accuracy, and quality through the collection and management of data at the point of care with such innovations as online communication and electronic prescribing. Clinical interventions performed after the fact can be inefficient and less effective, potentially resulting in patient dissatisfaction. New technologies offer concurrent information, complete access to patients' medical and prescription history, contraindications, as well as providing instant eligibility status at the clinician's fingertips. Although they are still in the seminal stages, online POC systems have the potential to provide clinicians immediate access to:

- Patients' complete prescription record from all prescribers
- Drug information
- Allergies
- Generic alternatives
- Formulary and preferred drug lists with a cost comparison to nonformulary alternatives
- Patient's eligibility and plan specifications
- Automatic warning of contraindications or questionable doses, with hyperlinks to relevant clinical guidelines, research findings, and product information
- Patient education material

Additionally, the prescriber can transmit prescription orders electronically to the pharmacy's computer system, thus reducing the potential for errors from interpretation of handwriting or manual entry. The pharmacist benefits by receiving a prescription that is complete and ready to fill because problems with insurance coverage and potential drug interactions are resolved at the point of care. It is estimated that 26% of pharmacists' time is spent on insurance-related issues, and the use of electronic prescribing can free time for pharmacists to devote to providing pharmaceutical care and insuring better health outcomes.[11]

PHARMACOECONOMICS AND OUTCOMES RESEARCH

An "outcome" is a change in an individual's health status that can be attributed to some previous health care and is the result of that care.[12] Outcomes research involves data collection and analysis to assess the viability of various therapeutic interventions. The results from outcomes research is then used to manage the overall health status of patients over time.

Pharmacoeconomics is a component of outcomes research. Pharmacoeconomics is the study of costs and consequences of pharmaceutical products and services. The results of these studies are then used to formulate best-use plans for health management. The most common pharmacoeconomic studies include cost–benefit analysis, cost-effectiveness analysis, cost-minimization analysis, and cost–utility analysis, as described below.

Cost–Benefit Analysis (Evaluation)

Cost–benefit is an analytic method in which a program's cost is compared to the program's benefits for a period of time as an aid in determining the best investment of resources. Cost–benefit analysis expresses the outcomes of therapy in terms of dollars rather than physical units. Because all outcomes are measured in dollar units, this can be used to compare a variety of alternative courses of action with different outcomes. For example, it would be possible to compare the cost of expanding a community-based hypertension clinic to the cost of adding the latest antihypertensive medication to a managed-care formulary.[13]

Cost–Effectiveness Analysis

A cost–effectiveness analysis or CEA evaluation relates the cost of a drug or procedure to the health benefits resulting from it. The efficacy of a program in achieving given intervention outcomes is measured in relation to the program costs. This is usually expressed as a ratio, as the cost per life-year saved, or as the cost per quality-adjusted life-year saved. Follow-up studies, outcome studies, and various management programs attempt to assess treatment efficacy, while cost–effectiveness analysis provides a ratio of this measurement in relation to expenditures.

Cost-Minimization Analysis

As its name implies, cost minimization analysis (CMA) is method of determining the least costly option among several alternatives that will yield an equivalent outcome. CMA is used when outcomes for all alternatives are known or accepted to be identical. Such analyses are useful, for example, when determining patient-to-caregiver ratios or when creating formularies.

Cost–Utility Analysis

Cost–utility analysis compares two or more treatments in which costs are measured in dollars and outcomes are measured in quality-adjusted life years. Cost utility analysis is used to attribute monetary values to quality-of-life issues or patient preferences. Because quality of life is difficult to quantify, this method is rarely seen in healthcare literature outside of very specific follow-up studies of cancer patients.

EXPANDING OPPORTUNITIES IN MANAGED-CARE PHARMACY

This is a propitious time for managed-care pharmacists. The market for managed-care pharmacy is growing at a phenomenal pace. Economic opportunities for pharmacists in managed care are accompanying that growth. HMOs and other MCOs provide pharmacists with established practice settings nationwide as well-paid clinicians, managers, and administrators. Increasing numbers of pharmacists are being employed by PBMs to assist with drug formulary management, contract negotiations with pharmaceutical manufactures, and prescription claims processing. Pharmacists are also finding employment as consultants to managed-care companies and large self-insured corporate employers. As consultants, their responsibilities include such diverse roles as examining existing pharmacy benefits plans, developing strategies for improvement, as well as program and compliance oversight.[14]

The pharmaceutical industry has established managed-care divisions to participate in pharmacy benefits programs and managed-care activities. Opportunities in government include such agencies as the Indian Health Service, Veterans Administration, and National Institutes of Health along with Medicare and Medicaid programs. States are employing managed-care pharmacists to assist in the implementation of their new statewide UR (utilization review) programs. Colleges of pharmacy are incorporating didactic and experiential courses in managed care, which opens the door for managed-care pharmacists interested in practicing in academia.[15]

Optimizing health care relative to drug therapy in the managed-care environment is a complex task that involves state-of-the-art fiscal and clinical management skills. Given the need for today's managed-care pharmacists, the need for pharmacists to train for practicing in managed-care settings is as great or greater than for any area of practice.

PREPARING FOR YOUR MANAGED CARE CLERKSHIP

The fundamental goal of the clerkship in managed-care pharmacy is to provide a structured educational and training experience for pharmacy students whose ability, motivation, and career aspirations suggest potential for creative and innovative leadership. The focus of the clerkship is geared toward the education and training of fiscal, human resource, and clinical managers who can serve as creative and innovative leaders in assuring high standards in managed-care pharmacy practice. Advancing those standards of practice means serving the drug therapy needs of society in the most efficient and effective manner. Managed-care pharmacists are viewed as individuals leading the way in assuming a major responsibility for advancing and redefining the evolving interprofessional system of healthcare management and delivery.[16]

Your managed-care experiential clerkship will vary depending on the practice setting and organization. However, the essential managed-care survival skills involve the same basic competencies. They include developing and using the following:

1. Communication skills: written, oral, and active listening
2. Critical thinking/problem solving
3. Deductive reasoning/analytic skills
4. Teamwork/collaboration
5. Negotiation skills
6. Influence/persuasion skills
7. Project management
8. Time management
9. Computer skills.[17]

In addition to these general skills, you should be aware of and incorporate specific organizational protocols and basic business etiquette in your quest for excellence. The managed-care clerkship may be your first experience in a nontraditional pharmacy setting, but it is an opportunity to develop skills that will serve you for a lifetime. Often you will be working out of administrative offices in close association with non–healthcare professionals. This requires that professionalism be scrupulously maintained. Professional conduct and appropriate dress are essential. In a nontraditional pharmacy setting, a consultation jacket or smock will not suffice. Meetings, business lunches, and presentations with various departments require that the student be dressed appropriately at all times.

Attendance at meetings may make up a large portion of the managed-care clerkship, just as it does in the corporate world. This unique experience will expose you to the larger context of providing health services and nonpharmacy issues in managed care. This is often a student's first exposure to professionals in marketing, contracting, quality assurance, and information technology. Ask your preceptor to explain the job requirements of those in attendance or provide you with an organizational chart. It may also help to review previous minutes so that you are better able to understand the projects and issues being discussed. If during any meetings you should have questions, write them down. After the meeting, discuss with your preceptor any terms or concepts that are unfamiliar to you. Following this advice will make meetings more meaningful and allow you to contribute insight and information that are valuable.

In any business environment, you may have access to data that are proprietary. This is especially true in the health industry. The same rules of respect and confidentiality that apply in a hospital or community pharmacy setting also apply in a managed-care setting. You would not want a patient's family member to overhear you discussing their loved one's medical condition in the hospital elevator. Likewise, you would not want a competing organization to be privy to contract prices or innovative programs that are being implemented at your organization.

There are several resources available that provide in-depth information on healthcare reform and managed-care principles in pharmacy that can help prepare you for your clerkship. An excellent online resource is provided by the Academy of Managed Care Pharmacy (AMCP) found at *www.AMCP.org*. Their Web site provides late-breaking industry news, internship opportunities, and information on managed-care residencies as well as links to a wide variety of published sources of information. Their publication, *The Journal of Managed Care Pharmacy,* is considered a leader in the field. The American Society of Health-System Pharmacists (ASHP) also provides a Web site with unique insight for pharmacists employed by HMOs, PBMs, and other managed-care operations. Their Web site, found at *www.ashp.org/managedcare/*, provides information, resources, and links to articles on patient care, monitoring patient outcomes, design management of pharmacy benefits, and participation in a pharmacy and therapeutics (P&T) committee to establish the types of drugs used by health maintenance organizations.

Other sources for guidance are the many knowledgeable pharmacists already practicing in the field of managed care. Building relationships with experienced managed-care practitioners can provide practical insight and perceptiveness that is often not obtainable from Web sites, books, or even a college-level course of instruction.

In view of the drug information explosion, emerging reimbursement trends, changing healthcare delivery patterns, functional differentiation and specialization in health care, and the increased recognition of the need to improve drug therapy management, it is essential that educational and training activities be "responsive to the needs of the professional marketplace and the health needs of society."[16] This training experience should develop an appreciation and desire to advance your knowledge and skills in the delivery of pharmaceutical services within the managed-care setting.

QUESTIONS

1. What is the role of PBMs in today's healthcare system?
2. What are the common drivers of pharmacy costs?
3. Provide examples of a cost–benefit analysis, cost-effectiveness analysis, cost-minimization analysis, and a cost–utility analysis.
4. Which online resources offer students information on industry news, internships, and residency opportunities?

5. How would you distinguish utilization review (UR), utilization management (UM), and drug utilization review (DUR)?

6. How are managed-care principles present in nonmanaged-care pharmacy clerkships?

REFERENCES

1. Hughes EFX. Foreword. In: Nash D, ed. The physicians guide to managed care. Gaithersburg, MD: Aspen, 1994.
2. History of managed care. Available at www.ncmic.com/NCMIC_Ins/DoctorsOfChiro/Practice Tools/managed_care_sln/history.asp. Accessed August 1, 2001.
3. Eisenberg JS. Will the HMO beast grow new fangs? Rev Optom OnLine 2000;April 15. Available at www.revoptom.com/Features/ro0400f4.htm. Accessed August 2, 2001.
4. Mullen MJ. Testimony on the impact of managed care on the delivery of health services before the Department of Health Interim Budget Committee on Health Care, June 27, 2000. Available at: www.health.state.nd.us/testimony/interim/ManagedCare062700.pdf/. Accessed August 2, 2001.
5. Kuttner R. The American health care system—employer sponsored health coverage. N Engl J Med 1999;340(3):248–252.
6. Iglehart JK. The American health care system—expenditures. N Engl J Med 1999;340(1):70–76.
7. Teitelbaum F, et al. Express scripts. Drug Trend Rep June 2000. Available at www.express-scripts.com/other/#. Accessed August 3, 2001.
8. Point of View. Direct to consumer advertising. POV Rep 1998;36.
9. Pohly P. Pam Pohly's net guide: glossary of terms in managed health care. Available at: www.pohly.com/terms_u.html. Accessed August 2, 2001.
10. Managing pharmacy benefit costs—new insights for a new century, 2000 edition. Merck-Medco Drug Trend Rep 2001.
11. Hunter TS, Kost TM. The Internet—a new way to communicate. In: Hunter TS, ed. E-pharmacy—a pharmacist's guide to the internet CareZone. Washington, DC: APhA, 2001.
12. Schug SH. Choosing a health outcome instrument. European Research Group on Health Outcomes Policy Statement, March 4, 1996. Available at: www.meb.uni-bonn.de/standards/ERGHO/ERGHO_Instruments.html. Accessed August 3, 2001.
13. Reeder CE, Kozma CM, McCollam AR. Overview of pharmaceutical outcomes, pharmacoeconomics, and quality of life. In: Ito S, Blackburn S, eds. A pharmacist's guide to principles and practices of managed care pharmacy. Alexandria, VA: Foundation for Managed Care Pharmacy, 1995:103.
14. Ito S, Blackburn S, eds. A pharmacist's guide to principles and practices of managed care pharmacy. Alexandria, VA: Foundation for Managed Care Pharmacy, 1995:103.
15. McCarthy RL, O'Connor PJ, Fossen MS. How to start a managed care pharmacy residency program, AMCP. Available at http://64.226.220.36/residency/index_residency.asp. Accessed August 2, 2001.
16. Academy of Managed Care Pharmacy. Starting a residency program in managed care pharmacy. Available at www.amcp.org/residency/body.asp. Accessed August 2, 2001.
17. Mednick DM. The essential skills needed for managed care pharmacists. Pharmacy Times Career Suppl 2001.

C H A P T E R 1 4

COMMUNITY PHARMACY EXPERIENTIAL ROTATION

Dan Krinsky

Goals: After reviewing the information in this chapter, you should be able to:

1. Explain at least three methods for dispensing prescriptions in the community setting and how problem solving for patients in each of these environments differs.
2. Describe how third parties and gross margins (pharmacy and front end) affect a community pharmacy's financial status and ability/desire to develop new nondispensing programs.
3. List at least five factors used to facilitate optimal patient counseling sessions.
4. Describe at least six questions you would ask a customer during an over-the-counter medication consultation before making a product recommendation.
5. Briefly describe seven steps that must be completed when monitoring and evaluating the effectiveness of a patient's drug therapy regimen in the community pharmacy setting.

INTRODUCTION TO THE COMMUNITY PHARMACY EXPERIENTIAL ROTATION: AN OVERVIEW

Welcome to community pharmacy! Community pharmacy is facing some very challenging and exciting times. Chain pharmacies continue to expand into many untapped markets. Independent pharmacies appear to have held their own against many of their much larger competitors. Other retailers have entered the pharmacy business, trying to capture market share and bring a new type of customer into their stores. Most recently, the internet pharmacies have entered the fray, creating a whole new look for the way health care is delivered and medications are dispensed. Finding ways to constantly balance the complex issues of health care and retail sales makes the community pharmacist position one of the most challenging and rewarding in the entire industry.

The goal of the community pharmacy clinical experiential rotation is to provide you with experience in contemporary pharmacy practice in the community setting. Under the direction of your pharmacist preceptor, you will be expected to demonstrate effective pharmacy practice skills such as dispensing, patient education, disease-state management, problem solving, and communications. In addition, you will be expected to display the interpersonal dimensions appropriate for a professional working with the public and other healthcare providers.

In this chapter we review all important aspects of medication order processing, dispensing, and patient care as they relate to community pharmacy practice. In this practice setting, you will learn how to address patients' medication needs to help them improve their quality of life. You are expected to perform activities focused on identifying and solving drug-related problems. Some of this may involve work that includes filling prescriptions, accepting phone orders, and consulting with patients and other healthcare workers. In the case of prescription filling, you should not be engaged simply for the sake of filling prescriptions but in order to learn the skills and techniques of problem solving as they relate to this function. Activities may also include participating in any clinical services the pharmacy currently provides, seeing manufacturers' sales representatives, attending important meetings, and other functions the pharmacist may perform as part of his or her daily routine. All objectives must be met and completed to the preceptor's satisfaction by the end of the rotation, and fulfillment of these objectives will typically make up a portion of your grade. You should look for and become involved in any activities requiring judgment. Whenever possible, utilize the seven steps to solving problems and apply these in judgmental and decision-making situations related to the eight types of drug-related problems. Table 14.1 lists both the categories of drug-related problems and the steps to problem solving. It is important to recognize that the principles of pharmaceutical care apply in the community setting.

TABLE 14.1. DRUG-RELATED PROBLEMS AND STEPS TO PROBLEM SOLVING

EIGHT CATEGORIES OF DRUG-RELATED PROBLEMS	SEVEN STEPS TO PROBLEM SOLVING
1. Untreated indication	1. Recognize and define the problem
2. Improper drug selection	2. Gather or access the information
3. Subtherapeutic dose	3. Define all reasonable alternatives
4. Failure to receive drug	4. Identify risks and benefits of each alternative
5. Overdosage	5. Select approach to resolution
6. Adverse drug reaction	6. Implement plan
7. Drug–drug interaction	7. Evaluate success of problem resolution
8. Drug use without an indication	

The pharmacist is a respected and involved member of his or her community. In keeping with this tradition, as a part of the experiential rotation, you may be expected to participate in at least one community service activity. The definition of "community" is quite flexible and will vary depending on the location of an assigned site. For example, if the site is located in a small town or neighborhood with an elementary, junior high, or high school nearby, you may be asked to provide educational talks to students. If the site is located near a high-rise apartment complex with a large elderly population, you may be asked to do a "brown-bag" educational program for the residents. The particular activity is typically assigned by the preceptor, and any activities must be reviewed and approved by the preceptor in advance. Remember that all your actions are being performed as a representative of the pharmacy organization and the university. The preceptor must have the final authority over each of these activities.

There are different types of preceptors with whom you will work. Clinical community rotations are a relatively new entity, and each relationship between a university and pharmacy organization is unique. Each will also have a different scope of responsibilities for both student education and work in the pharmacy. The types of preceptors seen in the community pharmacy setting include shared faculty, full-time academia, and a full-time pharmacy employee. Shared faculty have responsibilities for both organizations, and both organizations typically share in the compensation of this individual. Any of these types of faculty could be based either on campus, at the pharmacy site, or divide time between the two locations. Regardless of the official title, position, and location, community pharmacist preceptors will be extremely committed to an optimal educational experience for you.

Community Pharmacy Business Issues

Historically, community pharmacy was synonymous with independent pharmacy. One can picture the traditional pharmacist standing behind the counter pouring medicine from a large stock bottle into a patient's prescription bottle, with the patient looking on. The pharmacist was the chemist, "Doc" to all his customers and patients, someone who would share counsel with and gain the confidence of all his patrons. Often, the pharmacist was the first stop on the healthcare circuit, with his opinion sought on how to treat anything from a sore throat to an ingrown toenail. Times have certainly changed since those days.

Community pharmacies now encompass everything from the mass merchandiser pharmacies, such as Target and Wal-Mart, to the supermarket pharmacies (Topps, Giant Eagle), the national chain drug stores (CVS, Rite Aid, Walgreens, Eckerd), and the remaining single-owner independent pharmacies. Each type of organization has a unique environment in which its professionals dispense medications and work with patients, yet there are many similarities in practices. Each type of pharmacy organization is briefly reviewed to provide the student with important background information in preparation for community pharmacy

practice rotations. The following descriptions are offered for the different types
of pharmacies seen in the community setting:

Traditional Chain

These are pharmacy operations with multiple locations, similar physical designs,
one primary management/leadership team, and a varied mix of merchandise to
offer their customers. Chains can be as small as three stores or as large as 4000
stores. Examples of some of the larger chains include Walgreens, Eckerds, CVS,
and Rite Aid, and some of the regional chains include Kerr Drugs, Longs, and
Happy Harrys.

Independent Pharmacy

These include the traditional type of pharmacy with a single store and owner,
whose primary product line is the prescription department.

Mass Merchant

This is a retail outlet whose primary goal is generating traditional retail sales,
not pharmacy business. Mass merchants have recently entered into the pharmacy
market in a more serious fashion, primarily to attract new types of customers to
their stores and grow the sales of their traditional products. Most have entered
this market with the pharmacy department being a loss leader, meaning they are
willing to lose money in this department because losses are more than offset by
sales to these customers in other departments. Example of these types of organizations include Wal-Mart, KMart, and Target.

Supermarket

Again this is a retail outlet whose primary goal is to generate sales of their traditional product lines, primarily groceries and related items. Only recently have
they too entered into the pharmacy business in a more serious way, and again,
it's primarily as a loss leader. Examples of supermarket organizations that are in
the pharmacy business include Tops, Giant Eagle, Ukrops, and H-E-B Supermarkets.

Mail-Order Pharmacy

Many of the larger chain pharmacies and pharmacy benefits managers (PBMs)
have developed a mail-order division in order to try and maximize efficiencies,
address the insurance companies and third party payers' demands for less costly
prescription processing, and to meet some customer needs. Examples of organizations with mail-order pharmacies include Merck-Medco, PCS, DPS, and some
of the larger chain pharmacies.

Internet

With the explosion of the Internet and the growth of the "dot-com" world, entrepreneurial professionals and businesspersons have developed systems to obtain the necessary information to be able to process and dispense prescriptions using internet technology. These "on-line" pharmacies began to take shape in 1999, and it has been interesting watching their progress. The typical scenario for prescription processing on line would be the following: a customer would complete an on-line intake form, including demographic and insurance information. If the customer's health plan allows for direct billing, the prescription can be transmitted by fax to the internet pharmacy or mailed to them. Other options would be electronic transmission of the prescription from the doctor's office to the pharmacy, or the prescription could be transferred from a retail pharmacy. Once received, the prescription is processed by the Internet pharmacy's facility and shipped to the patient. If the patient's insurance does not allow the Internet pharmacy to direct bill, the patient will be responsible for initial payment, and then will submit the necessary paperwork to receive reimbursement. The National Association of Boards of Pharmacy (NABP) has developed a seal of approval program for Internet pharmacies known as the VIPPS (Verified Internet Pharmacy Practice Sites), identifying the sites with proper processes and procedures.

Prescription Costs

Today's Americans have more contact with their community pharmacist than they do with any other healthcare providers. For 10 consecutive years, pharmacists were selected by the public as America's most trusted professionals. This achievement is unprecedented in any industry and speaks volumes to the value of pharmacists in today's society. The public relies on the pharmacist for timely, precise filling of their prescriptions as well as accurate, reliable information about their medications. They also exhibit frustration at the cost of their prescriptions and often point an accusatory finger at the pharmacy for these rising prices. What many have a difficult time understanding is that the pharmacist is just as frustrated, as a great majority of these cost increases are a result of issues outside the pharmacist's control. Some of these factors include managed-care formularies, copays, more new medications, and increased access to prescription drugs. Over the past 5 years, spending on prescription drugs increased twice as fast as spending on overall healthcare. Although the overall cost of prescription drugs represents approximately 10% of total healthcare spending, many employers and managed-care organizations see this rate of increase as a concern. Some of the specific factors affecting prescription volume, drug costs, and reimbursement include:

1. Development of new medications. Increased development costs are passed on to consumers, as evidenced by the more than 8% increase in the cost of a brand-name prescription from 1997 to 1998 (to $53.51), while the average cost of a generic medication increased by only 2% (to $17.33).

2. Aging population. Medications are still the least expensive option for treating disease, and as the population ages, more prescriptions will be written and dispensed for the ailments and conditions of this group.

3. Access to medications. As more employers offer healthcare benefits to their employees, and managed care continues to grow, more individuals have access to prescription drugs.

4. Direct-to-consumer advertising. Manufacturers spent over $1.5 billion during a 12-month period in 1998–1999 promoting their medications directly to consumers.

5. Decreased reimbursement from managed-care plans. Rates are constantly being negotiated to reduce expenses to the payer.

6. An increased percentage of prescriptions covered by managed-care plans. This goes hand in hand with what is described above.

The average percentage of total revenues generated from the prescription department for the different types of pharmacies varies significantly. This number ranges from approximately 6% for the mass merchandisers to 10% for the supermarkets, 50% for the average large chain, and around 90% for the typical independent pharmacy. What does this mean? The independent pharmacy is at the greatest risk from decreasing reimbursement rates for prescriptions, whereas the other organizations have many more options for sales and revenue generation. However, the smaller pharmacy organizations and the independents are creative in establishing new services, with the dual purpose of helping their patients and increasing their bottom line. These are discussed later in this chapter. One last interesting piece of financial data relates to who gets what percentage of the payment pie. The average cost for a prescription in 1998 was $38.64, and this amount was divided in the following manner: 74% to the manufacturer of the medication; 23% to the retailer (community pharmacy); and 3% to the wholesaler. As the retailer piece of the pie continues to dwindle (because of many reimbursement issues outside the control of the retailer), independent pharmacies will continue to be in jeopardy of having to sell or close their doors because of insufficient operating revenue.

Pharmacy Employees

Who works in the pharmacy? Who are the people in the front of the store? What are each of these employees' responsibilities? It is important for you to have a clear understanding and appreciation of the individuals with whom you will be working, what they do, and how they contribute to the success of the business. Some of these employees include the pharmacist, pharmacy technician, cashier, general manager, other management staff, and other nontechnical support staff. Depending on the size and type of store, there may be various specialists in departments such as greeting cards, gifts, health and beauty aids (HBA), over-the-counter medications (OTC), durable medical equipment (DME), cosmetics, photo, food/groceries, natural products, vitamins and minerals, the information area, and diagnostic/home testing products.

The individuals with whom you will be spending most of your time will be in the pharmacy department. The pharmacist is the licensed professional responsible for the safe, effective, accurate processing and dispensing of prescriptions. Requirements for licensure vary by state, but in every state this individual must sign off on every prescription before it is dispensed from a community pharmacy. Pharmacists may hold many titles and have additional responsibilities, such as store or department manager, general manager, or may be responsible for just the prescription department. Support personnel in the pharmacy may have many job titles and responsibilities. Job titles for other individuals who may work in the pharmacy department are the pharmacy technician and the pharmacy clerk. The technician is usually competent in many areas of prescription processing, insurance issues, third-party reconciliation, and inventory management. Many types of training and education programs are available to help develop these and other competencies, and most are available through local, state, and national organizations and schools. The role of the pharmacy technician is to support the pharmacist with prescription processing, to help manage all tasks not requiring a pharmacist's direct participation or judgment, and to free the pharmacists so they can manage and perform their professional responsibilities. One of the areas where pharmacies typically try to maximize technician support is with insurance claims and documentation. The pharmacy clerk manages certain tasks in the store, such as the sales transaction, responding to questions about general merchandise, and directing the customers to the correct department. Clerks usually work the cash register in the pharmacy and may assist with taking in new prescriptions, triaging customer inquiries, and possibly helping with prescription processing and insurance questions.

Pharmacy Department Setup

The prescription intake area is where patients present their prescriptions for filling. Establishment of correct patient information forms is required for a complete database. This is discussed in more detail on page 356. Prescriptions are reviewed for completeness, and patients are informed about wait times and other possible products and services that may complement their care and the specific condition for which the prescription is being filled.

The prescription entry area is the workstation where the pharmacy computer is located, where information is input into the computer system, and where profiles are maintained and updated. This is usually located in close proximity to the intake area, and it's possible that the same person would work in both areas. Once prescriptions are ready for filling, they are classified into "waiters" (the patient will wait for their prescription), "returners" (the patient will return for pickup), or "delivery." Each pharmacy will have a method of prioritizing prescriptions to minimize wait times and maximize the use of pharmacy personnel.

Prescriptions for patients who are waiting require immediate entry into the computer system. Once prescriptions have been entered, they must be filled in the proper order based on priority. It is important to understand the system for the particular pharmacy where you are working in order to be of some assistance, and not a hindrance, to patient care.

The setup area is where all the parts of the prescription come together to be assembled: the written prescription, patient medication container with label, stock bottle, patient information leaflet (PIL), and any adherence aids (such as dosing spoon, medication calendar). The dispensing area is the space on the pharmacy counter where medications are packaged and prepared for checking by the pharmacist. It is very important to keep everything organized so prescriptions aren't misfilled. Equipment and resources that may be used in this area include counting devices, calculator, computer, textbooks, prescription containers, auxiliary labels, and a distilled water dispenser.

The pickup area is where prescriptions that have been filled and are ready for patient pickup are stored in the pharmacy. There are usually baskets or bins where these prescriptions are arranged in alphabetical order according to the patient's last name. This is also where prescriptions are dispensed and patient counseling takes place, so there should be an area where a confidential conversation can take place.

There are other areas in the pharmacy with which you should become familiar. Medications are usually stored on shelving units called "bays." These are typically horseshoe-shaped units with adjustable shelves to accommodate different bottle sizes. These bays are typically directly behind the pharmacy counter, and the medications may be arranged in one of many ways. The most commonly used system has medications arranged alphabetically according to the brand name. Generic medications are stored on the shelves next to the brand name product or are kept in a separate section designated for generic medications. Because generic medications are being prescribed with greater frequency, the generics may be stocked directly behind the filling counter for easy access. There may also be what is referred to as a "quick mover" shelf. This section contains the fastest moving prescription items, usually located directly above the filling counter, and is designed to save pharmacy employees time in retrieving medications. Because some stock medications require refrigeration for storage, a full-sized or compact refrigerator is typically kept in the dispensing area. This may also be used to store prescriptions that have been filled for medications requiring refrigeration, with a notice placed in the prescription pickup bin that the medication is being kept there.

Financial Data in Community Pharmacy

Another important aspect of community pharmacy is the financial structure of the business. Although most of your activities are focused on patient care, an understanding of the finances will assist in making sense of many of the organizational decisions, such as staff and resource allocation, product mix, and program development. There are two general sides to the balance sheet: income and expenses. Income into the pharmacy is primarily generated through three sources: sales of prescription medications, sales of nonprescription products, and other income (which varies considerably among organizations). On the expense/cost side of the ledger, there are many items for which a company has to pay out monies, including costs of goods sold (both prescription and over-the-counter products), interest on loans/line of credit, and the general operating expenses associated with most businesses (including human resources, marketing and advertising, rent and leases, and professional services).

The average gross margin in the pharmacy department (the difference between sales and the cost of goods sold) is typically in the range of 18–24%, while the gross margin in the nonprescription departments averages in the 30–40% range. A typical expense structure in the pharmacy, including all departments, is approximately 15–24%. Net operating income or loss before taxes is calculated by totaling sales and income, then subtracting all expenses. When one looks at the numbers discussed above, it is obvious there is a fine line between making a profit and taking a loss. This is why pharmacies are looking to grow sales in their nonprescription departments that offer more margin dollars and greater chances for improved profits.

Professional Organizations and Community Pharmacy

Many professional organizations serve the needs of community pharmacy. The National Association of Chain Drug Stores (NACDS), American Pharmaceutical Association (APhA), and National Community Pharmacists Association (NCPA), along with local, state, and other national organizations, offer many programs and services to support community pharmacy. Each has their own slant toward the practice and how they approach the business and patient-care aspects, but all are valuable in their own way. These organizations very active politically, and they use their ties to affect policy decisions that impact this business. You are encouraged to learn more about these organizations and how they might offer some benefits.

COMMUNITY PHARMACY—MORE THAN COUNTING, POURING, LICKING, AND STICKING

The Dispensing Process

Medication dispensing involves much more than counting by fives with a spatula and putting pills in a bottle. The dispensing process incorporates many very important steps, each offering an opportunity to identify a potential or actual drug-related problem. You should work closely with the pharmacy staff during the dispensing process so these problems are addressed appropriately.

The initial step in this process is to obtain the prescription. This may be in person or via telephone, facsimile machine, e-mail, or the internet. Verify that all information on the prescription is legible, review for omissions, and if any part of the prescription is not legible, do not guess and do not assume. Make the necessary calls to verify information and clarify any discrepancies before processing and dispensing the prescription. It is critical to review prescriptions for completeness and to use the prescription as a starting point for identifying potential or actual drug-related problems. Taking the written prescription into the pharmacy should be uncomplicated, as it is an original, hard-copy document from the prescriber. Prescriptions called into the pharmacy must be reduced to writing immediately. Pharmacists or, in some states, licensed/registered interns, are allowed to receive called-in prescriptions. Some states allow doctors' offices to leave call-in prescriptions on a recorder, which are then transcribed to writing. It is important to distinguish between physicians and their agents/representatives when prescriptions are called in to the pharmacy. These agents/representatives (who could be clerks, administrative assistants, or nurses) may not be as familiar with medical terminology and word pronunciation. All information called in from the doctor's office should be repeated back to the caller to verify all facts. This practice will minimize errors and problems. Also, all the same information for written prescriptions must be included for the ones that are phoned in to the pharmacy.

Electronic transmission of prescriptions via electronic mail (e-mail), directly through the computer, and by facsimile machine will continue to grow in popularity. With each process comes a new set of potential opportunities and problems. Regardless of how the prescription gets to the pharmacy, the information in Table 14.2 must be reviewed and verified.

The next step is to gather all patient information necessary for dispensing and counseling. Determine who is presenting the prescription: is it the patient, a family member, a caregiver, another individual? Knowing this will help assess the validity of any information, how the counseling session will go, and what other calls might be necessary to address all concerns and issues. When obtaining patient information it is important to have a document to record these data, one that patients and staff could complete. You will find in Appendix E an example of one type of form that is used for documenting patient medical information. There are seven sections of information that, when completed, provide a comprehensive database. (A more detailed description of this process is included later in this chapter.) This information allows for more involvement in problem solving and greater opportunities to assist with improving outcomes. Often, these are the types of data collected when disease state management programs, which are also discussed later in this chapter, are operated. It's also important to determine if the patient will wait for the prescription, return, or want it delivered or mailed.

At this time, once the initial interaction with the patient has taken place, it is time for the behind-the-counter processes to begin. A patient profile will be created or updated, and the prescription information will be entered. Verify

TABLE 14.2. INFORMATION TO VERIFY ON THE PRESCRIPTION

1. Prescriber's name and address
2. Patient name (and address for controlled substances)
3. Other patient information, where necessary (age, weight—important for children; also important to have a date of birth for all patients in their profile)
4. Drug indication, whenever possible; many medications used for many reasons; critical for appropriate patient counseling ("Mrs. Smith, why did your doctor prescribe this medicine?")
5. Date of issuance of the prescription
6. Drug name/strength/dosage form
7. Total quantity of medication to dispense
8. Instructions/directions for the medication (SIG), such as amount or units per dose, frequency, route of administration
9. Number of refills remaining
10. DAW (Dispense as Written) line: indicates whether a generic medication may or may not be dispensed; requirements are state-specific; there may be a check box or additional prescriber signature on the blank to address this issue
11. Prescriber signature and address
12. Prescriber DEA number for controlled substance prescriptions, and recently, it's a required piece of data for filing insurance claims for prescription (Rx) payment
13. There may also be a length of therapy, or a reason for the therapy, indicated on the prescription. This information can be very useful when reviewing a profile, monitoring for drug-related problems, and counseling patients. Pharmacists and other healthcare professionals are encouraging physicians to include the indication for the medication on the prescription. This helps the pharmacist determine how to counsel the patient, what to say, and how to help patients determine if they are receiving the greatest benefit from the therapy. This information is also useful because some medications have more than one approved, and some unapproved, indications.

insurance/payment method and address any DUR (drug utilization review) alerts (reviewed later). The system will update files and print a label and patient information leaflet (PIL). The stock package will be retrieved from the shelf, and the prescription will be filled, ensuring the dosage, dosage form, and other aspects of the medicine are appropriate for the patient.

There are additional issues related to medication dispensing in a community pharmacy that are important for patient care. Determining the appropriate drug delivery system (i.e., dosage form) for a patient based on individual patient needs and characteristics is very important. Evaluate patient characteristics that may influence the selection of a drug delivery system. Solid (capsules, tablets), liquid (solutions, suspensions, syrups), and topical (creams, lotions, ointments, gels, patches, inhalants) dosage forms are available. Determining the appropriate dosage form can greatly facilitate positive patient outcomes.

Select a system that will provide optimal therapeutic benefit to the patient and, if realistic, investigate the possibility of an extemporaneously compounded prescription for drug administration. Prescription compounding offers the pharmacist an opportunity to develop a patient-specific product to meet a unique need. Compounding is an aspect of pharmacy practice making a comeback in the community setting. A multitude of resources are available to provide training and support for pharmacists interested in becoming compounding specialists. Patient groups such as those taking difficult-to-find medicines, individuals with swallowing problems, children who desire more tasteful flavors, and hospice patients with administration challenges all have special needs that can be met by entrepreneurial pharmacists. You are encouraged to participate in these types of services whenever possible.

Each medication approved by the Food and Drug Administration (FDA) has a brand (or trade) name and a generic name. The generic name is the official, chemical name for the product's active ingredient. Typically, for a particular brand-name product, there is only one generic name; however, on rare occasions, there is more than one brand-name product for a particular generic drug. For example, there are two brand name products for generic glyburide (a medicine used for diabetes), and there are multiple brand-name nitroglycerin patches available. Brand-name products will usually become available as generics once the patent on the brand-name product has expired. Patents expire 17 years from the time the drug is discovered, not from the time the drug is commercially available. Generic drugs are almost always less expensive than the brand-name product, which affords pharmacists an opportunity to offer their patients options to reduce drug costs and possibly improve compliance.

Generics may also raise questions about quality, and pharmacists and students must be ready to address and alleviate patient concerns. The FDA approves generic products, and they must meet the same stringent requirements as brand-name products. There are isolated circumstances where brand-name products are preferred over generic products. This would be when medications have a narrow therapeutic index or a narrow range between subtherapeutic, therapeutic, and toxic levels. Examples include Dilantin® (phenytoin sodium), Lanoxin® (digoxin), and Synthroid® (levothyroxine). These medications are commonly referred to as narrow-therapeutic-index drugs, or NTIDs.

Another issue affecting whether or not a generic drug is dispensed is what type of insurance the patient has and what the requirements are for a specific plan. Some insurance companies mandate generic dispensing, but others incentivize generics based on lower copays. In addition, some state laws require that the pharmacist offer generics to patients when generics are available. The pharmacist/

TABLE 14.3. INFORMATION SUPPLIED BY AUXILIARY LABELS

1. How and when to take the drug
2. What to avoid when taking the medication (such as foods, other medications)
3. The number of refills remaining
4. If the product is a new generic drug for the same medication dispensed previously
5. Possible side effects
6. The expiration date for the medication, especially if it is a reconstituted antibiotic
7. How to store the medicine

pharmacy student must address all pertinent issues related to generic medications so patients receive the greatest benefit from the drug prescribed.

One of the next steps in the dispensing process is applying the appropriate auxiliary labels to the prescription vial. These are usually applied in a conspicuous place without interfering with the prescription label. The types of additional patient information and instructions for medication use, for which auxiliary labels are used, are listed in Table 14.3.

Once the prescription is completely assembled, all work should be rechecked by comparing information on the label with what is written on the prescription and with what is written on the stock bottle. The best verification for ensuring that the correct product is in the prescription container is through the use of the NDC (National Drug Code) number. The NDC number is assigned by the manufacturer for each specific product. The NDC code has 11 numbers, which provide three pieces of information about each product: manufacturer (first five digits), drug name, strength, dosage form (next four digits), and package size (last two digits). An important part of checking prescriptions and verifying drugs prescribed for patients is matching the NDC number on the stock bottle with the product number printed on the label. NDC numbers are also used for billing prescriptions through third parties and insurance companies.

The final check of the prescription must be conducted by the pharmacist. Once it is ready for dispensing, all pertinent pieces are placed together: the prescription, the PIL, any other information necessary for the prescription, and everything is placed in a bag. If filling more than one prescription for a patient, be sure the correct information is kept with the respective prescription. If filling prescriptions for more than one family member, be sure to bag only those prescriptions intended for a particular patient. Do not put more than one patient's prescriptions in a bag; this practice increases liability if the pharmacy were to mistakenly dispense a prescription to the wrong individual. Also, if filling prescriptions for someone with a common name who will return to pick them up,

---

TABLE 14.4. COMMONLY RECOMMENDED
ADHERENCE DEVICES

1. Pill boxes—Seven day with one compartment per day, or up to four compartments per day for the doses commonly given during the day: morning, noon, evening, and bedtime.
2. Dosing spoons—important for accurate measurement of liquid medications; ordinary household teaspoons do not measure liquids accurately.
3. Droppers—important for administration of small doses of liquid medications
4. Dial-a-dose containers—there is usually a dial, and when it is twisted to a specific spot, the medication drops out of a compartment for administration. Commonly used for oral contraceptives.
5. Medication calendars—calendar with the necessary medication information written into the appropriate boxes to help patients remember what to take and when.
6. Beeping devices—these fit on top of the medication vials and are programmed to emit a sound when it is time to take a dose of medicine
7. Telephone calling services—there are services available (usually a programmed computer) that will place a call to a patient's home to remind him or her when it is time to take a dose of medicine.

---

be sure to verify the correct patient and the medications when they come back. An easy way to do this is to verify their birthday or address.

Patient adherence with prescribed therapy is important for patients to realize positive outcomes. The term "adherence" is selected for this chapter, as it reflects a more participatory action on the part of the patient. Oftentimes, one will see the term "compliance" used to reflect an action taken by the patient to follow directions. However compliance is more of a directive action from one to another, rather than the relationship-building action, adherence. Many adherence devices are available to assist patients with their medications. Table 14.4 lists the most frequently used devices. Each has benefits and should be selected because of specific patient needs. Costs for these aids are usually very reasonable and should not be a barrier to use.

Your level of experience, training, and education, along with the pharmacist's level of comfort with your skills and competencies, will dictate the extent to which you will be involved in these dispensing activities.

Patient Confidentiality

Laws vary from state to state, but everyone, including legislators, is taking this issue very seriously. Organizations will strive to change to electronic medical records. The attention of health care administrators, legislators, and lobbying groups will be directed at maintaining and limiting access to these data to individuals with the proper credentials. The levels of security and who will have access to specific types of data have not been outlined completely. It is very important for pharmacists to support the position of access to information so they can advance their practices, collect outcomes data, improve patients' lives, and document their value to third-party payers.

Confidentiality in the community pharmacy during day-to-day operations is a constant challenge. There are many situations where confidentiality can be unknowingly/accidentally violated, so it is critical for everyone in the pharmacy to be aware of these situations and to act appropriately. Some examples of situations where confidentiality might be jeopardized are described in Table 14.5.

Third-Party Issues

The growth of third-party prescriptions over the past 10 to 15 years has been amazing: from less than 10% in the late 1980s to over 65% by the year 2000. What are third-party prescriptions? These are prescriptions paid for by someone other than the patient. There are three parties involved in the payment of these prescriptions: the patient, the pharmacist, and the payer. Payers may be private insurance companies, government programs, or any other organization paying for prescriptions. Third-party prescriptions are a love–hate issue for most commu-

---

TABLE 14.5. SITUATIONS IN THE COMMUNITY PHARMACY WITH POTENTIAL FOR BREACH OF CONFIDENTIALITY

1. Telephone communications. When taking a telephoned prescription, calling for a prescription copy, or providing a copy to another pharmacy, repeating the information for verification purposes. It would be very easy to repeat the patient name and medication loud enough for a customer or patient to overhear the information.
2. When counseling a patient on his or her medication, it would be easy to share information loud enough for someone to overhear what was being discussed. Management must work with their staff when designing pharmacies and work flow to take this issue into consideration so pharmacists have the opportunity to speak with customers in an area that addresses the confidentiality needs.
3. Some patients will present to the pharmacy for refills of their prescription, yet not remember which medication they need. Typically, someone on the pharmacy staff would check the patient's computer profile, and list off for the patient those medications ready for refill. This practice of voicing the medication list to the patient has the potential to violate confidentiality if other customers/patients are in the store.

nity pharmacies. While they have helped to increase the number of prescriptions written, they have had a significant effect on profits and the role of the pharmacist and other employees. A key issue with third-party prescriptions is the amount of payment received by the pharmacy. Typically, third-party prescriptions are paid for in the following manner: patients pay a premium for a prescription card through their medical insurance program. This entitles them to obtain prescriptions from an approved pharmacy under a shared-payment structure. The insurance company pays for part of the prescription cost (under a discounted payment plan they have negotiated), while the patient pays either a deductible or copay. In many cases, the pharmacy organization has had no impact on the payment they receive for the prescription. Often, the total reimbursement is barely sufficient to allow the pharmacy to make a profit on the prescription.

To demonstrate how large a role third parties play in community pharmacy, the National Association of Chain Drug Stores recently hired the Arthur Andersen consulting group to evaluate this issue. Their findings documented the variety of activities performed by pharmacy personnel and also showed quite clearly that our profession has a long way to go before we can focus even a majority of our time on nondispensing professional activities. Their analysis of 36 activities revealed that pharmacists spend most of their time processing and presenting prescriptions and preparing and delivering orders. Disease-state management occupied only 1.6% of the pharmacist's time. What is interesting about the report submitted by Arthur Andersen is a statement in their Executive Summary: "We think pharmacists need to be involved with reviewing and interpreting the prescription, assessing patients' drug therapy (including drug interactions), resolving clinical conflicts, contacting doctors concerning approvals or prescription clarification, and counseling patients about prescriptions. Pharmacists spend only 31% of their time on these activities. . . ."

Discovery of a way to decrease the time spent taking care of third-party insurance claims will allow pharmacists to move toward this recommendation.

Communications

Development of verbal, nonverbal, and written communication skills is a challenging yet necessary exercise for you. Communications with patients, physicians and their staff, insurance companies, and others will be key to relationship development and ultimately, patient care. For in-depth discussion of required communication skills for pharmacists, refer to Chapter 3 of this handbook. This section is designed to emphasize a few of the basic aspects of communication skills in the community pharmacy setting and areas where you should focus your attention.

One of the most important aspects of prescription dispensing is the interaction with the patient. The Omnibus Budget and Reconciliation Act of 1990 (commonly referred to as OBRA 90), legislation passed by the federal government, mandates certain professional responsibilities by the pharmacist specific for Medicaid patients receiving prescription medications. These include:

1. OBRA-90 mandates that pharmacists make the offer to counsel all of these patients on the correct use of their medications.
2. This legislation also requires that pharmacists maintain patient profiles for these particular individuals that includes information such as allergies, medications, and adverse events caused by medications.

The reason for this requirement is to help reduce the incidence of drug-related problems such as side effects, poor adherence, duplication, or allergies, which worsen patient outcomes and increase costs. Many states have expanded these responsibilities to include all patients so outcomes and costs can be improved in the entire population of medication users. It is important to understand the state-specific patient counseling requirements applicable for the practice site where you are based.

In my previous practice, for all new prescriptions and for those refills about which the pharmacist wants to be sure to speak with the patient, an OFFER COUNSELING sticker was applied to the outside of the prescription bag. When the patient, caregiver, or designated representative comes in to pick up the prescription, whoever waits on the individual summons the pharmacist to go meet with the individual and counsel/educate/discuss pertinent issues. Students in our practice are active observers of this activity and gain as much experience as early as possible participating with the pharmacist in counseling patients on the proper use of their medications.

Written communications are necessary at times to share information or to request information. When communicating with patients in writing, make sure they can understand what is written. It is suggested that writing at the fourth to sixth grade reading level will ensure most patients will comprehend the document. One doesn't want to use scientific terminology that only healthcare providers will understand, as this will alienate patients very quickly.

Verbal communications can take place either over the telephone or in person. When answering the phone, be sure to identify yourself. Triage calls, distinguishing those that can be answered by you from those that must be referred to staff in the pharmacy and other departments. Examples of calls that should be transferred to the pharmacist, who is an employee of the organization, include questions about possible prescription errors, emergency calls, and calls from another pharmacy. If a patient is calling to check on the status of a refill, never assume things are completed without verification. If a patient is calling in a refill, obtain all important information, including pick-up procedure.

Face-to-face dialogue is usually prompted through the need for patient counseling (share information), or to obtain information. Make sure it is clear who is present to pick up the prescription, as the conversation will take on a different tone if it is someone other than the patient. There are many actions a pharmacist can take to facilitate optimal counseling sessions. Muldary has described six key factors, his CLOSER actions, to help meet this goal. These include:

C: Control distractions, such as nervous habits
L: Lean toward the patient. Try to stay between 1.5 and 4 feet from the patient
O: Open body posture. Keep legs and arms uncrossed, maintaining an approachable style
S: Squarely face the patient. Don't turn to one side or away
E: Eye contact. Maintain eye contact with the patient for at least half the counseling session, preferably at least three-fourths of the time.
R: Relax, use your knowledge, interpersonal, and communication skills to share information, answer questions.

Other factors to promote effective patient counseling include:

1. Counsel the patient in a comfortable, confidential setting
2. Allow sufficient time for the consultation
3. Utilize optimal counseling techniques, such as being empathetic, accepting, nonjudgmental, sincere, specific, clear, and concise
4. Provide accurate, relevant information and be sure to avoid information overload
5. Adapt information to the patient's level of understanding
6. Provide supplemental memory aids, devices, pictograms, or other informational materials
7. Whenever possible include family members, caregivers, or others who may be assisting the patient
8. Reinforce key topics and ask the patient to restate important information to ensure his or her understanding of the information shared
9. Ask open-ended questions, such as the ones listed in Table 14.6. The information patients share when responding to these questions will assist you and the pharmacist in your understanding of the situation, and the specifics to share to complete the counseling process.

The last step in the counseling process is final verification. Final verification is when the pharmacist/student has the patient repeat the information that was just shared in order to verify the patient's understanding. A key prompt to ask the patient is "Just to make sure that I did not forget to tell you anything important, please describe how you are going to use the medicine."

Customer Conveniences

There are additional issues that are difficult to classify, yet may have a profound effect on the pharmacist–patient relationship as well as the dispensing and counseling processes. For lack of a better term, these will be called "customer conveniences," and they are listed below:

TABLE 14.6. KEY QUESTIONS TO ASK PATIENTS DURING A COUNSELING SESSION

1. What did the doctor tell you the medication is for?
   a. What problem or symptom is it supposed to help?
   b. What is it supposed to do?
2. How did your doctor tell you to take the medication?
   a. How often did your doctor say to take it?
   b. How much are you supposed to take?
   c. How long are you to continue taking it?
   d. What did your doctor say to do when you miss a dose?
   e. How should you store this medication?
   f. What does three times a day mean to you?
3. What did your doctor tell you to expect from the medication?
   a. What good effects are you supposed to expect?
   b. How will you know if the medication is working?
   c. What bad effects did your doctor tell you to watch for?
   d. What should you do if a bad reaction occurs?
   e. What precautions are you to take while on this medication?
   f. How will you know if it is not working?
   g. What are you to do if the medication does not work?

Drive-Through Pharmacies

They are certainly a convenience for patients, especially parents with sick kids who don't want the aggravation of having to haul the kids out of the car again to get a prescription filled. It's also a convenience for folks such as the elderly or disabled who may have difficulty getting in and out of the car. However, the lack of direct patient contact with the pharmacist has the potential to jeopardize optimal outcomes and address patient concerns.

Extended Hours

Many of the larger chain and mass merchandiser pharmacies have extended pharmacy hours to try to meet the needs of our time-conscious society. This can be an opportunity for pharmacists to interact with patients at times when the pharmacy may not be quite as busy.

Prescription Delivery

This is a service to offer patients who can not get to the pharmacy, for whatever reason. There are both pros and cons to this. For refills, where the patient has at least a general understanding of the medication, it could be a benefit because of improved adherence. However, for a new prescription, there probably won't be any face-to-face contact with the pharmacist, again reducing the chances of optimal outcomes.

Managing the Clinical Messages/DUR Messages/Computer Checks

Almost every pharmacy dispensing computer system, and most third parties, incorporate programs designed to alert the staff about various types of issues. These are commonly referred to as DUR alerts or messages. They include situations such as interactions, allergies, and early or late refills. These alerts are designed to create awareness of potentially risky situations should the medication in question be dispensed. It is imperative that someone in a position to render judgment on these issues (i.e., pharmacist, student with supervision) reviews each message, takes the appropriate steps, and documents these actions. An article describing a process where this practice has been implemented and how it works has been published.[5] The goals when taking action on these alerts are to increase patient safety with their medications, improve patient care, and decrease liability. An example of the type of issue one may see, and the importance of review and communication, is described in Table 14.7.

TABLE 14.7. DESCRIPTION OF THE PROCESS FOR MANAGING A DUR MESSAGE/ALERT

An example of an issue that arises in community pharmacy is when patients present for refills at a time different from what the dispensing computer would predict. One reason may be that there may have been a change in the dosing schedule that was not communicated to the pharmacy. For example, a patient presents for a refill for their glyburide 5 mg almost 2 weeks early. Dialogue with the patient reveals that his doctor told him to take two tablets per day for a few weeks to see if his blood sugar would come down (versus one daily previously). This was communicated verbally from the doctor to the patient, with no communication to the pharmacy. Therefore, the pharmacy had no idea to expect the patient 2 weeks early. However, the pharmacy initiated communication with the patient, verified the information with the doctor's office, obtained a new prescription with the new SIG, and updated their records. The opposite situation occurs too, when decreases in doses or frequency of administration are ordered by the physician but not communicated to the pharmacy. This often results in the pharmacy assuming (incorrectly) inappropriate adherence with the medication regimen. Again, the interaction with the patient, the physician, and other providers is critical for optimal outcomes. The pharmacist/student must look at more than just the numbers when evaluating a DUR message.

Over-the-Counter (OTC) Medications

One of the unique aspects of community pharmacy practice is the opportunity to interact with the public and offer assistance regarding OTC medications. Sales of traditional OTC products are greater than $30 billion annually, and it is predicted that growth will exceed 10% per year. Traditionally, sales of OTC products have been in the community pharmacy stores. However, with the growth in general retail outlets (i.e., mass merchandisers) and expansion of their product lines to include more healthcare-related items, a majority of OTC products are now sold in these outlets. The key areas where the pharmacist/pharmacy student should focus there time include cough/cold, allergy, pain/analgesia, GI (antacids, laxatives), dietary aids, vitamins, minerals, supplements, herbs, other natural products, self-testing/diagnostics, and feminine hygiene. Other areas include first aid, eye/ear, foot care, oral care, home health care, and baby needs.

The primary goal of the OTC consult process is to assist the customer in determining the best approach to their particular situation. This will result in one of three types of recommendations: for a product, referral to their physician, or nothing at all. Certain patients with specific disease states will require special attention, as their status will have a significant impact on your decision. Special patient groups include neonates/infants/pediatrics, breastfeeding mothers, pregnant women, certain elderly folks, and some patients who are disabled. Often a very conservative approach is necessary to avoid increasing the risk to these individuals by self-treatment. Consumers must be made aware of as many risks and benefits as possible about their OTC product selection. Use of effective questions, listening, and assessment of the nonverbal cues will result in an educated, satisfied customer. The communication skills described elsewhere in this handbook should be utilized.

Tremendous opportunities exist for pharmacists to improve their professional position by counseling about OTC medications. The elderly population (those over 65 years of age) purchase and use over a third of these products. Currently, over four dozen prescription products are in various stages of consideration for change from prescription to nonprescription status. Over half of all health problems experienced by Americans are self-treated with OTC medications. Pharmacists are the most accessible healthcare professional and are uniquely trained to be able to address self-limiting conditions and potential application of OTCs and to know when to refer individuals to their doctors.

When counseling on OTC medications, remember that these chemicals deserve the same respect as prescription agents. They have pharmacologic, pharmacokinetic, and toxicologic properties, and they have side effects, precautions, interactions, and contraindications that must be taken into consideration in discussions with patients. You should pay special attention to opportunities to become involved as either an observer or an active participant in OTC consults. Some guidelines to follow when performing an OTC consult are included in Table 14.8. If follow-up to assess response is indicated, ensure that this will take

---

TABLE 14.8. GUIDELINES FOR OTC CONSULTS

1. Obtain information from the patient sufficient to help make an informed decision
2. Assist the patient in selecting a product, taking into consideration factors such as dosage form, frequency, goals and desired outcome, cost, and taste.
3. Advise the patient about possible side effects
4. Assist the patient in reading the package labeling
5. Inform the patient about when to expect results and what to do if there's no response or a negative response
6. Where appropriate, advise about storage, especially if there are children in the home

---

place by documenting the interaction and making a note to contact the patient. An example of a "question and answer" session with an individual about an OTC product is included below.

EXAMPLE OF A QUESTION-AND-ANSWER SESSION DURING AN OTC CONSULTATION

Situation: You are back in the pharmacy and notice a woman in the cough/cold section. You approach her, introduce yourself, and ask "How may I help you today?" (Remember to ask open-ended questions.) Your customer replies that she is looking for a product for her daughter. You obtain the following information to help you determine your action steps:

Student/RPh questions	Mother's response
Who is the patient?	Daughter
What are her symptoms?	She has a low-grade fever (100–101°F), cough, congestion, malaise
How have these symptoms affected her drinking, eating?	She's drinking fine but not eating much
How long has she had these symptoms?	Approximately 2 days
How old is she?	Seven years old
What is her weight?	Approximately 54 pounds
What are her allergies/reactions?	Penicillin—she had a rash and hives

What are her medical conditions?	She doesn't have anything chronic, but she has a history of ear infections four times between ages 2 and 5
Have you called your doctor about this yet?	Not yet
Do you have access to medical care?	Yes, we have a pediatrician
What medications is your daughter taking?	Right now she is only taking a vitamin, and I've given her Children's Motrin for 36 hours
How has the Motrin worked?	It's brought her fever down some
Are there other kids in the house?	Yes, but none are sick (a 3-year-old and a 9-month-old)
Is your daughter in school/ day care?	Yes, in school (second grade). She does go to daycare after school for a couple of hours a day. There has been some flu going around over the past week or so.
May I have your telephone number so I can call in a couple days to check and see how your daughter is doing?	Sure, that would be great . . . it's 555-1212.

There are other issues to discuss with this person. Based on the information provided, the pharmacist may have recommended the mother purchase a liquid decongestant and call the pediatrician within 24 hours if her daughter is still febrile or experiencing malaise. Mom would also have been told when to expect a response to this medication and what to do if her child has no response or gets worse. Mom should also be educated on how to determine the amount of medicine to administer by reviewing the package labeling. Ensure her understanding of the product and what she's going to do when she gets home.

Certainly there will be situations where this much depth is not necessary. However, you should always be prepared to enter into an OTC consult with this systematic approach in mind so all patient concerns are addressed appropriately.

Third Class of Drugs

As of mid-2000, there was renewed interest in this issue, as some major drug manufacturers with products soon to come off patent approached the FDA about changing the status of their products. This is not a new idea, but one that has been discussed by organizations on both sides of the issue for quite some time. This third class of drugs would create a group of medications available without a prescription, but that would be stocked behind the pharmacy counter and be sold through the pharmacist. The thought is that these medications have a higher risk profile than readily available OTC medications, yet the safety profile suggests a prescription might not be required. The pharmacist would be required to counsel the patient on the use of the medication before making the sale. Other countries have this process in place, and most report mixed results.

There are a couple variations on this concept. One would be a permanent third class of medications where, once included, they would stay there indefinitely. The other is termed a transitional class, where medications would be classified here for a certain period of time while the FDA reviews safety and efficacy data. Once enough data have been generated and evaluated, a decision would be made to either move the product to OTC status or send it back to prescription status. Creating a third class or a transitional class of drugs would require an act of Congress. You should gain an understanding of the dynamics of this situation because it will continue to generate significant interest. Categories of medications being considered for a change from prescription status, as of Fall 2000, include cholesterol-lowering medications, oral contraceptives, some types of antibiotics, other classes of ulcer-reducing medications, and ophthalmic medications used to treat glaucoma and cataracts.

Disease-State Management Programs

The desire to increase the number of nondispensing activities, to become patient care providers, and to integrate this with the need to fill a sufficient quantity of prescriptions to generate revenues to support the business, creates a very challenging dynamic for today's community pharmacists. Disease-state management (DSM) programs offer pharmacists professional challenges in helping patients to manage diseases. The most commonly monitored conditions in community pharmacy are diabetes, hypertension, dyslipidemia, and asthma. Some of the community pharmacies where you will have your rotations will have disease-state management programs in place. These will vary considerably depending on any number of factors, but the one thing they should all have in common is their goal to improve patient outcomes. Often it is the independent pharmacist, with more flexibility in his or her practice (who also must create ways for alternate revenue generation), who implements these types of programs. However, many of the regional and national chain pharmacy organizations are piloting programs in targeted geographic areas with the hope that success leads to additional channels of revenue and better relationships with employers, managed-care organizations, and the community in general.

Establishing DSM programs is very similar to setting up a medical practice in that a policy and procedure must exist for patient visits, documentation, follow-up, outcomes assessments, and communications. The key steps for implementing and managing DSM programs are writing, maintaining, and updating all policies and procedures; assessing work flow in the pharmacy to decide how DSM will fit into the existing processes; identifying equipment and resource needs; developing an updated clinical database; assessing the financials; developing a marketing and advertising plan; implementing; monitoring progress, and making changes to improve. Many state and national organizations offer training and education programs to assist pharmacists in developing DSM services. DSM programs may be as simple as a more focused approach to educate patients on the use of certain devices. In addition, they may be extremely complicated, with many detailed processes outlined to help patients manage the many complexities of diseases such as diabetes. Most community pharmacies are probably involved in a version of a simple program, such as teaching patients how to use their metered-dose inhalers or blood glucose meters. The next step is to get more involved with these patients to measure the results of the teaching and education.

Getting paid for disease-management nondistributive patient care programs is a challenging task. Pharmacists have a couple of choices: first, we can wait until insurance companies and third parties decide we are qualified as primary care providers and they become willing to pay us for these services. Alternatively, pharmacists can take the initiative to develop these programs, document their value, then present scientifically sound data to the decision makers within these payer organizations to request provider status, thus becoming qualified to receive direct payment. Many pharmacists/pharmacies have chosen the latter option, with the biggest challenge being the generation of the type of data these payers are willing to consider for compensating pharmacists. As a profession, the future does not look very promising if we continue to place most of our efforts into processing and dispensing prescriptions. Automation and technology have developed to the point where robotics can work more efficiently than humans at processing prescriptions, so we must look at different venues for helping our patients.

MANAGING YOUR ROTATION HOURS

Specific Student Activities and Documentation Processes

Up to this point the information in this chapter has been devoted primarily to describing the major who's, what's, where's, when's, and how comes of community pharmacy practice. The remainder of the chapter is devoted to describing specific activities in which you will most likely participate while in the community pharmacy setting. You will have day-to-day responsibilities, some longer-term projects, and many core skills to develop and objectives to meet. Appendix F outlines examples of learning objectives for this type of rotation. These are offered as a detailed description of what students might experience during their advanced community pharmacy experiential rotation. Those of you earlier in your academic career may be asked to achieve a more basic level of these learning

TABLE 14.9. PROPOSED OUTLINE FOR COMMUNITY PHARMACY EXPERIENTIAL ORIENTATION

1. Philosophy and purpose
2. The pharmacy organization and site description
3. Dress code, parking, other logistical issues
4. Confidentiality of information, communications
5. Attendance
6. Tour of facilities
7. Computer systems to access the pharmacy dispensing system, drug information data
8. Student's expectations and goals
9. Preceptor's expectations and goals
10. Conference and meeting schedule
11. Student evaluation and grading process
12. Overview of assignments

objectives. The list is only a guide and should be customized based on your year of education and the rotation site.

When you begin your rotation, it is very possible you will be exposed to many new sights and sounds of pharmacy practice. The preceptor should be expected to conduct an orientation to the site and activities, which will set the stage for a successful experience for both of you. Table 14.9 is a list of suggested items that should be discussed during this orientation.

As you spend time in the pharmacy, various situations and opportunities will be identified to evaluate drug-related problems (DRPs). A systematic approach to this exercise will allow you to organize information and develop a process for problem resolution. This process, a care plan document based on solving DRPs, is an abbreviated version of the seven steps to problem solving described earlier in this chapter. Appendix G is an example of this tool that can be used for monitoring more complex patients seen in the community setting. Patient profiles and other data are reviewed and DRPs identified and prioritized. For each problem a plan is devised and implemented, and all of this is documented on this form. These data would be reviewed with the preceptor and decisions made about patient care.

How to Conduct a Medication History Interview in the Community Pharmacy Setting

The medication history interview is a goal-directed communication. Its purpose is for one person to obtain information from another. The degree of success of the interview is a measure of the effectiveness of communication between the pharmacist/pharmacy student and the patient. The goals in conducting a medication history interview should include the following:

1. Obtain information from the patient to establish a more comprehensive database than what exists in the pharmacy computer.
2. Establish a positive patient–pharmacist relationship.
3. Identify any potential or actual drug-related problems.
4. Observe the patient's behavior for trends that may affect outcomes.

The following is a description of the content of a generalized medication history interview. Each interview must be tailored in emphasis and content to satisfy the needs of the particular patient. In the community setting, a great majority of medication history interviews will take place "blind"; that is, the only information the pharmacist will have in advance is the patient profile and whatever he or she knows about the patient from previous visits and discussions. If any additional information is available before the medication history interview, it should be reviewed and used to augment the interview process.

In most cases, you will be supervised by a pharmacist during the interview process. The level of your participation will vary based on experience and the particular situation. Before an interview is attempted, you should become familiar with as much of the patient's social, medical, and drug information as possible. Introduce yourself to the patient and explain your purpose. It is important to seek the patient's approval to conduct the interview. Attempt to conduct the interview in a comfortable area with a limited number of, or no, outside distractions. Establish professional rapport with the patient and keep social conversation to a minimum. It is important to get to the point of the interview, and the patient should feel as though he or she has your complete attention and interest. Allow the patient to speak without interruptions unless the patient begins to digress. Verbal and nonverbal cues may be used to keep the patient on track without significant interruption.

Begin the interview with a general question about the patient; then obtain the necessary demographic information. Follow the format on the Patient Medication History Form (Appendix E). Review the specific information obtained about the patient's medications, such as indication, dosing schedules, duration of therapy, and reasons for discontinuing. Remember to include information about both prescription and over-the-counter medications and products. Special care should be taken when interacting with women to ensure issues such as possible medication effects in pregnancy and during lactation are addressed appropriately. Ask the patient if he or she has ever had an adverse effect to a medication and obtain as many details as are available if this has occurred. Closing the interview should be done as smoothly as possible. A summary of the information obtained allows the interviewer to check information for accuracy and may remind the patient or caregiver of other significant information that may have been overlooked. A statement that you may contact the patient later to ask for more details leaves this option open to you in case you have forgotten something.

There are various ways information may be obtained from patients. The comprehensive patient medication history interview will accomplish this goal; however, there may not be too many patients willing to spend the necessary time with the student/pharmacist. An alternative to the face-to-face interview is to provide patients with a Patient Medication History Form to take home. The benefit of allowing patients to complete these on their own is that they don't feel the pressure of completing the document while in the pharmacy. They can fill it out on their own in the comfort of their home. Disadvantages are that the form may never be returned, it may be returned incomplete, and the pharmacist/student doesn't have the opportunity to evaluate body language and nonverbal cues as he or she would during the face-to-face interview. Each patient should be assessed and a determination made regarding the optimal method of obtaining additional information.

Drug Information Assignments

During your experience in the community pharmacy setting, numerous opportunities to answer drug information questions will be identified. Questions will be asked by patients, other healthcare professionals, and even the preceptor. It's important to always identify the actual question. Attempt to keep the topic narrow enough so that a brief review is possible—work with the preceptor to define the appropriate focus. Do not get involved in answering very general questions such as "can you tell me about steroids and what they do?" All statements of fact must be referenced. All references used to answer a question, regardless of the perceived significance, must be documented. A sample document used for recording responses to drug information questions is included as Appendix H. This will be used for documenting all information related to the question and the response provided. Answers to these requests must be approved by the preceptor or another registered pharmacist.

Case Presentations

During the course of this rotation, you may be required to complete at least one formal case presentation. Many structures are used for presenting cases, but the one that appears to work best in the community setting is where the primary focus is on a drug-related problem. The following are suggested guidelines to be used in the preparation of the case presentation. In addition, Appendix I is a suggested outline for the format of these presentations.

1. The focus of the case presentation should be on a patient-specific drug-related problem.
2. Include relevant information useful for patient education, counseling, and outcomes assessment.

3. Do not try to include information that is not routinely available to community pharmacists (for example, some laboratory data such as renal function or liver function studies).
4. If issues such as general health education are important for the presentation, these should be included.
5. There should be a defined period of time for the case presentation (for example, 30 minutes, including time for questions).
6. A handout should be prepared, with copies for all attendees, that includes all pertinent information about the patient, his or her DRPs, therapeutic and clinical data, and the plan for problem resolution. In addition, a list of references should be included.

Student Performance

Evaluating your performance during this type of rotation is an extremely challenging process. Many of the activities are subjective in nature, and there are no specific criteria to use to evaluate performance. However, collectively, each of the specific activities fits in with at least one of the primary learning objectives (reviewed earlier), so student performance is commonly measured against meeting the objectives. Weighting factors may be assigned to each objective that suggest where the efforts should be focused during the rotation. Each preceptor/site will determine the best process for measuring and evaluating your performance, and it is important for you to have an understanding of the grading process early in the rotation.

SUMMARY AND CONCLUSION

Tremendous opportunities exist for you in community pharmacy practice. In this chapter we have reviewed the different types of pharmacies where you may be placed, who works in them, many of the business issues related to community practice, and financial considerations in this environment. We've also discussed issues related to dispensing prescriptions, patient counseling, confidentiality and third parties, OTC medications, and disease-state management programs. As a student in this environment, you will be exposed to each of these issues and activities, some to a greater degree and in more depth than others. You will also be asked to participate in many assignments that will build knowledge and skills to help you become a more effective community pharmacy practitioner. Take advantage of every opportunity to learn as much as possible, especially about the nondispensing activities, because this is where the future of pharmacy is moving in the community setting. If you challenge your preceptor and challenge yourself, you will obtain the best possible experience during your community pharmacy rotation.

CASE STUDY

The following case is representative of a situation that presents itself during a typical day in a community pharmacy. The approach to these situations should be to search for DRPs and use the problem-solving approach. Describe in as much detail the process to determine prescription and overall patient profile appropriateness. Create a prioritized problem list, assess each problem, develop a theoretical plan, and define your desired outcome(s) for the patient. Also list the questions that should be asked of the patient before filling the prescription, and who should be contacted to obtain some of this information (i.e., patient, other family member, other healthcare professional).

CASE EXAMPLE

A 58-year-old woman presents a prescription for the following on April 11, 1996:

Diabeta 5 mg   Disp. # 90

Sig: Take one tablet ½ hour prior to each meal

5 refills

Dr. Jack Smith

When you check the patient's profile, you see the following information:

Drug Regimen	Refill Dates
HCTZ 50 mg 1 QD, #30	2/22/96, 1/23/96, 12/10/95, 11/1/95, 9/20/95
Procardia XL 90 mg 1 QD, #90	1/23/96, 9/20/95, 6/5/95
Zoloft 100 mg, 1 QHS, #30	2/27/96, 1/12/96, 12/11/95
Lopid 600 mg, 1 TID, #90	3/1/96, 1/30/96, 12/28/95, 11/30/95
Cimetidine 400 mg, 1 BID, #60	3/1/96, 1/23/96, 12/11/95, 11/10/95
Coumadin 2.5 mg, U.D., #30	1/30/96, 12/16/95, 11/14/95, 10/5/95

QUESTIONS

1. Which of the following statements are true regarding community pharmacy business and financial issues?
    A. Gross margins in the pharmacy department are typically lower than the gross margins for the front-end merchandise
    B. Mass merchandisers are willing to lose money in the pharmacy because it is such a small percentage of the business and it attracts new customers to their store.

    C. Third parties have effectively decreased the amount of profit a pharmacy can make dispensing medications.

    D. All the above are true.

2. All of the following are pieces of information on the prescription to verify *except:*

    A. Prescriber name and address, signature, and DEA number

    B. Patient name, address, allergies, age, and sometimes weight

    C. Patient method of payment, delivery preference, what counseling took place at the doctor's office

    D. Medication dose, SIG, quantity to dispense, and number of refills

3. Which of the following are key factors to promote effective patient counseling?

    A. Counsel the patient as close to the pharmacy as possible in case another question comes up

    B. Be empathetic, sincere, and nonjudgmental

    C. Ask closed-ended questions so the counseling session doesn't take up much of the patient's time

    D. If a family member is present, ask them to stay in the waiting area so they don't disrupt the session

4. The primary goal of the OTC consult process is to:

    A. Assist the customer in determining the best approach to the situation

    B. Select the least expensive product in the shortest amount of time, so you can wait on other customers

    C. Allow one of the clerks to manage the situation unless it's an emergency

    D. Don't ask too many questions so as to upset the customer

5. The key steps to establishing disease-state management programs in the community pharmacy setting include:

    A. Write, maintain, and have up-to-date policies and procedures

    B. Assess work flow in the pharmacy to determine how these programs will fit in with the dispensing process

    C. Develop a marketing and advertising plan

    D. All the above are important steps

REFERENCES

1. Bluml BM, McKenney JM, Cziraky MJ. Pharmaceutical care services and results in Project Im-PACT: hyperlipidemia. J Am Pharm Assoc 2000;40:157–165.
2. Fuller C. Weekly memorandum to NACDS chain members via Mondaymorning@NACDS.com, Aug 20, 2000.
3. Gardner M, Boyce RW, Herrier RN. Pharmacist–Patient Consultation Program PPCP–Unit 1. An interactive approach to verifying patient understanding. An educational service by Pfizer, Inc. sponsored by the US Public Health Service and Indian Health Service, 1994.
4. Hepler CD, Strand LM. Opportunities and responsibilities in pharmaceutical care. Am J Hosp Pharm 1990; 47:533–543.
5. Krinsky DL. How pharmaceutical care can work in your pharmacy. US Pharmacist 1997;3:124–128.

6. Muldary TW. Interpersonal relations for health professionals: a social skills approach. New York: Macmillan, 1983.
7. "Pharmacy Activity Cost and Productivity Study," performed by Arthur Andersen LLP, for NACDS, November 1999.
8. Rodriguez de Bittner M, Haines ST. Pharmacy-based diabetes management: a practical approach. J Am Pharm Assoc 1997;NS37:443–455.
9. Rupp MT, McCallian DJ, Sheth KK. Developing and marketing a community pharmacy-based asthma management program. J Am Pharm Assoc 1997;NS37:694–699.
10. Strand LM, Cipolle RJ, Morely PC. Drug-related problems, their structure and function. Drug Intell Clin Pharm 1990;24:1093–1097.
11. Schafermeyer KW, and Hobson EH, eds. The Community Retail Pharmacy Technician Training Manual. Alexandria. National Association of Chain Drug Stores and National Community Pharmacists Association, 1997.
12. The State of Community Pharmacy: An Educational Publication. East Hanover. Supported by Novartis Pharmaceuticals Corporation, 1999.

C H A P T E R   1 5

HOSPITAL PATIENT CASES

Stephanie D. Garrett

After reviewing the information in this chapter, you should be able to:

1. Identify the critical data in a patient chart or profile.
2. Prioritize patient problems and plan for correction.
3. Work with the healthcare team to solve therapeutic problems.
4. Work with the patient to identify missing pieces of data from history.
5. Write a SOAP note.
6. Present the patient case to the preceptor in an organized manner.

NOTE TO STUDENTS

The information provided in the following hospital cases is quite similar to what you might find on review of a typical patient chart in a teaching hospital. When evaluating the cases, you may find that not all necessary data are present. If you feel that additional information is necessary in order to make decisions about the medication regimens provided in this chapter, you should be prepared to elicit this information from your preceptor in the setting of a "role-playing" exercise. Formulate questions that you might theoretically ask the patient, physician, or nurse in order to obtain the information that you feel is lacking.

After reviewing the cases, you should be able to use the methods described in previous chapters to assess each patient problem (i.e., SOAP). You may identify additional patient problems (need for counseling regarding smoking cessation, inhaler technique, medication compliance, weight loss, etc.). These tend to be patient problems that only a pharmacist will identify and thus are not generally included in the physician's problem list. These problems should, however, be part of the pharmacist's problem list for that particular patient.

The patient's laboratory results and progress notes for the entire hospital course are available, but the student should try to formulate a plan for each day (as you would in clinical practice) *before* looking ahead to the labs and notes for the following day. Remember, there may be several correct ways to approach each patient problem.

Laboratory tests and medication profiles are provided in table format following each case. Additional tests (i.e., ECG, x-rays, etc.) are discussed in the daily progress notes.

NOTE TO PRECEPTORS

We have chosen to omit some information from the following cases in order to challenge the student to consider all aspects of the cases and to use his or her knowledge to develop a more appropriate therapeutic plan. When the student feels that additional information is necessary, try to engage him or her in a "role-playing" exercise (with the student playing the role of the pharmacist and the preceptor playing the role of patient, physician, or nurse). Ask the student to phrase questions in the same manner that would be used to address the patient or other caregivers.

For each case, the student should try to use the information provided in the "Progress Notes" and "Laboratory Results" to develop a rationale for medication changes made throughout the patient's hospital course. The student should be encouraged to identify additional patient problems (such as need for counseling on inhaler technique or smoking cessation) that were not identified in the case.

The patient's laboratory results and progress notes for the entire hospital course are available, but the student should try to formulate a plan for each day *before* looking ahead to the labs and notes for the following day.

Laboratory tests and medication profiles are provided in table format following each case. Additional tests (i.e., ECG, x-rays, etc.) are discussed in the daily progress notes.

HOSPITAL PATIENT CASE 1

Patient Name: Ewen, Mark	**Admission Date:** 7/16/00
Gender: M **Race:** White	**Weight:** 197 lbs **Height:** 6'1"
Allergies: NKDA	

Chief Complaint: "I'm having chest pain"

HPI:
ME is a 51-yo WM who presents to the ER complaining of stabbing chest pain with radiation to the left arm that woke him from sleep this morning. The pain has been constant since this morning and is rated an 8 of 10. He also complains of chest pressure, diaphoresis, and some shortness of breath. There has been no change in the pain (or associated symptoms) with activity or position.

PMH:	**PSH:**
MI and stent placement (11/99)	Stent placement (11/99 in Canada,
DVT and PE (11/99)	no records available)
CAD (? duration)	Multiple skin grafts to lower
Hyperlipidemia (? duration)	extremities
Lower extremity PVD	
(diagnosed 1980)	

Family History:	**Social History:**
Mother deceased at age 50, MVA	(−) tobacco
Father deceased at age 72, CHF	(−) illicit drug use
	occasional ETOH

Home Medications:	**ROS/PE:**
Lopressor 50 mg PO BID	GENERAL: WDWN WM with chest pain
Coumadin 5 mg PO QD	VITALS: BP: 111/76 HR: 82
Aspirin 325 mg PO QD	RR: 20 Temp: 98.4
Questran 1 packet QD	HEENT: no abnormalities
Darvocet N100 PRN	Neck: (−) JVD
Nitrostat SL PRN chest pain	CV: (+) CP, constant; (+) pain on chest wall with palpation
	LUNGS: (+) SOB; clear to auscultation bilaterally
	ABD: (+) BS; (−) tenderness or rebound
	GU: deferred
	EXT: multiple healed skin grafts on lower extremities; stage 2-3 stasis ulcer on LLE (2 cm diameter); vascular insufficiency
	Neuro: AAA × 3

Laboratory Results

Date:	7/16 Admission		7/17				7/18		7/19
Time:	1800	2400	0600	1200	1800	2400	0600	1800	0600
BP	142/83	115/75	116/75	110/76	112/77	115/76	110/75	115/77	112/78
HR	82	73	54	60	64	70	70	72	75
RR	20	19	20	19	19	20	19	20	20
Tmax	98.4	98.6	98.2	98.4	98.5	98.6	98.4	98.6	98.5
Na	141		139				140		
K	4.2		4.2				4.3		
Cl	108		106				105		
CO_2	27		26				26		
BUN	7		12				10		
SCr	0.9		1.0				1.0		
Glucose	101		84				95		
WBC	5.85		4.91						
HgB	15.7		14.9						
Hct	45.7		44						
Platelets	302		293						
MCV	96.1		96						
MCHC	33		34						
RDW	12.2		11.9						
PMN	51		50						
Lymphs	30		29						
Bands	2		2						
CK	76	74	58						
CKMB	0	0	0						
Troponin I	< 0.3	< 0.3	< 0.3						
PT	11.8								
INR	1.4								
PTT	27.8								
TC			509						
TG			841						
HDL			39						
LDL			—						

Hospital Medication Summary

Start Date	Medication Dose / Route / Frequency	D/C Date
7/16	Metoprolol 50 mg PO Q12	7/17
7/16	Famotidine 20 mg IV Q12	7/17
7/16	Baby aspirin 81 mg chew and swallow STAT × 1	7/16
7/16	Enoxaparin 90 mg / 0.9 ml SQ Q12	7/17
7/17	NTG Patch 0.2 mg / hr apply one patch QD	7/19
7/17	Enteric coated aspirin 325 mg PO QD	7/19
7/17	Famotidine 20 mg PO Q12	7/19
7/17	Metoprolol 50 mg PO QD	7/19
7/16	NTG 0.4 mg tab SL Q5 minutes × 3 PRN chest pain	7/19
7/16	NTG in D5W 50 mg / 250 ml IV PRN— titrate to relief of chest pain	7/17
7/16	Morphine 2 mg / 0.5 ml IV Q4 PRN chest pain	7/17
7/17	Alprazolam 0.25 mg PO Q8 PRN anxiety	7/18

Progress Notes

7/16

Admission ECG: rate 95; NSR; nonspecific ST-T abnormalities

Problem #1—Unstable angina, rule out MI

- Admit to telemetry bed; vitals Q6 hours
- Start NTG drip PRN for chest pain not relieved by SL NTG
- Start O_2 via nasal cannula
- First cardiac enzymes (−); subsequent cardiac enzymes pending; awaiting cardiology consult for further plan
- ECG PRN chest pain and in AM
- Chem 7 and CBC in AM

Problem #2—History of hyperlipidemia

- Fasting lipid panel in AM

Problem #3—Left leg stasis ulcer

- Wound care; monitor for infection

7/17

ECG: rate 59; sinus bradycardia; nonspecific ST-T abnormalities

Problem #1—Unstable angina, rule out MI

- Cardiac enzymes (−) × 3
- Chest pain only 4 of 10 today
- Sinus bradycardia on AM ECG; patient lightheaded

- Patient extremely anxious about catheterization; having difficulty sleeping
- Scheduled for cardiac catheterization today per cardiology

Problem #2—History of hyperlipidemia
- TC 509; TG 841
- Discuss treatment with cardiology after catheterization

Problem #3—Left leg stasis ulcer
- Unchanged; no evidence of infection; continue wound care

7/18
Problem #1—Unstable angina, rule out MI
- Cardiac catheterization revealed two-vessel disease (45% and 50%) without significant involvement of the LAD
- Cardiology recommends medical management
- Patient ready for discharge from cardiac standpoint

Problem #2—Hyperlipidemia
- Draw baseline liver function tests
- Schedule patient with dietician for heart-healthy diet counseling
- Discuss exercise

Problem #3—Left leg stasis ulcer
- Continue home wound care

HOSPITAL PATIENT CASE 2

Patient Name: Vaughan, Susan	**Admission Date:** 9/15/00
Gender: F **Race:** Black	**Weight:** 150 lbs **Height:** 5'8"
Allergies: NKDA	

Chief Complaint: "My legs have been swelling up"

HPI:
SV is a 78-yo BF who presents to the ER with swollen and tender legs × 3 days. She states that the swelling and some tenderness started in the morning several days ago. She states that she has tried to elevate her legs and stay off her feet, but the pain and swelling are getting worse.

PMH:	**PSH:**
GERD	Greenfield filter placement (11/98)
Chronic iron deficiency anemia	
PE (11/98)	

Family History:	**Social History:**
Mother deceased; age 85;	(−) tobacco
heart attack	(−) ETOH
Father deceased; age unknown;	(−) illict drugs
cancer	

Home Medications:	**ROS/PE:**
Acetaminophen PRN	GENERAL: WDWN BF in NAD
Multivitamin PO QD	VITALS: BP: 126/65 HR: 70
Pepcid 20 mg PO QD	RR: 24 Temp: 97
(Pepcid prescribed QD, but patient	HEENT: No abnormalities
"takes it when she needs it")	CV: RRR; borderline
	bradycardia
	Lungs: clear to auscultation
	bilaterally
	ABD: (+) BS × 4
	GU: deferred
	EXT: bilateral pain and ten-
	derness with touch; (+)
	Homan's sign; decreased
	strength and ROM; (+)
	edema with R > L; good
	pulses
	Neuro: AAA × 3

Laboratory Results

Date:	9/15 Admission			9/16	9/17	9/18	9/19
Time:	1200	1800	2400	0600	0600	0600	0600
BP	126/65			120/57	135/74	111/57	105/62
HR	70			66	80	75	73
RR	24			20	20	20	18
Tmax	97			99.2	98.5	98.6	98
Na	139			140	139		
K	3.9			3.9	3.9		
Cl	100			102	101		
CO_2	28			29	29		
BUN	10			9	9		
SCr	0.8			0.9	0.9		
Glucose	111			99	105		
WBC	7.6			6.5			
HgB	12.3			11.3			
Hct	36.8			36.1			
Platelets	200			211			
MCV	31.3			35			
RDW	45			44			
PMN	65.7			68			
PT	12.1	12.3	13.3	13.3	15.3	17	17.5
INR	1.07	1.2	1.29	1.29	1.7	2.09	2.48
PTT	25.8	30.2	57.4	59.9	61.2	65.5	68

Hospital Medication Summary

Start Date	Medication Dose / Route / Frequency	D/C Date
9/15	Heparin drip 250,000 units / 250 ml D5W	
9/15	Ferrous sulfate 325 mg PO TID with meals	
9/15	Multivitamin tablet PO QD	
9/15	Famotidine 20 mg PO BID	
9/16	Warfarin 7.5 mg PO X 1 today	9/16
9/17	Warfarin 5 mg PO X 1 today	9/17
9/18	Warfarin 5 mg PO X 1 today	9/18
9/19	Warfarin 5 mg PO X 1 today	9/19
9/15	Docusate sodium 100 mg PO PRN constipation	
9/15	Acetaminophen 500 mg PO Q4-6 hours PRN pain or headache	
9/15	Propoxyphene 100 mg / acetaminophen 650 mg take 1-2 tablets PO Q4 hours for pain not relieved by acetaminophen	

Progress Notes

9/15

Problem #1—LE pain and swelling; rule out DVT
- Start heparin drip per standing orders
- Schedule for bilateral LE doppler
- Have RN measure circumference of both LE

Problem #2—History of GERD
- Start scheduled BID famotidine

Problem #3—History of iron deficiency anemia
- Continue multivitamin QD
- Start ferrous sulfate TID

9/16

Problem #1—LE pain and swelling; rule out DVT
- Heparin drip per standing orders
- Doppler (+) for bilateral DVTs
- Start warfarin today
- Edema somewhat improved today

Problem #2—History of GERD
- Continue famotidine

Problem #3—History of iron deficiency anemia
- Continue multivitamin QD
- Continue ferrous sulfate

9/17
Problem #1—DVT
- Heparin drip per standing orders
- Call pharmacy for warfarin counseling
- Dietary counseling on warfarin
- Edema significantly improved this a.m.
- Less pain

Problem #2—History of GERD
- Continue famotidine

Problem #3—History of iron deficiency anemia
- Continue multivitamin QD
- Continue ferrous sulfate TID

HOSPITAL PATIENT CASE 3

Patient Name: Jones, Nathan	**Admission Date:** 1/27/00
Gender: M **Race:** Hispanic	**Weight:** 174 lbs **Height:** 5'9"
Allergies: Aspirin, codeine	

Chief Complaint: "I threw up blood"

HPI:
NJ is a 57-yo Hispanic male with a LeVeen shunt and reported history of liver disease, who presents to the ER complaining of hematemesis (X 1, two hours before arrival) and melena (X 2 the day before arrival). Patient denies other complaints; specifically he states he has no abdominal pain, no fever, and no chest pain. Upon arrival in the ER, the patient experienced emesis again with blood clots and bright red blood (witnessed by ER staff).

PMH:	**PSH:**
Umbilical hernia	LeVeen shunt placement 5/99
History of "liver disease"	

Family History:	**Social History:**
Mother deceased at age 57,	(+) ETOH approx. 8 beers/week
rectal cancer	(+) tobacco (20 pack years)
Father deceased at age 80, "old age"	(−) illicit drug use

Home Medications:	**ROS/PE:**
Not currently taking any medications	GENERAL: WDWN Hispanic male
History of taking potassium and a	VITALS: BP: 96/67 HR: 96
"water pill"	RR: 32 Temp: 99.4
	HEENT: no abnormalities
	Neck: (−) JVD; (−) goiter
	CV: tenderness with palpation
	on chest wall
	LUNGS: clear to auscultation
	bilaterally
	ABD: (+) BS; mild distention;
	(+) ascites
	GU: (−) gross blood; occult
	blood (+)
	EXT: Bilateral 1+ edema
	Neuro: AAA X 3

Laboratory Results

Date:	1/27 Admission	1/28			1/29	1/30	1/31
Time:	2400	0600	1200	2400	0600	0600	0600
BP	96/57	136/79			129/76	137/82	154/89
HR	96	95			111	72	80
RR	32	18			32	20	21
Tmax	99.4	99.3			102.5	101	102.5
Na	140	142			144	143	137
K	4.2	3.5		3.1	3.8	3.4	3.7
Cl	109	122			116	116	113
CO_2	25	20			24	24	23
BUN	27	25			26	19	13
SCr	0.7	0.5			0.7	0.6	0.6
Glucose	124	166			119	134	114
WBC	8.77	4.78	5.01	5.89	6.06	3.11	5.53
HgB	9.9	7.3	6.2	10.8	12.3	10.9	10.1
Hct	29.7	21.2	17.8	31.7	36.3	32.5	29.6
Platelets	91	40	43	43	38	28	42
MCV	101.4	96	93.2	93.2	93.3	91.9	94.8
RDW	56.7	55.4	54.3	54.6	56.1	55.9	56
PMN	72	84.8	85	84.6	85.5	85.6	84.1
AST		40			52		
ALT		39			39		
Alk Phos		53			63		
Bilirubin		1			1.7		
Albumin		1.2			2.1		
Ammonia		16			56	37	18
Mg			0.7	1.8			1.6
Ca	8.9	5.6			7.4		7.4
PT	16	19.3			15.3		
INR	1.72	2.49			1.58		
PTT	30.9	41.7			30.4		

Hospital Medication Summary

Start Date	Medication Dose / Route / Frequency	D/C Date
1/27	Famotidine 20 mg IV Q12	1/30
1/27	Multivitamin IV QD (added to first liter of IVF QD)	1/30
1/27	Thiamine 100 mg IV QD (added to first liter of IVF QD)	1/30
1/27	Folate 1 mg IV QD (added to first liter of IVF QD)	1/30
1/27	NS at 150 ml/hr	1/29
1/28	Vitamin K 10 mg SQ QD × 3 days	1/30
1/28	Magnesium sulfate 2 grams in 400 ml NS over 2 hours × 1	1/28
1/29	Cefotaxime 1 gm IV Q6	
1/29	Lactulose 30 ml PO BID	
1/29	Spironolactone 50 mg PO BID	
1/29	NS at 75 ml/hr	
1/30	Famotidine 20 mg PO Q12	
1/30	Multivitamin PO QD	
1/30	Thiamine 100 mg PO QD	
1/30	Folate 1 mg PO QD	
1/27	Lorazepam 0.5 mg IV Q4-6 PRN anxiety or agitation	
1/27	Acetaminophen 650 mg PR Q6 PRN pain / fever	
1/27	Promethazine 25 mg IV Q4-6 PRN nausea	
1/27	Furosemide 20 mg IV PRN (after each transfusion)	

Progress Notes

1/27
Admission ECG: rate 94; NSR
Serum and urine toxicology screen (−)
CXR: clear

Problem #1—Upper GI bleed
- Admit to ICU; vitals per protocol
- NPO
- GI consult for endoscopy
- Transfuse 2 units PRBC, FFP, and platelets
- CBC, Chem 7, and hepatic panel in a.m.

Problem #2—History of liver disease
- Coagulopathy - check PT/INR daily
- Check ammonia

Problem #3—Alcohol abuse
- Monitor for alcohol withdrawal syndrome

1/28
Problem #1—Upper GI bleed
- No further emesis
- Patient to remain NPO
- Patient received a total of 4 units PRBC, 2 units FFP, and 10 units platelets throughout night
- GI consult ordered another 2 units PRBC this am; endoscopy scheduled for this afternoon

Problem #2—History of liver disease
- Patient difficult to arouse or unwilling to cooperate; refuses to answer questions this a.m.

Problem #3—Alcohol abuse
- Monitor for alcohol withdrawal syndrome

1/29
Problem #1—Upper GI bleed
- Endoscopy revealed grade 4 esophageal varices with bleeding present
- Band ligation procedure performed
- (+) melena this a.m.
- Patient may resume oral intake (liquid diet only)

Problem #2—History of liver disease
- T_{max} 102.5 with normal WBC; draw blood cultures $\times$ 2
- Ascites and peripheral edema; start spironolactone PO

Problem #3—Alcohol abuse
- Monitor for alcohol withdrawal syndrome

1/30
Problem #1—Upper GI bleed
- Stable from GI standpoint

Problem #2—History of liver disease
- Diarrhea $\times$ 3 yesterday
- Patient still uncooperative
- T_{max} 101; blood cultures (−) $\times$ 24 hours

Problem #3—Alcohol abuse
- Monitor for alcohol withdrawal syndrome

1/31
Problem #1—Upper GI bleed
- Stable

Problem #2—History of liver disease

- T_{max} 102.5; blood cultures (−) × 48 hours
- Patient resting comfortably today and more willing to cooperate
- Eating well

Problem #3—Alcohol abuse

- Monitor for alcohol withdrawal syndrome

HOSPITAL PATIENT CASE 4

Patient Name: Lewis, Jack **Admission Date:** 7/14/00	
Gender: M **Race:** White **Weight:** 250 lbs **Height:** 5'10"	
Allergies: NKDA	

Chief Complaint: "I can't stop coughing"

HPI:
JL is a 34-yo WM who presents to the ER complaining of a cough with some brown-tinged sputum and right upper quadrant pain × 7 days. He also complains of subjective fever, chills, and decreased appetite for about one week. He has been short of breath, but denies dyspnea on exertion. JL had one episode of hemoptysis the evening prior to admission.

PMH:	**PSH:**
Asthma since childhood	Arthroscopic knee surgery (1993)
Hyperlipidemia × 2 years	

Family History:	**Social History:**
Mother alive no known medical problems	(−) ETOH
Father alive with arthritis and HTN	(+) tobacco (1 pack per week)
	(−) illicit drug use
	Occupational exposure to bleach

Home Medications:	**ROS/PE:**
Albuterol inhaler PRN	GENERAL: Obese WM with cough
Zocor 20 mg PO QD	VITALS: BP: 136/78 HR: 109
	RR: 18 Temp: 100.6
	HEENT: no swollen lymph nodes or glands; nares patent
	CV: (−) CP; tachycardic (NSR)
	LUNGS: decreased breath sounds at right base; dullness to percussion at right base; (+) egophany; bilateral ronchi; no wheezes noted
	ABD: (+) BS; nontender
	GU: deferred
	EXT: good capillary refill; muscle strength 5/5 in all extremities; no rashes or lesions noted
	Neuro: AAA × 3

Laboratory Results

Date:	7/14 Admission	7/15			7/16	7/17
Time:	2200	0600	1200	2400	0600	0600
BP	136/78	129/82	130/81		129/78	133/80
HR	109	108	110		105	101
RR	18	20	19		19	19
Tmax	100.6	101	100.8		99.5	99.2
Na	137	137			142	143
K	3.2	4.5			4.0	4.1
Cl	94	103			102	104
CO2	28	26			28	28
BUN	10	7			7	6
SCr	0.9	0.8			0.8	0.8
Glucose	110	88			90	92
WBC	19.8	13.9			12.8	12.1
HgB	15	13			13.1	13
Hct	42.6	40			40	41
Platelets	199	201			213	308
MCV	90	91			89	90
RDW	45	42			42	44
PMN	89	82			76	68.7
Lymphs	6.1	9.2			10.4	13.1
Bands	3	2			3	2
AST	30					
ALT	22					
Alk Phos	98					
Bilirubin	1.1					
Albumin	4.2					
Mg		2.3				

Hospital Medication Summary

Start Date	Medication Dose / Route / Frequency	D/C Date
7/14	D5 ½ NS + KCL 40 mEq/L at 125 ml/hr	7/15
7/14	Ceftriaxone 1 gram IV Q12 hours	7/16
7/14	Clarithromycin 500 mg PO BID	
7/14	Simvastatin 20 mg PO QD	
7/15	D5 ½ NS + KCL 20 mEq/L at 100 ml/hr	7/17
7/16	Cefuroxime 250 mg PO Q12 hours	
7/14	Guaifenesin 100 mg / dextromethorphan 10 mg; use 2 tsp PO Q4-6 hours PRN cough	
7/14	Acetaminophen 650 mg PO Q4-6 hours PRN temp > 101	
7/14	Albuterol MDI PRN SOB	

Progress Notes

7/14

Problem #1—Cough / SOB; rule out pneumonia
- CXR with (+) infiltrate in RLL; no pleural effusion
- Temp 100.6
- Admit to medical floor; vitals per protocol
- Continue medications as at home
- Obtain sputum culture
- Start antibiotics

Problem #2—Asthma
- Continue albuterol MDI

Problem #3—Hyperlipidemia
- Stable; continue simvastatin

Problem #4—Hypokalemia
- Add 40 mEq/L of KCl to maintenance IVF

Problem #5—Elevated BP
- Monitor

7/15

Problem #1—Pneumonia
- Tolerating antibiotics well
- Unable to obtain sputum culture
- Requesting cough medication from RN every few hours
- Still febrile today

Problem #2—Asthma
- Continue albuterol MDI

Problem #3—Hyperlipidemia
- Stable; continue simvastatin

Problem #4—Hypokalemia
- Improved; reduce KCl in IVF

Problem #5—Elevated BP
- Monitor

7/16 and 7/17
Problem #1—Pneumonia
- Pneumonia much improved
- Less SOB and cough overnight

Problem #2—Asthma
- Continue albuterol MDI

Problem #3—Hyperlipidemia
- Stable; continue simvastatin

Problem #4—Hypokalemia
- Resolved

Problem #5—Elevated BP
- Consider treatment

Patient Name: Earnright, Richard	Admission Date: 8/5/00
Gender: M Race: Jamaican	Weight: 174 lbs Height: 5'10"
Allergies: NKDA	

Chief Complaint: "I can't breathe, and I feel really tired"

HPI:
RE is a 65-yo Jamaican male with a significant history of repeated inpatient admissions for heart failure exacerbations. He presents to the ER with a 4-day history of increasing SOB and fatigue. He is presently using three pillows to sleep comfortably at night (increased from his normal of two pillows). He complains of cough, difficulty walking without getting short of breath, weakness, and swollen feet and ankles. He also admits to a 10-pound weight gain over the last month. RE is also quick to admit that he rarely remembers to get his prescriptions refilled when they run out and doesn't follow the diet that was suggested to him.

PMH:	PSH:
Heart failure (diagnosed 1993)	Glaucoma laser surgery (right eye)
Glaucoma (right eye)	× 3
Hypertension (since age 30)	
Hyperlipidemia (? duration)	
Hemorrhoids (since 1995)	
Diverticulitis (diagnosed 1995)	

Family History:	Social History:
Mother deceased age 50, heart attack	(+) history of tobacco (2 packs/day since age 18)
Father deceased age 78, Parkinson's disease	(+) history of ETOH (since age 18; heavy alcohol use in the past, but only social drinking now per patient) (−) illicit drug use

Home Medications:	ROS/PE:
Lipitor 10 mg PO QD	GENERAL: WDWN male with significant SOB
Enteric coated aspirin 325 mg PO QD	VITALS: BP: 146/80 HR: 100 RR: 26 Temp: 97
Lasix 20 mg PO QD	
Vasotec 5 mg PO QD	HEENT: Blind in right eye
Pred Forte 1 gtt OD QID	Neck: (+) JVD
Atropine 1 gtt OD BID	CV: (+) mild CP; heart regular rate and rhythm; (+) S3 gallop
Timolol XE 1 gtt OD QD	
Alphagan 1 gtt OD TID	LUNGS: inspiratory rales bilaterally
Truspot 1 gtt OD TID	ABD: (+) BS; nontender, mildly distended
	GU: (+) hemorrhoids; (−) occult blood
	EXT: 2+ pitting edema to ankles bilaterally
	Neuro: AAA × 3

Laboratory Results

Date:	8/5 Admission		8/6		8/7	8/8
Time:	1500	2100	0300	0600	0600	0600
BP	146/80			153/92	142/83	140/83
HR	100			99	98	96
RR	26			25	25	24
Tmax	97			98.1	97.9	98.2
Na	133			134	135	136
K	3.3			3.5	3.6	3.6
Cl	101			100	100	102
CO2	28			26	26	25
BUN	20			19	19	19
SCr	1.1			1.3	1.2	1.1
Glucose	98			100	101	99
WBC	8.7					
HgB	15.2					
Hct	43.6					
Platelets	350					
MCV	87					
MCHC	33					
RDW	14.2					
CK	43	47	45			
CKMB	–	–	–			
Troponin I	< 0.3	< 0.3	< 0.3			
Ca			9.2			
Mg	1.8					
PO4	3.5					

Hospital Medication Summary

Start Date	Medication Dose / Route / Frequency	D/C Date
8/5	All eye drops as per home doses	
8/5	Atorvastatin 10 mg PO QD	
8/5	Enteric coated aspirin 325 mg PO QD	
8/5	Enalapril 5 mg PO QD	8/6
8/5	Furosemide 40 mg IV BID	8/6
8/5	Potassium chloride extended release 20 mEq PO QD	
8/6	Furosemide 20 mg IV QD	8/7
8/6	Enalapril 10 mg PO QD	
8/7	Furosemide 20 mg PO QD	
8/5	NTG 0.4 mg tab SL Q5 minutes X 3 PRN chest pain	
8/5	Morphine 2 mg / 0.5 ml IV Q4 PRN chest pain	8/6
8/5	Acetaminophen 650 mg PO Q4-6 PRN fever/pain/ headache	

Progress Notes

8/5

EKG: NSR with significant LVH

Old charts from prior admissions show last echocardiogram done 6 months ago (EF 23%)

CXR: cardiomegaly, ? right-sided pleural effusion

Problem #1—Heart failure exacerbation; rule out MI; rule out pneumonia

- Cardiac enzymes
- Na restriction (1 gram daily)
- Discussed with patient the need to limit fluid intake
- Start IV furosemide
- Chem 7 in a.m., monitor fluid I/O

Problem #2—HTN

- Uncontrolled at present
- Continue Vasotec; same dose

Problem #3—Hypokalemia

- Potassium replacement
- Check K in a.m.

Problem #4—History of glaucoma, hyperlipidemia, and diverticulitis
- All stable
- Continue home management

8/6
Problem #1—Heart failure exacerbation
- Fluid I/O for previous 24-hour period:
    ○ In: 1200 mL
    ○ Out: 2475 mL
- Ankle swelling diminished
- Chem 7 in a.m., monitor fluid I/O
- Consult pharmacy for medication teaching (emphasis on medication compliance)

Problem #2—HTN
- Uncontrolled
- Increase Vasotec dose

Problem #3—Hypokalemia
- K 3.5 today; continue replacement

Problem #4—History of glaucoma, hyperlipidemia, and diverticulitis
- All stable
- Continue home management

Hospital Patient Case 6

Patient Name: Bowen, Francine	**Admission Date:** 3/2/00
Gender: F **Race:** Black	**Weight:** 96 lbs **Height:** 5'4"
Allergies: PCN	

Chief Complaint: "My leg hurts, and it isn't getting better"

HPI:
FB is an 83-yo BF who presents to the ER with complaints of a swollen and painful left lower extremity. She noticed that her leg seemed swollen about 1 week prior to arrival. For the past 3 days, however, the swelling has worsened and is painful. The leg is also extremely red and warm to touch.

PMH: HTN × 10 years DM × 20 years	**PSH:** TAH at age 56
Family History: Mother deceased at age 80; "ulcer" Father deceased at age 78; HTN/DM	**Social History:** (−) ETOH (+) tobacco (1 pack per week) (−) illicit drug use

Home Medications:
Cardizem CD 240 mg PO QD
Insulin 70/30 30 units in the a.m.
Insulin 70/30 20 units in the p.m.
	ROS/PE:
	GENERAL: Thin BF in NAD
	VITALS: BP: 165/92 HR: 75
	               RR: 18 Temp: 100.6
	HEENT: (+) cataracts bilaterally
	Neck: (−) JVD; (−) goiter
	CV: RRR
	LUNGS: Clear to auscultation
	               bilaterally
	ABD: (+)BS
	GU: occult blood (−)
	EXT: significant peripheral
	               neuropathy present
	               bilaterally; LLE swollen to
	               mid calf, warm to touch,
	               diffuse redness, no
	               obvious abrasions or
	               cuts; poor nail and foot
	               care
	Neuro: AAA × 3

Laboratory Results

Date:	3/2 Admission	3/3			3/4	3/5	3/6	3/7
Time:	1800	0600	1200	2400	0600	0600	0600	0600
BP	165/92	157/89	139/90	160/90	156/87	143/82	140 /82	141/79
HR	75	87	79	82	80	75	77	77
RR	18	20	20	20	19	19	19	20
Tmax	100.6	100.4	99.8	100.1	99.6	99.2	98.9	99.1
Na	136	136			134	135	135	135
K	4.4	4			3.9	4	4.1	4.1
Cl	98	100			100	101	99	100
CO_2	26	28			28	27	27	28
BUN	16	15			10	11	11	10
SCr	1.4	1.3			1.3	1.3	1.3	1.2
Glucose	146	130	170	110	122	113	110	111
WBC	12.2	12			11.2	10.9	9.8	9.2
HgB	13.2	13			13.1	13.2	12.9	13
Hct	40.3	39.8			40.2	39	40.1	40.3
Platelets	272	270			275	300	289	288
PMN	87	86			86	82	73	74
Lymphs	9.7	8.5			8.2	8.1	7.6	7.5
Bands	2	3			2	2	3	2
Albumin	3.8							
HgBA1C		9.2						

Hospital Medication Summary

Start Date	Medication Dose / Route / Frequency	D/C Date
3/2	Clindamycin 600 mg IV Q8	3/3
3/2	Diltiazem CD 240 mg PO QD	
3/2	Insulin 70/30 30 units SQ QAM (30 minutes before meal)	
3/2	Insulin 70/30 20 units SQ QPM (30 minutes before meal)	
3/3	Lisinopril 2.5 mg PO QD	
3/3	Vancomycin 1 gram IV Q12	3/3
3/4	Vancomycin 750 mg IV Q24	3/5
3/4	Potassium chloride extended release tablet 20 mEq PO QD	3/5
3/7	Vancomycin 750 mg IV Q48	
3/2	Sliding scale regular insulin per protocol	
3/2	Acetaminophen 500 mg PO Q4-6 PRN fever/pain	

Progress Notes

3/2
Problem #1—Cellulitis
- Start clindamycin IV
- Vitals per protocol

Problem #2—DM
- Continue home insulin regimen
- Order glycosylated hemoglobin
- Fingerstick glucose measurement Q6 with sliding scale coverage

Problem #3—Hypertension
- Continue Cardizem home dosage
- Monitor

3/3
Problem #1—Cellulitis
- Minimal improvement; T_{max} this a.m. 100.4
- Upper trunk rash noted this a.m. (covering face, chest, and upper arms); ? clindamycin allergy
- Start vancomycin 1gram IV Q12 (first dose 1500 today); pharmacy consult on dosing and levels

Problem #2—DM
- $HgbA_{1C} = 9.2\%$

Problem #3—Hypertension
- Uncontrolled
- Start lisinopril

3/4
Problem #1—Cellulitis
- T_{max} and WBC improved
- Less painful today per patient report, but no change in size of cellulitis area
- Vancomycin 750 mg Q24 per pharmacy consult (dose scheduled for 1500 today)

Problem #2—DM
- D/C finger sticks

Problem #3—Hypertension
- Still elevated, continue to monitor

3/5
Problem #1—Cellulitis
- Improvement in size of swollen area today
- Less pain, T_{max} and WBC normalizing
- Vancomycin 750 mg IV administered at 1500 today
- Vancomycin trough level 32.3 @ 1300
- Vancomycin peak level 52.4 @ 1730
- Consult pharmacy for dosage adjustment

Problem #2—DM
- Continue home insulin regimen
- Order glycosylated hemoglobin
- Fingerstick glucose measurement Q6 with sliding scale coverage

Problem #3—Hypertension
- Continue Cardizem home dosage
- Monitor

AMBULATORY CARE PATIENT CASES

Ming Wang and Karen Daniel

After reviewing the information in this chapter, you should be able to:

1. Identify the critical data in an outpatient profile and prescription history.
2. Prioritize patient problems and discuss a plan for correction.
3. Work with a physician to solve therapeutic problems.
4. Educate a patient on the plan for correcting a problem.
5. Write a note in a medical chart.
6. Present the case to the preceptor in an organized manner.

NOTE TO STUDENTS

The following cases contain information similar to what you will find in an outpatient clinic setting. You should treat the information as if these are real patients and you are now in charge of their care. They have been assigned to see you, the pharmacist. You may ask your preceptor questions to get a better patient history, as not all of the information you need may be found in the chart. Your preceptor will play the role of the patient, while you play the role of the pharmacist. You must also, in some cases, approach your preceptor as "the patient's physician" to get further information. You will then proceed to complete a SOAP note and a patient case presentation for your preceptor.

In addition to determining the patient's problems and developing a plan, you should look at your patient's social history. Knowing the social history may help you develop an education plan to assist the patient in attaining your goals. You should also determine if you and the patient can come to an agreement on the goals of therapy and the plan for getting there. Sometimes the best plan can go awry if a patient can not or is not willing to follow your advice and plan. You should be prepared to present your patient education materials to your preceptor as if he or she is the patient.

NOTE TO PRECEPTORS

These cases should be approached by the student as patient charts. One example is available to the student at the beginning of the chapter. This has the patient data listed, then goes through the writing of an entire SOAP note, with assessment and plan included. You can guide your student through the critical thinking skills required to formulate the plan and write the note for this patient. Following that example are six more cases with various histories and laboratory values included. These are designed for you to role play with the student, as either the patient or a physician, in order to provide other information they need to solve the patient problem(s) and move on to therapeutic planning.

You control the outcome of these cases, depending on how you role play with the student. Data can be changed or added to guide the student in the direction of disease states and toward information they need to learn on your rotation. You can modify these cases as needed from student to student. Once they have completed these cases, you should feel comfortable sending them out to look at charts in your clinic. The student should have an improved ability in reviewing patient records and ascertaining pertinent information. They should be able to communicate the important information to the physicians and nurses.

AMBULATORY PATIENT CASE EXAMPLE

Pt. Name: Sweet, Melissa		Date: 9/05/00	
Ht: 5'6" Wt: 160 lbs Gender: F		Age: 53	Race: Black
Allergies: NKDA MD: Dr. B. Sugar			Insurance: Medicaid
CC/HPI: MS presents to clinic for diabetes f/u. Pt c/o continued cramps in feet and hands × 3 months and cut on L big toe.			
PMH: Type 2 DM, HTN, PVD, OA, hyperlipidemia, peripheral neuropathy, postmenopausal (1997)		PSH:	
FH: Noncontributory		SH: No tobacco or ETOH	
Home Meds: 1. Prinivil 10 mg PO QD 2. Humulin 70/30 35 U a.m., 15 U p.m. 3. Glucotrol XL 10 mg PO QD 4. Trental 400 mg PO QD 5. Zocor 10 mg PO QD 6. Elavil 50 mg PO QHS 7. Motrin 600 mg PO TID PRN		Problem List: 1. Type 2 DM 2. Diabetic foot ulcer 3. HTN 4. PVD 5. Hyperlipidemia	

ROS/PE

GEN: 53-yo obese bf in NAD.
HEENT: Pt experiences occasional blurry vision (~3 × week) – last eye exam in 1998. PERRLA, EOMI, nares patent, neck supple without adenopathy.
CV: Denies CP, chest tightness, palpitations; RRR, no M/R/G.
LUNGS: CTA bilaterally
ABD: Denies N/V/D/C, abd pain.
GU: Denies polyuria
EXT: Pt experiences painful cramping in feet and hands (× 3 months) mainly in the evening. Cramping in feet relieved by sitting down. Denies numbness and tingling in hand, legs, and feet. Patient does not wear shoes in her house. 1.5 cm ulcerative lesion on L great toe.
NEURO: Grossly intact

Vitals and Labs

Date	7/07/00	8/10/00	9/05/00
BP	158/96	150/94	148/92
HR	76	72	76
RR	24	20	20
Temp			
Glucose	250	233	225 (PP)
SCr	0.8		0.8
HbA1c	10.3		
PT/INR			
ALT	45		
AST	20		
Alk Phos	84		
LDH			
Tot Bili	0.8		
TC	270		208
HDL	45		55
LDL	187		119
TG	190		170
Urinary albumin (24 hour)	30		

Progress Note

1. Type 2 DM—BS not controlled. Patient states BS was 76 this a.m. before breakfast.
2. Foot ulcer—L great toe
3. HTN—BP not controlled.
4. PVD—Cramps in hands and feet × 3 months relieved only by sitting, currently on Trental 400 mg PO QD.
5. Hyperlipidemia—Lipids have improved, on Zocor 10 mg PO QD.

Example Ambulatory Care Soap Note

Subjective

CC/HPI: MS is a 53-yo obese bf who presents to the clinic for diabetes f/u. She states that she continues to have painful cramps in her feet and hands in the evening. Pt states she has been experiencing these cramps × 3 months. MS also states that she has a cut on her left big toe.

PMH: Type 2 DM
HTN
PVD
Peripheral neuropathy
Hyperlipidemia
OA
Postmenopausal (1997)

SHx: (−) tobacco and ETOH

FH: Noncontributory

ROS: Denies any s/s of hypoglycemia. Pt states experiences occasional blurry vision ~3 × week.

Objective
Home Meds: Prinivil 10 mg PO QD
Humulin 70/30 35 U a.m., 15 U p.m.
Glucotrol XL 10 mg PO QD
Trental 400 mg PO QD
Zocor 10 mg PO QD
Elavil 50 mg PO QHS
Motrin 600 mg PO TID PRN

Vitals: BP 148/92   HR 76   RR 20

PE: 1.5-cm ulcerative lesion on L great toe

Labs:
9/05/00:
Glucose (finger stick) 225
TC 208   HDL 55   LDL 119   TG 170

7/07/00:
HbA$_{1c}$ 10.3
24-hour urinary albumin 30

Assessment
1. Type 2 DM. Not controlled as evidenced by fingerstick glucose, HbA$_{1c}$, blurry vision and presence of long-term complications (i.e., microalbuminuria and PVD). Today, fingerstick blood sugar (postprandial) was 225 (pt states BS was 76 before breakfast this a.m.). Pt's HbA$_{1c}$ not at goal of < 7 (10.3 on 7/07/00). Pt has been experiencing occasional blurred vision (~3 × week) possibly secondary to uncontrolled BS.
2. Foot ulcer. Pt has ulcer on L great toe. Pt does not wear shoes inside her house.
3. PVD. Cramps in hands and feet × 3 months relieved only by sitting down. Currently on Trental 400 mg PO QD.

4. HTN. Not at BP goal of < 130/80. Currently on Prinivil 10 mg PO QD
5. Hyperlipidemia. LDL has decreased from 187 on 7/07/00 to 119 today. However, still not at LDL goal of < 100. Currently on Zocor 10 mg PO QD.
6. Microalbuminuria. Currently on Prinivil 10 mg PO QD for HTN and renal protection.
7. Postmenopausal. Pt is a candidate for HRT.

Plan
1. Type 2 DM. Increase Humulin 70/30 to 37 U a.m., continue 15 U p.m. Explain importance of yearly eye exam to monitor for retinopathy. Refer to optometry for eye exam. Reassess BS control when RTC. Begin ASA 325 mg PO QD for cardioprotection.
2. Foot ulcer. Refer pt to podiatry for L great toe ulcer. Instruct pt to wear shoes inside and outside the house. Educate pt on importance of keeping feet clean, dry, and moisturized daily. Instruct pt to check feet for cuts/lesions daily.
3. PVD. Refer to primary care physician for evaluation. Recommend increasing Trental to 400 mg PO BID with meals to relieve pain.
4. HTN. Increase Prinivil to 20 mg PO QD. Reassess BP control when RTC.
5. Hyperlipidemia. Increase Zocor to 20 mg PO QHS. Reassess lipids in 3 months.
6. Microalbuminuria. Continue Prinivil for HTN and renal protection.
7. Postmenopausal. Counsel pt and pt's family on indications, risks, and benefits of HRT. Provide pt with educational pamphlets.

AMBULATORY PATIENT CASE 1

Pt. Name: Oliver, Ellen	**Date:** 8/28/00

Ht: 5'4" **Wt:** 175 lbs **Gender:** F	**Age:** 60	**Race:** Black

Allergies: NKDA **MD:** Dr. W. Davis	**Insurance:**

CC/HPI: EO is a 60-yo bf presenting to the clinic for f/u of lab results. Pt states that she was prescribed Bactrim DS PO BID X 3 days for a UTI last week. She stopped treatment after 2 days because she could not swallow the tablets. She states that her sx have lessened but are not resolved.

PMH: Type 2 DM, hyperlipidemia, carpal tunnel syndrome, allergic rhinitis, GERD, HTN	**PSH:** None
FH: Father ↓ 62, MI Mother ↓ 88, CVA	**SHx:** Denies tobacco and ETOH
Home Meds: 1. Zestril 10 mg PO QD 2. Procardia XL 60 mg PO QD 3. Glucotrol XL 10 mg PO HS 4. Zyrtec 10 mg PO HS 5. Zocor 10 mg PO HS 6. Glucophage 500 mg PO BID 7. Zantac 150 mg PO BID PRN	**Problem List:** 1. Unresolved UTI 2. Type 2 DM 3. HTN

ROS/PE

GEN: 60-yo bf in NAD.
HEENT: Denies vision changes
NECK:
CV: Denies CP, chest tightness, palpitations; RRR, no M/R/G
LUNGS: CTA bilaterally
ABD: Denies N/V/D and abd pain
GU: Pt c/o dysuria, urgency, frequency, nocturia with decreasing severity X 1 week; suprapubic tenderness on palpation
EXT: Denies cramping, tingling, numbness in hands, legs, and feet; feet clean and dry, no cuts or lesions
NEURO: Grossly intact

Vitals and Labs: EO

Date	8/21/00	8/28/00	
BP	120/80	122/82	
HR	76	80	
RR	20	20	
Temp			
Glucose	251	194	
SCr	1.0		
HbA1c	10.4		
PT/INR			
Tot Prot	8.1		
Alb	4.3		
ALT	35		
AST	30		
Alk Phos	84		
LDH			
Tot Bili	0.6		
TC		196	
HDL		50	
LDL		105	
TG		206	
TSH		1.2	
Urinary albumin (24 hour)	< 30		

Urinalysis 8/28/00

Color	Amber	Appearance	Hazy
SP Gravity	1.020	pH	6.5
Protein	Trace	Glucose	+ 3
Ketones	Negative	Bilirubin	Small
Blood	Negative	Urobilinogen	0.2
Nitrite	Negative	WBC Esterase	Trace
WBC	1-2	RBC	None
UA Crystals	Few		

Progress Note:
1. Unresolved UTI. Give Rx for Cipro 500 mg BID × 7 days.
2. Type 2 DM. Uncontrolled; pt needs education on disease, complications, diet, exercise, and foot care; refer to Pharmacy for management. Pt does not have glucose meter.
3. HTN. Controlled

AMBULATORY PATIENT CASE 2

Pt. Name: Dale, Joyce	**Date:** 9/21/00	
Ht: 5'4" **Wt:** 130 lbs **Gender:** F	**Age:** 48	**Race:** Black
Allergies: NKDA **MD:** Jones		**Insurance:** BCBS

CC: JD is a 48-yo bf c/o vaginal itch × 3 weeks.

HPI: Patient states that she is experiencing constant vaginal itch with an odor, which started ~ 3 weeks ago. JD states that she has used Neosporin without relief. Patient also c/o of polyuria, nocturia, polyphagia, polydipsia, and weight gain, which she has never experienced in the past.

PMH: Thyroid nodule 1993	**PSH:** Hysterectomy 1995
FH: Father ↓ 　　　Mother ↓ 75, cancer 　　　(−) FH of Type 2 DM, HTN	**SHx:** (−) Tobacco 　　　(−) ETOH 　　　(−) Drug abuse 　　　(−) Sexually active, 　　　　　　married 15 years
Home Meds: None	**Problem List:** 1. Type 2 DM 2. HTN 3. Vaginal candidiasis

ROS/PE

GEN: 48-yo bf in NAD
HEENT: + blurred vision × 1 month
NECK: Nonswollen, nontender
CV: Denies CP, chest tightness, palpitations, RRR, no M/R/G
LUNGS: CTA bilaterally
ABD: Denies N/V/D and abd pain
GU: Intense itching in vaginal area, thick vaginal discharge; + polyuria
EXT: Denies cramping, numbness, tingling in hands, legs, and feet; feet clean and dry, no lesions or cuts
NEURO: Grossly intact

Vitals and Labs: JD

Date	9/01/00	9/21/00	
BP	146/94	150/96	
HR	72	72	
RR	16	20	
Temp			
Glucose	280	282	
SCr	0.8		
HbA1c	11.6		
PT/INR			
ALT	15		
AST	10		
Alk Phos	71		
LDH			
Tot Bili	0.4		
TC	262		
HDL	56		
LDL	188		
TG	88		
TSH	1.58		
Urinary albumin (24 hour)	34		

Urinalysis 9/21/00

Color	Yellow	Appearance	Clear
SP Gravity	1.01	pH	7
Protein	Trace	Glucose	+ 3
Ketones	Negative	Bilirubin	Negative
Blood	Negative	Urobilinogen	0.2
Nitrite	Negative	WBC Esterase	Negative
WBC	None	RBC	1-2

Urine Culture: No growth
Wet mount: Yeast

Note

1. Type 2 DM. Newly diagnosed with evidence of long-term complications, refer to Pharmacy for education and management.
2. HTN. Stage I, begin Zestril 5 mg PO QD. Reassess when RTC in 2 weeks.
3. Vaginal candidiasis. Diflucan 150 mg PO QD × 1.

Ambulatory Patient Case 3

Pt. Name: Joints, Sarah	**Date:** 9/07/00

Ht: 5'6" **Wt:** 272 lbs **Gender:** F		**Age:** 48	**Race:** Black

Allergies: PCN and sulfa	**MD:** Dr. H. Knee	**Insurance:**

CC/HPI: 48-yo bf c/o swollen and extremely painful knees. She states that she cannot walk because of the pain.

PMH: HTN, angina, Type 2 DM, OA, GERD	**PSH:** None
FH: Mother ↑ 76, Type 2 DM Father ↓ 72, HTN and lung cancer	**SHx:** (+) tobacco, drinks tea/coffee
Home Meds: 1. Glucotrol XL 10 mg PO BID 2. Glucophage 500 mg PO QD 3. Pepcid 40 mg PO QD 4. Celebrex 200 mg PO BID 5. Isosorbide mononitrate ER 30 mg PO QD	**Problem List:** 1. OA 2. Type 2 DM 3. Obesity

ROS/PE

GEN: 48-yo bf in some discomfort
HEENT: Denies changes in vision
NECK: Nonswollen, nontender
CV: Denies CP, chest tightness, palpitations; RRR, No M/R/G
LUNGS: CTA bilaterally
ABD: Denies N/V/D and abd pain
GU: Denies polyuria
EXT: Denies cramping, tingling, numbness in hands, legs, and feet. Knees swollen and painful to touch.
NEURO: Grossly intact

Vitals and Labs: SJ

Date	8/31/00	9/7/00	
BP	122/76	120/80	
HR	76	72	
RR	20	16	
Temp	98.9	98.9	
Glucose	207	180	
SCr	0.7		
HbA1c	8.9		
PT/INR			
Alb	3.3		
Tot Prot	9.1		
ALT	15		
AST	18		
Alk Phos	130		
LDH			
Tot Bili	0.4		
TC	290		
HDL	40		
LDL	212		
TG	190		
TSH	1.3		
Urinary alb (24 hour)	< 30		

Note

1. OA. Currently on Celebrex 200 mg BID. Give Kenalog, Marcaine, and Xylocaine injection in both knees. RTC in 1 week.
2. Type 2 DM. Uncontrolled BS, increase Glucophage to 500 mg PO BID with meals. Reassess BS and tolerability of Glucophage in 1 week.
3. Obesity. Need to lose weight, would help OA and DM.
4. Hyperlipidemia. LDL is not at goal of < 100. Begin Lipitor 10 mg QD. Reassess lipids in 3 months.

Ambulatory Patient Case 4

Pt. Name: Huff, Pam	Date: 9/05/00

Ht: 5'5" Wt: 288.5 lbs Gender: F	Age: 45 Race: White

Allergies: Sulfur MD: McIntyre Insurance:	

CC/HPI: PH is a 45-yo wf who presents to the clinic for f/u of asthma exacerbation (secondary to a URI), which required hospitalization. She states her asthma is not relieved by Ventolin treatments. She also states "I want to get off the Vicodin" because she does not want to be on something that is addicting. She states that she would rather have Tylenol with codeine.

PMH: Asthma, Type 2 DM, HTN, diabetic neuropathy, lower back pain 2° OA, hyperlipidemia, URI, bronchitis, kidney stones, anxiety, hypothyroid, CHF	**PSH:** C-section, kidney stones

FH: Sister: viral meningitis Grandfather: HTN, stroke Aunt: Type 2 DM	**SHx:** (+) tobacco, 1ppd No ETOH

Home Meds:	**Problem List:**
1. Glucophage 500 mg PO BID	1. Otitis media
2. Glucotrol 5 mg PO QD	2. Asthma
3. Humulin N 35 U am	3. CHF
4. Humulin R SS	4. Type 2 DM
5. Ventolin MDI 2 puffs TID	5. Diabetic neuropathy
6. Ventolin TX w/ nebulizer PRN	6. Lower back pain
7. Flonase 2 puffs QD	7. Hot flashes/ amenorrhea
8. Accolate 20 mg PO BID	X 3 mos
9. Vasotec 10 mg PO BID	8. Hyperlipidemia
10. Lasix 80 mg PO QD	
11. K-Dur 20 meq PO QD	
12. Tofranil 75 mg PO HS	
13. Soma 350 mg PO BID	
14. Tricor 67 mg PO QD	
15. Atacand 16 mg PO QD	
16. Vicodin ES 1 tab PO Q8H PRN	

ROS/PE

GEN: 45-yo wf slightly anxious but in NAD
HEENT: Left TM slightly bulging w/ mod. injection/erythema; nares patent w/o discharge; mild pharyngeal erythema; no syncope, dizziness; + coughing, allergic rhinitis; + vision changes recently
NECK: Nonswollen, nontender, no JVD
CV: Tachycardia w/o murmur, regular rhythm
LUNGS: + faint expiratory wheezes bilaterally; + SOB w/ exertion, + orthopnea (3–4 pillows),
ABD: Obese, + BS × 4, soft and nontender; no N/V/D and abd pain, + constipation
GU: Amenorrhea × 3 mos, + hot flashes
EXT: 2+ pitting edema bilaterally in LE, +2/4 pulses bilaterally in LE, DTR intact; + tingling/numbness in LE
NEURO: Grossly intact

Vitals and Labs: PH

Date	8/22/00	8/29/00	9/05/00
BP	136/84	140/90	138/86
HR	88	80	108
RR	24	20	24
Temp			99.3
Glucose	150	151	124
SCr	0.7		
HbA1c	7		
Alb	4.0		
Tot Prot	8.2		
ALT	45		
AST	40		
Alk Phos	80		
LDH			
Tot Bili	0.6		
TC	211		
HDL	39		
LDL	102		
TG	352		
TSH	0.653		
Urinary alb (24 hour)	< 30		

Progress Note

1. OM of left ear. Begin amoxicillin 500 mg PO TID × 10 days
2. Asthma. Uncontrolled
3. CHF. Symptomatic
4. Type 2 DM. Controlled as evidenced by glucose and HbA$_{1c}$
5. BP. Not at goal of < 130/80
6. Diabetic neuropathy. C/O tingling and numbness in legs and feet, currently on Tofranil 75 mg PO HS
7. Lower back pain 2° OA. Pt wants Tylenol #4 vs. Vicodin
8. Hot flashes + amenorrhea × 3 months. May be candidate for HRT, encourage pt to implement life-style modifications for time being
9. Hyperlipidemia. Currently on Tricor 67 mg PO QD, reassess lipids in 3 months

AMBULATORY PATIENT CASE 5

Pt. Name: Poulec, Jada	**Date:** 6/26/00

Ht: 5'2"   **Wt:** 183.5 lbs   **Age:** 61   **Race:** White
Gender: F

Allergies: Sulfa   **MD:** Dr. B. Clot   **Insurance:**

CC/HPI: JP, a 61-yo wf, presents to clinic for routine PT/INR check. She states that she had unexplained bruising on the right leg a couple of weeks ago. The bruising resolved w/o treatment.

PMH: MV replacement 2° to rheumatic heart disease (12/98)
CABG (12/98)
Hyperlipidemia
CHF

PSH: Hysterectomy (1984)

FH: Father ↑ 81, CAD
Mother ↓, unknown cause

SHx: (−) tobacco, ETOH, illicit drugs

Home Meds:
1. Coumadin 5 mg PO QD except 2.5 mg Tues and Thurs
2. Digoxin 0.25 mg PO QD
3. Zocor 20 mg PO QD
4. Premarin 1.25 mg PO QD
5. Lasix 40 mg PO QD
6. K-Dur 10 meq PO QD
7. Atacand 16 mg PO QD
8. Isosorbide 10 mg PO BID
9. Coreg 3.125 mg PO BID
10. Zyrtec 5 mg PO QD PRN

Problem List:

ROS/PE

GEN:
HEENT: Denies any changes in vision
NECK:
CV: Denies CP, chest tightness, palpitations; RRR, no M/R/G + click
LUNGS: Denies SOB, orthopnea; CTA bilaterally
ABD: Denies N/V/D/C and abd pain
GU: Denies blood in urine or stool, denies nocturia
EXT: Denies unusual bruising or bleeding besides bruising on the right leg a few weeks ago, denies C/C/E
NEURO:

Vitals and Labs: JP

Date	2/16/00	3/6/00	4/26/00	5/24/00	6/26/00
BP	138/88	126/84	130/80	132/82	128/84
HR	76	72	72	70	70
RR	20	16	20	20	16
Temp					
Glucose	96	95	95	98	98
SCr	1.0		1.1		1.0
HbA1c					
PT/INR	20.5/2.9	20.9/3.1	23.7/3.8	20.7/3.0	20.1/2.5
Alb	4.3				
Tot Prot	7.1				
ALT	40				
AST	35				
Alk Phos	90				
LDH					
Tot Bili	0.8				
TC		266			248
HDL		103			101
LDL		109			96
TG		270			257
TSH					

Note

1. Anticoagulation—PT/INR is on the low end of the therapeutic range. Pt has been therapeutic on current Coumadin regimen for past 4 months. Pt states that she has not missed any doses, but did eat a lot of "greens" at a family picnic over the weekend. She also states that she has been eating leftover "greens" all week.
2. Hyperlipidemia—Lipid levels have decreased since 3/6/00 on Zocor 20 mg PO QD. At LDL goal < 100 and HDL goal > 40.

Ambulatory Patient Case 6

Pt. Name: Cohen, Betty	**Date:** 7/19/00
Ht: 4'10" **Wt:** 183.5 lbs **Gender:** F	**Age:** 70 **Race:** Black
Allergies: PCN, Quinine **MD:** Brittle	**Insurance:**

CC/HPI: BC is a 70-yo bf who presents to the clinic to pick up her osteoporosis medications. The pt. was diagnosed by bone densitometry about 1 week ago with osteoporosis of the left hip. Today she states that her "right leg hurts."

PMH: Osteoporosis, GERD, HTN, DVT/PE (5/14/95), bilateral carpal tunnel syndrome, OA, depression, gastritis w/hx of H. pylori, anemia, benign abdominal mass (8/25/99), fibrinous breast tissue	**PSH:** None
FH: Noncontributory	**SHx:** No tobacco, ETOH, illicit drug use
Home Meds: 1. Fosamax 70 mg PO QWEEK 2. Oscal + Vit. D 1200-1500 mg/d 3. Prilosec 20 mg PO BID 4. Ziac 2.5 mg PO QD 5. Neurontin 100 mg PO TID 6. Celebrex 200 mg PO QD 7. Zoloft 10 mg PO QHS	**Problem List:** 1. Right leg pain 2. HTN 3. Osteoporosis 4. GERD

ROS/PE

GEN: 70-yo obese bf c/o pain in right lower extremity.	
HEENT: Denies cough	
NECK:	
CV: Denies CP, chest tightness, palpitations; RRR, no M/R/G	
LUNGS: Denies SOB, tachypnea; CTA bilaterally	
ABD: Denies N/V/D/C and abd pain	
GU:	
EXT: Pain, tenderness, swelling in right calf area; + Homan's	
NEURO:	

Vitals and Labs: BC

Date	6/21/00	7/19/00	
BP	160/100	154/92	
HR	70	72	
RR	20	20	
Temp	98.9	97.9	
Glucose	93	76	
SCr		1.0	
HbA1c			
PT/INR			
Alb		4.0	
Tot Prot		7.0	
ALT		30	
AST		25	
Alk Phos		89	
LDH			
Tot Bili		0.5	
TC			
HDL			
LDL			
TG			
TSH			

Note

1. Right leg pain. Pt has hx of DVT/PE, R/O DVT.
2. HTN. BP not controlled on Ziac 2.5 mg PO QD.
3. Osteoporosis. Pt on Fosamax and Oscal w/ Vit D. Counsel pt on importance of correctly taking Fosamax since pt has hx of GERD. Will need
   to monitor GERD sx closely.

COMMUNICATIONS ROLE-PLAYING SCENARIOS

The following pages contain 15 examples of pharmacy-related communication scenarios.* They are designed for pharmacy students to practice their communication skills through role playing.

For each scenario, two alternative approaches are proposed for the exchange. As a student we suggest you try them both ways and get feedback from your friends. Additionally, discussion questions for each scenario are included. Reviewing such situations before you encounter them will be helpful.

The exercises may also be used as learning tools for study groups or for rotation exercises. In addition to the discussion questions, for each scenario, consider what communication tools would be most helpful in working through the issues presented. It will be helpful to have others provide feedback on the interactions and offer suggestions for improvement; a discussion of different perspectives can reveal new methods of approaching communication.

SCENARIO I

While the pharmacist (student 1) is busy filling a prescription for a surgical patient waiting at the counter, another patient (student 2) comes into the pharmacy to ask for advice concerning her medications. She has been started taking a new drug called Euphoravil for the treatment of depression. In addition to this prescription, she wants to take St. John's wort because she knows that it worked for a neighbor. This patient is older and just wants to feel better; she has diabetes and is already on many medications. She is impatient and interrupts you many times while you are trying to finish filling the surgical patient's prescription.

Version 1

The pharmacist drops everything to help the patient and counsels her immediately. Complicating the interview is the patient's confusion about her medica-

---

* These scenarios were developed by Dr. Ruth Nemire at Nova Southeastern University, College of Pharmacy for use in the classroom component of early experiential education.

tions and inability to fully answer the pharmacist's questions. This counseling session requires patience on the part of both parties.

Version 2

The patient is in a hurry and wants the pharmacist to answer her questions before finishing with the surgical patient. The pharmacist asks the patient to wait for a moment, at which point the patient begins to get belligerent. The pharmacist agrees to counsel her at that point.

Discussion Questions

1. As the patient, how did you feel?
2. As the pharmacist, what were your frustrations?
3. What could have improved the communication better in each scenario?

SCENARIO II

The pharmacist (student 1) in a really slow pharmacy is talking on the phone with her boyfriend. A patient (student 2) comes to the counter and wants to have a prescription filled. The pharmacist hangs up and comes to help the patient, but the drug is not in stock.

Version 1

The pharmacist tries to be helpful, but the patient is very upset because the prescription is for a baby. Further, the patient does not know what to do because he came to the pharmacy by bus and does not have enough money for transportation to another pharmacy.

Version 2

The pharmacist hangs up the phone and comes to the counter to help. The patient cannot find the prescription but is certain he has it. After receiving the prescription from the patient, the pharmacist reviews it and says it's not available. The patient wants to know what it is for (antibiotic) and what he is supposed to do now. It is now 8:45 p.m., and the pharmacy closes in 15 minutes.

Discussion Questions

1. How might you improve the communication in each version?
2. What factors are important to recognize in dealing with this type of situation?
3. What might the pharmacist be feeling that interferes with her communication with this patient?
4. What might the patient be feeling?

SCENARIO III

A physician (student 1) calls the pharmacy to ask for advice. The physician has a patient who needs to be started on two inhalers but does not have sufficient time to teach the patient how to use them. The doctor wants the pharmacist (student 2) to fill the prescriptions and teach the patient how to use the inhalers, with an aerochamber (device to help use inhalers) if necessary. The pharmacist is working alone today because the pharmacy technician called in sick. It is early in the day, and he has already filled 40 prescriptions. The doctor is a friend of the pharmacist and is always asking for favors such as this. The pharmacist has been considering asking the physician for a fee for providing these service and decides to do that today.

Version 1

The pharmacist agrees to spend time with the patient today.

Version 2

The pharmacist says it cannot be done today.

Discussion Questions

1. What feelings does the physician need to validate for the pharmacist?
2. Should the pharmacist have asked for a fee from the physician, or should the pharmacist provide the education at the physician's request for free?
3. Is the physician taking advantage of his friendship with the pharmacist?

SCENARIO IV

A patient (student 1) comes to the pharmacy seeking advice regarding the choice of a vitamin supplement. The patient is elderly and is living on a fixed income. The patient confides in the pharmacist (student 2) that she has lost 20 pounds in one month and attributes this weight loss to an improper diet. In addition to the weight loss, she is thirsty all the time and has spells when she cannot remember where she has been. The pharmacist listens patiently and then offers suggestions to the patient.

Version 1

The patient is hard of hearing.

Version 2

The pharmacist is hard of hearing.

Discussion Questions

1. What advice would you offer the pharmacist to improve the communication?
2. As the patient, what information did you want from the pharmacist? Did you get it?
3. As the pharmacist, what information would have been helpful to have from the patient?
4. What did this conversation look like from the perspective of a customer waiting to pick up a prescription?

SCENARIO V

A nurse (student 1) calls the pharmacy to find out the store's hours and if the pharmacy offers a delivery service. She also tells the pharmacist (student 2) she wants to call in a prescription for a patient. The patient, who does not have transportation, is the physician's mother. The prescription is for Nopain, a schedule II medication for which a hard copy of the prescription is required by law. The nurse tells the pharmacist she will mail the prescription today. The pharmacist must handle this. Both times, the pharmacist will not fill the prescription.

Version 1

The rationale for not filling the prescription is that the pharmacy does not offer a delivery service for anyone.

Version 2

The rationale for not filling the prescription is that, legally, the pharmacist cannot fill a prescription for Nopain without a valid prescription in hand.

Discussion Questions

1. What communication skills are important to utilize in such situations?
2. What is of particular concern for the pharmacist in either scenario?
3. What should be expected of the pharmacist in this situation? What should be expected of the nurse in this situation?

SCENARIO VI

A patient (student 1) calls the pharmacist (student 2) requesting a refill of a heart medication but cannot recall its name. The profile in the computer says that she is on Heartache once daily. The patient usually gets a 30-day supply but has not had a refill for 90 days. The patient is still on the phone. There are no other medications on file. The patient does not speak English very well, and the pharmacist speaks only English. The pharmacist needs to know why the patient has not been taking the Heartache and/or if there is a new medication.

Version 1

The patient has a prescription for another medication that was filled by a mail-order company. Unfortunately, the prescription was lost in the mail. When the pharmacist tries to fill this prescription with the patient still on the phone, it is rejected by the insurance company as an early refill. The pharmacist will have to call the insurance company.

Version 2

The patient was feeling better, so she stopped the medication. Now she feels bad and thought she should start again because she has a doctor's appointment in 2 days and has to get a blood level drawn.

Discussion Questions

1. What is the problem for the pharmacist in either case?
2. What is the problem for the patient?
3. What should the pharmacist do?

SCENARIO VII

It is 5:30 p.m. on Sunday afternoon, and the pharmacy will close in half an hour. A cardiologist (student 1) calls in a prescription for an allergy medication for a patient who is the son of one of the physician's friends. The doctor mentions that the parent cannot get to the pharmacy until after 6:00. Because the manager will not allow the pharmacist (student 2) to leave the pharmacy open even 1 minute after 6:00, the pharmacist must explain to the doctor that the parent must get there before 6:00 or the pharmacy will be closed.

Version 1

The cardiologist gives the wrong directions for the allergy medication because it is not something she normally prescribes. She then asks you about the hours. The cardiologist tells you that you will have to stay open past closing because you are a healthcare professional. The pharmacist thinks that this should have been taken care of earlier in the day and that it is not an emergency situation. Based on this, the pharmacist refuses to stay open.

Version 2

The cardiologist gives wrong directions for the medication and then adds that the patient also needs an antibiotic. Because the physician does not know the patient

but does know that the child has some allergies, the physician tells the pharmacist to give the patient the same prescription as the antibiotic bottle the mother
brings in. The pharmacist must explain why she will not do this. The cardiologist reminds the pharmacist that she is the doctor and that the pharmacist has to
do what she is told.

Discussion Questions

1. What is the problem here, and what makes communication so difficult?
2. What suggestions do you have for improving the potential outcomes of the
   scenarios?
3. What are you going to do when this happens to you?
4. Did the pharmacist or physician get defensive, abusive?
5. How should those issues be dealt with?

SCENARIO VIII

A pharmacist (student 1) is working in a hospital. There is a survey team coming from the accreditation body, and really all you can think about is all the work
and paperwork that there is to do. Because the other clinical pharmacist called
in sick, you have to cover rounds on the Internal Medicine floor and the intensive care unit (ICU). In the ICU, a medical student (student 2) asks you to tell
him how to mix total parenteral nutrition (TPN). You do not do that routinely in
your practice, so you are unsure yourself. The pharmacist believes that the medical student should have to do this as an exercise, but the student thinks it is the
pharmacist's job to take care of this.

Version 1

The medical student is a brash, overconfident person who believes the other
healthcare professionals at the hospital are there to serve the needs of the medical students. The pharmacist is a responsible professional who will not have patients suffer as a result of the lack of involvement from the medical student.

Version 2

The pharmacist believes the medical students are in the hospital for learning and
will not do the TPN orders.

Discussion Questions

1. What is happening when these two healthcare professionals communicate?
2. When power struggles occur, is there always a communication problem?
3. Who will suffer if this is not worked out?
4. What do you think *should* occur in the scenario?

SCENARIO IX

A patient (student 1) with diarrhea comes to the pharmacy in distress. The patient wants the pharmacist (student 2) to make a recommendation for an over-the-counter product. The patient tells the pharmacist that it is bloody diarrhea, and because it is Saturday night, she cannot see her doctor. This patient should be seen by a doctor, so the pharmacist attempts to suggest that the patient go to the emergency room (ER). The patient does not have insurance and will not go to the ER because it costs too much. The pharmacist must make a decision about whether to tell the patient to get Imodium AD or not.

Version 1

The patient plans to buy an over-the-counter product such as Pepto Bismol. The pharmacist knows that may not really help the diarrhea and that a bloody stool is a sign of a larger problem because the patient says it is bright red blood. The patient is wishy-washy and reluctantly agrees to go to the ER.

Version 2

After the pharmacist learns that the diarrhea is tinged with bright red blood she insists that the patient seek medical attention. The patient says she will die before going to the ER.

Discussion Questions

1. Were there any problems in communication in either scenario?
2. What do you think is the best way to handle this?
3. Did the patient feel she was being counseled well in either scene?
4. What could have made the interaction better?

SCENARIO X

The pharmacist (student 1) at this pharmacy has just started charging for counseling sessions for patients who want to know about their medications that have been purchased elsewhere (i.e., mail order). The usual fee for "brown bag" counseling is $10.00 per half-hour. A patient (student 2), who had been a regular patron of the pharmacy until insurance required her to receive her prescriptions by mail order, enters the pharmacy with a bag of pills. She mentions that she has several questions about each of the medications. The patient has not been in the pharmacy for over a year and hopes the pharmacist will take the time necessary to counsel her. The pharmacist is upset because the insurance company will not pay him to dispense the medications, and yet the patient wants to discuss them.

Version 1

The patient does not understand how health care has come to this. The patient argues with the pharmacist, saying that it is the responsibility of pharmacists everywhere to help anyone with questions free of charge.

Version 2

The pharmacist tells the patient about the fee, and the patient agrees to pay for the counseling session.

Discussion Questions

1. What dilemma does the pharmacist face?
2. What dilemma does the patient face?
3. Did both pharmacists communicate effectively? What improvements could be made in each case?

SCENARIO XI

A pharmacist (student 1) is working in a nursing home reviewing charts. A patient's family member (student 2) demands to know why his 98-year-old relative is on Tranquil. He understands that it is an awful drug and that it is very addicting. The pharmacist feels that although the drug is addicting, the addiction potential is irrelevant when the patient is 98 years old. The patient was prescribed Tranquil because she has been getting out of bed in the middle of the night and wandering the halls of the nursing home. The drug was given in hopes that it would keep the patient from waking up during the night and wandering to where she should not. The family member is screaming at the pharmacist to get her off of the drug.

Version 1

The family member does not calm down until the pharmacist does something to get his attention such as yelling back. After that, the pharmacist can explain her perspective, and the family member asks questions appropriately.

Version 2

The family member is willing to listen to the pharmacist, but the pharmacist seems glib about the entire situation because of the patient's age. The family member threatens to report the pharmacist to her supervisor.

Discussion Questions

1. What did the first pharmacist do that was effective? What was not effective?
2. What happened in the second version that was probably not an effective form of communication?
3. What important factors should be considered when communicating with any family member or patient?

SCENARIO XII

A person (student 1) telephones the pharmacy to ask a question about the prescription drug Nodrinky. She asks the pharmacist (student 2) what will happen if one drinks alcohol with the prescription. Drinking with this drug will cause her to vomit and to have flu-like symptoms, a high fever, and a rapid heart rate. She tells the pharmacist that she has already had a drink and now feels quite sick. The person blames the pharmacist. The pharmacist clearly recalls telling a patient earlier in the day about Nodrinky's interaction with alcohol.

Version 1

The person who calls the pharmacy is not the patient. By law, the pharmacist cannot discuss the patient's medications with anyone but the patient. After some discussion, the patient (student 3) gets on the phone and is angry that the pharmacist would not talk to her friend. This issue should be resolved with the patient agreeing to go to the hospital.

Version 2

The person on the phone is the patient. She wants to drink and attempts to get the pharmacist to agree that it is okay to have a drink and that nothing will happen. The pharmacist tells the patient the potential outcome of consuming alcohol while taking the medication and that she should not drink. The pharmacist resorts to trying to scare the patient.

Discussion Questions

1. What could help the pharmacist more effectively convey the message?
2. What should the pharmacist have done when the prescription was picked up?
3. Does the pharmacist have a responsibility to make sure the patient does not drink, or does the pharmacist's responsibility end with counseling?
4. What was good about the communication that went on? What could be improved?

SCENARIO XIII

A busy pharmacist (student 1) in the hospital notices that an order has been written for a dose of Apedrug that will kill a child. The pharmacist knows that the physician (student 2) is always hard to get hold of and has a reputation for being rude and disrespectful. The pharmacist places a call to the physician, who happens to be in the hospital on the floor writing orders and answers right away.

Version 1

The pharmacist asks the doctor if what has been written is really what the doctor wants. The pharmacist repeats the dose and the age of the patient, says that the patient will die, and refuses to fill the prescription. This is said in such a way as to anger the doctor. Tempers flare, but the pharmacist still refuses to fill the prescription. The doctor hangs up.

Version 2

The pharmacist reaches the doctor as in scene 1 but finds a better way to tell the doctor the dose is wrong. The doctor, who starts out the conversation abruptly, thanks the pharmacist in the end.

Discussion Questions

1. What elements of Version 1 and Version 2 made a difference in the outcome?
2. What else could the pharmacist have done?
3. How can pharmacists change other healthcare professionals' perception of their role on the healthcare team from watchdog to team member?
4. How might the pharmacist best approach the physician: on the phone, in person, or ask the nurse?

SCENARIO XIV

A patient (student 1) brings in 10 prescriptions and tells the pharmacist (student 2) that he will return in 15 minutes exactly to pick them up. This patient is a young person who does this every month. The patient also wants the pharmacist to fill out insurance paperwork in that amount of time.

Version 1

The pharmacist tells the patient that it will be at least 2 hours or more before the prescriptions are filled, and the paperwork will not be done until the next day. The pharmacist is able to present this information in such a manner that the patient accepts the answer readily.

Version 2

The patient is not willing to accept anything the pharmacist says and insists that the prescriptions and paperwork be ready in 15 minutes.

Discussion Questions

1. In the first scene, did the pharmacist really appease the patient with the answer? Or did the patient just accept it because he thought he had to?
2. What if the patient started screaming and yelling? How would that be handled?
3. Is there ever a time when it is okay to tell the patient that the pharmacist is a professional and deserves some courtesy?
4. What about the pharmacist's actions made the patient accept that the prescription would not be available right away?

SCENARIO XV

A patient (student 1) arrives in the pharmacy with a question about a prescription she received. The bottle says Artemis 10 mg; take one tablet daily. The problem is that the pill on the inside is usually green with yellow stripes. The pill inside now is red with white dots. The patient wants to know what has happened. The pharmacist (student 2) looks at the bottle and notices that it was not filled at this particular pharmacy. The pharmacist does not recognize the pill in the bottle but does recognize that it is not Artemis 10 mg.

Version 1

The patient is very upset to learn that the prescription was misfilled. She is not screaming but is on the verge of yelling. The pharmacist is very calm and explains that the he does not recognize the pill in the bottle. Ultimately, the pharmacist makes a comment about the pharmacist who filled the prescription and tells the patient to get a lawyer.

Version 2

The patient is not yelling or screaming but wants to know the number of the Board of Pharmacy because she is going to file suit against the pharmacist who filled the prescription. The pharmacist is careful not to comment on the misfill. Further, the pharmacist is helpful in determining what is in the bottle. After some investigation, it is revealed that the medication in the bottle is one of the patient's vitamin supplements.

Discussion Questions

1. What is the appropriate way to handle a prescription when it has been misfilled?
2. What communication techniques would be the most appropriate and professional for handling this situation?
3. How would you improve on the pharmacist's communication in either version?

A P P E N D I X B

ADDITIONAL READINGS

GENERAL

Northouse PG, Northouse LL. *Health communication: strategies for health professionals.* Norwalk, CT: Appleton & Lange, 1992.

Tindall WN, Beardsley RS, Kimberlin CI.. *Communication skills in pharmacy practice.* Malvern, PA: Lea & Febiger, 1994.

CULTURE

Huff RM, Kline MV. *Promoting health in multicultural populations.* Thousand Oaks, CA: Sage Publications, 1999.

Kreps GL. *Effective communication in multicultural health settings.* Thousand Oaks, CA: Sage Publications, 1994.

Spector RE. *Cultural diversity in health and illness.* Stamford, CT: Appleton & Lange, 1996.

WRITING

Lynch BS. *Writing for communication in science and medicine.* New York: Van Nostrand Reinhold, 1980.

Navarra T. *Toward painless writing: a guide for health professionals.* Thorofare, NJ: Slack, 1998.

A P P E N D I X   C

EXAMPLE OF STUDY ABSTRACT FOR POSTER PRESENTATION SUBMISSION: ANALYSIS OF DIRECT-TO-CONSUMER ADVERTISING IN MAGAZINES TARGETED AT WOMEN AND TEENS

Karen L. Kier, Crystal R. Hall, and Sara B. Jutte

OBJECTIVES

Pharmaceutical companies have used direct-to-consumer prescription advertising (DTC-Rx) as a means to stimulate consumer interest. This continues in the 1990s with companies increasing the number of DTC-Rx. The objective of the study was to evaluate DTC-Rx claims in consumer magazines with an emphasis on families, women, and teens and to use a pharmacy review group to evaluate their educational value and balance. Other objectives included looking at reference use and availability as well as publication of telephone numbers, web sites, and consulting a pharmacist.

DESIGN

The study was an observational design.

SETTING

The study included 19 consumer magazines.

PARTICIPANTS

Consumer prescription ads were reviewed.

RESULTS

There were 66 DTC-Rx ads in the 19 magazines, with 36 ads for herbal products and 57 for OTC products. In subgroup analysis, the teen magazines had significantly fewer ads and fewer DTC-Rx ads than either the family or the women's magazines. Women's magazines targeted had a similar quantity of ads as did the family magazines. Sixty-two (94%) of the ads gave the name of the product. Only nine ads provided references to support their claims. Fifty-five (83.3%) provided a telephone number. A dismal six (9%) mentioned a pharmacist. The review panel were asked to analyze information as to indications, benefits, risks, consumer terminology, balance, educational level, and fairness (reliability = 0.923). The means were statistically lower (less fair) for the ads targeted at teens than for those aimed at women and families. The weaker areas included poor explanations of risk and low educational value.

CONCLUSIONS

The ads targeted at women appear to provide a good balance of benefits to risks. Few magazines target teenagers with DTC-Rx. A concern is that the ads were less balanced and fair. A discouraging note is the ads that did not mention a pharmacist.

REFERENCES

1. Host TR, Kirkwood CF. Computer-assisted instruction for responding to drug information requests. Paper presented at the 22nd Annual ASHP Midyear Clinical Meeting, Atlanta, December 1997.
2. Malone P, Mosdell KW, Kier KL, Stanovich J. Drug information: a guide for pharmacists, 2nd ed. New York: McGraw-Hill, 2000.

MONITORING FORM EXAMPLE FOR PATIENTS ON CARDIOLOGY/MEDICINE SERVICE

Patient: _John Doe_   **Room:** _401_   **Date of Admission:** _01/20/00_

Age: _60_   **Gender:** _M_   **Allergies:** _penicillin-rash_

Ht (in): _71_   **Wt (kg):** _96_   _ibuprofen-stomach pain_

Diagnosis: _CP/Rule out MI_

CC:

"My chest is hurting and it is hard to breathe"

HPI:

Presented to ED with substernal CP described as squeezing sensation.
Radiation down left arm. Pain began 2 hours ago while working in the yard.
Pain not relieved w/rest or SL NTG

PMH:

HTN × 15 yrs. h/o MI 7 yrs. ago, hyperlipedemia × 7 yrs, cardiac cath
w/PTCA 7 yrs ago

SH:

hyperlipdemia

2-3 glasses of iced tea/d,

occas. yard work. 40-pack yr

tobacco hx 8–10 cups coffee/d

Retired, married with 2 kids, insurance

w/ prescription plan, ⊕ ETOH–3–4

12 oz. beers/d,

FH:

Father died of MI age 54,

Mother age 82,

HTN, CMP, 2 brothers ⊕ CAD

PE:

General: Moderately obese WM, somewhat anxious, A&O × 3

Heart: RRR, w/o MRG. C/o SOB, denies orthopnea, DOE, or PND, no JOD

Lungs: CTA bilaterally. No rales or rhonchi , c/o nausea associated with CP,

denies N/O

CXR: Heart is slightly enlarged. Clear lung fields

ECG: NSR, HR 75, nonspedific ST segment changes in inferior leads

ECHO:

Medication History:

ECA SA 81 mg qd, pravastatin 20 mg qd, NTG patch 5mg qd, atenolol
50 mg qd, amlodipine 5mg qd, SLNTG prn, APAP prn

Current Medications

Start Date	Medication/Route	Dose/Schedule	Stop Date	Start Date
1/20	EC ASA	81 mg qd		
1/20	Pravastatin	20 mg qhs		
1/20	NTG patch	5 mg /24 h qd		
1/20	Atenolol	50 mg qd		
1/20	Ambdipine	5 mg qd		
1/20	NTG SL	0.4 mg prn		
1/20	APAP po	1-2 tabs prn		
1/20	Lovenox SQ	100 mg bid		
1/20	Eptifibatide IO	2 μg/kg/min		

Vital Signs

Date	01/20							
WT (Kg)	96							
TEMP (F°)	98.1							
HR/RR	79/18							
BP	160/92							
I/O								

Chemistry Lab Values

Date	1/20					
Na	138					
K	3.6					
Cl	103					
HCO^3	26					
BUN	14					
SCr	1.1					
Glucose	132					
Ca	9.1					
Phos	2.6					
Mg	1.3					
Anion Gap						
Uric Acid	3.4					
Total Protein	7.0					
Albumin	4.0					
Alk Phos	102					
T. Bili	0.8					
D. Bili	0					
ALT	33					
AST	41					
Amylase						
Lipase						

Hematology Lab Values

Date	1/20							
WBC	9.8							
Segs	62.9							
Bands	0							
Lymphs	33							
Monos	3							
Eosinophils	1							
Basophils	0.1							
Atypicals	0							
RBC	4.7							
Hgb	12.8							
Hct	44							
MCV	92							
MCH	29							
Plts	254							
PTT	36.6							
PT	11.1							
INR	1.01							
Warfarin Dose	N/A							

Miscellaneous Lab Values

Date	1/20	1/21					
CK	1930	0600					
CKMB	66	72					
Troponin I	5.0	5.0					
Total Chol		280					
Triglycerides		380					
HDL		30					
LDL		174					

Cultures and Sensitivities

Date			
Source			
Organisims			
Sensitivities			

PROGRESS NOTES:

01/21/2000 0900

S: Pt w/o any c/o CP this am. One episode of CP last pm relieved
w/ SL NTG 0.4 mg × 2

O: Cardiac enzymes are normal. Fasting lipid profile done this a.m

A: 60 year-old WM w/ unstable angina and a h/o HTN & hyperlipidemia.

P: Cardiac cath this a.m. Review medication profile for problems and counsel
patient on proper use of SLNTG. Follow up on lipid panel

A P P E N D I X E

PATIENT MEDICAL HISTORY FORM

The following categories of information should be obtained. The pharmacist/ student should meet with the patient to review this information to verify completeness and accuracy.

1. Patient information: name, birthdate, address, phone number, insurance company, gender, height, weight.
2. Life-style, social information: tobacco, alcohol, caffeine use; impairments; exercise; pregnancy/breastfeeding issues; diet.
3. Doctor information: determine if the patient is currently under the care of a physician, and if so, obtain a list of all physicians and their phone numbers, whenever possible, to facilitate communication.
4. Allergies: list, and have the patient describe any allergic reaction they have experienced and when it occurred.
5. Over-the-counter (OTC) issues: have the patient indicate which conditions they occasionally or regularly self-treat with nonprescription (OTC) medications, herbals, vitamins, minerals, or homeopathic remedies. Then have the patient identify the OTC products used occasionally or regularly, including the category of nutritional/natural products.
6. Medical conditions/diseases: identify all conditions for which the patient is receiving medical care or may be self-treating.
7. Prescription medications: the patient should list all prescription medications they are currently using. Patients should be sure to include any medications obtained via mail order, Internet pharmacies, or physician samples.

LEARNING OBJECTIVES FOR COMMUNITY PHARMACY EXPERIENTIAL ROTATION

1. Effectively communicate with healthcare professionals by:
   A. Obtaining and providing accurate and concise information in a professional manner.
   B. Using appropriate oral, written, and nonverbal language.
2. Effectively communicate with patients about prescription medications.
   A. Interview and counsel patients on medication usage, dosage, packaging, and storage.
   B. Discuss possible drug cautions, side effects, and interactions.
   C. Explain policies on fees and services based on the patient's specific prescription insurance coverage.
   D. Relate to patients in a professional manner.
   E. Interact with patients to confirm their understanding of the information.
3. Communicate with patients about nonprescription products and devices.
   A. Question a patient about his or her condition(s) and intended drug use.
   B. Assist in and recommend drug selection.
   C. Communicate OTC drug dosage, usage, storage, and side effects.
   D. Provide information about medical, surgical, and home health care devices and home diagnostic products.
4. Monitor and evaluate a patient's drug therapy.
   A. Establish and correctly interpret the patient's database. Refer to discussion later in this chapter regarding the Patient Medical History Form.
   B. Describe the symptomatology, physical findings, pathophysiology, diagnostic procedures, and laboratory tests for disease states encountered during the rotation.
   C. Intervene to prevent or identify the patient's drug-related problems (DRP's).
   D. Recommend an appropriate therapeutic plan and process for implementation. This should include:
      • Determining the appropriateness of the prescription.

Pharmacy Clerkship Manual

- Evaluating and selecting the most appropriate medications (prescription, nonprescription, natural products) for treating the patient's medical conditions or symptoms.
- Establishing a list of recommendations for dosage, dosage form, route of administration.
- Developing strategies for monitoring and assessing medication adherence.
- Devising a list of parameters for monitoring outcomes (efficacy, toxicity), and counsel patients on commonly prescribed/recommended devices (i.e. blood glucose meters, peak flow meters, home blood pressure monitors).
- Demonstrating proficiency in monitoring patients with various disease-states and in providing appropriate interventions, and document all interventions appropriately.
- Discussing various nationally-developed protocols in disease-state management (i.e. asthma, hypertension, diabetes, dyslipidemia).

E. Communicate the plan to the appropriate individual (physician, preceptor, patient, other healthcare provider, or any combination of these individuals).

F. Depending on the circumstances, either take the lead for, or support the preceptor/pharmacist with, plan implementation.

G. Devise a process for measuring and monitoring for plan success, including follow-up and re-evaluation for patient response to drug therapy.

H. Identify situations where patients must be referred to their physician for initial or additional follow-up.

I. Make sound decisions:
- Use good judgment in coming up with sensible, practical solutions to problems.
- Seek out and utilize important facts and information when making decisions.
- Recognize and evaluate available alternatives.
- Give thought to possible consequences of decisions.

5. Retrieve and evaluate drug information.
   A. Select the best available resource for answering a drug-related request in a timely manner.
   B. Evaluate the quality of information retrieved.

6. Review and gather an understanding for managing pharmacy operations.
   A. Gain exposure and a general understanding of the various departments within the organization that provide corporate structure (human resources, accounting, third-party reconciliation, marketing, systems, and technology).
   B. Describe how to control drug inventory.
   C. Establish mechanisms for maintaining quality assurance and improvement.
   D. Describe basic fiscal procedures, including financial management.

      E. Attend meetings related to operations.

      F. Describe the process for medication distribution and the responsibilities and limitations of ancillary pharmacy personnel (i.e., pharmacy technicians, clerks).

      G. Demonstrate a working knowledge of state and federal laws pertaining to community pharmacy practice.

  7. Demonstrate effective human relations skills.

      A. Display sensitivity to the needs, feelings, and concerns of others.

      B. Listen in a nonjudgmental manner and respond to the patient's problems.

      C. Act in the best interests of others.

      D. Deal professionally and ethically with colleagues and patients.

      E. Maintain confidentiality.

  8. Attend to detail when performing various tasks.

      A. Conscientiously follow established work procedures.

      B. Be attentive to details and technical issues and various relationships when completing tasks.

      C. Identify any discrepancies and irregularities and address these with your preceptor where appropriate.

      D. Keep accurate records and document actions.

      E. Take steps to ensure accuracy of work.

      F. Keep people informed and follow up on actions.

  9. Demonstrate effective time management by organizing and planning.

      A. Use own and others' time effectively and efficiently.

      B. Display a systematic and methodical approach when completing any activity.

      C. Establish meaningful goals and strategies for achieving these goals.

      D. Anticipate future needs.

10. Display independence and assertiveness in completing daily activities.

      A. Exhibit self-direction in undertaking responsibilities.

      B. Articulate your own viewpoint when dealing with others and in addressing controversial issues.

      C. Speak out against questionable tactics and practices.

      D. Act on self-identified strengths and weaknesses; develop a learning plan.

      E. Pursue further knowledge independently.

      F. Conduct self-assessment.

11. Develop an understanding of pharmacy-based patient care programs, such as preventive, wellness, and disease state management programs.

      A. Spend time reviewing policies and procedures that describe program details.

      B. Observe the pharmacist when he or she sees a patient in one of these programs.

      C. Be an active participant in one of these programs, providing the service and documenting all activities.

D. Describe and understand the general principle of immunizations, including appropriate schedules, as well as immunizations required and recommended in specific populations.

E. Demonstrate proficiency in recommending natural products (i.e., vitamins, herbals, supplements, etc.).

F. Become familiar with counseling patients about natural products and when to refer patients to their doctors.

A P P E N D I X   G

CARE PLAN
FOR COMMUNITY
PHARMACY PATIENT

Patient Name: **Phone #:**

Drug-Related Problem #1:

    Subjective/Objective Data:

    Assessment:

    Plan/Interventions/Goals/Monitoring/Follow-up:

Drug-Related Problem #2:

    Subjective/Objective Data:

    Assessment:

    Plan/Interventions/Goals/Monitoring/Follow-up:

Drug Related Problem #3:

    Subjective/Objective Data:

    Assessment:

    Plan/Interventions/Goals/Monitoring/Follow-up:

Note: Include a copy of the Patient Medical History Form and any other pertinent documents.

DRUG INFORMATION QUESTION DOCUMENTATION FORM

Date/Time of Inquiry: _____ / _____   RPh/student: _____

A. Inquirer:

   Pharmacist: _____

   Physician: _____

   Nurse: _____

   Other (specify): _____

   Phone #: _____

B. Type of Inquiry:

   ❏ Dosage/Administration   ❏ Pharmacokinetics

   ❏ Therapeutics   ❏ Pharmacology/Pharmaceutics

   ❏ Adverse Effects   ❏ Breast-Feeding/Teratogenicity

   ❏ Availability   ❏ Allergy

   ❏ Drug–Drug Interaction   ❏ General Information

   ❏ Compatibility/Stability   ❏ Drug ID/Pricing

   ❏ Other: Specify

C. Inquiry: If patient specific, obtain data such as age, gender, weight, medications, medical conditions, etc.

D. Response: (attach copy)

E. References Utilized:

F. Time required to answer question: _____

CASE PRESENTATION FORMAT

I. Introduction: statement of objectives

II. Discussion of patient: their medical and medication history, laboratory data, other pertinent data, and their drug-related problem list

III. Drug Information: Review of medications pertinent to the DRPs, including other possible medications available for treatment (prescription and OTC). Topics should include: pharmacology, pharmacokinetics, interactions, adverse effects, therapeutics, patient information and education, and economics

IV. Review of plan, outcomes assessment, and follow-up

V. Questions

RECOMMENDED RESOURCES FOR COMMUNITY PHARMACY PRACTICE

JOURNALS AND PROFESSIONAL MAGAZINES

Alternative Medicine Review
American Druggist
American Journal of HealthSystem Pharmacists
American Journal of Natural Medicine
Annals of Pharmacotherapy
Chain Drug Review
Computer Talk
Drug Store News
Drug Topics
Hospital Pharmacy
International Journal of Compounding
Journal of Alternative and Complementary Medicine
Journal of the American Medical Association
Journal of the American Pharmaceutical Association
Journal of Women's Health
Natural Pharmacy
Pharmacotherapy
Pharmacy Times
Retail Pharmacy News
US Pharmacist

SUBSCRIPTIONS/NEWSLETTERS

Drug Interactions Facts
Facts and Comparisons
The Green Sheet
Harvard Women's Health Watch
Medical Letter
Patient Drug Facts
Pharmacist Letter

Pharmacy Today
The Review of Natural Products
University of California Berkeley Wellness Letter

TEXTBOOKS

AHFS-Drug Information
Applied Pharmacokinetics
Drugs in Pregnancy and Lactation
German Commission E Monographs
Goodman and Gilman: The Pharmacological Basis of Therapeutics
Handbook of Clinical Drug Data
Handbook of Laboratory Data
Handbook of Nonprescription Drugs, 12th edition
Harriet Lane Handbook
Harrison's Principles of Internal Medicine
LexiComp Clinical Reference Library Handbooks
Martindale's
The Natural Pharmacy ("Lawrence Review" by Facts and Comparisons)
Nutritional Herbology
Poisoning and Toxicology Compendium
Prescription for Nutritional Healing
USP-DI vol II: Advice for the Patient

COMPUTERIZED INFORMATION

Drug Interactions Facts
Facts and Comparisons
LexiComp Clinical Reference Library (Online, For PDAs, handbooks, and CD-ROM)
USP-DI Plus for the Health Care Professional
Internet access for MEDLINE searches and other information

WEB SITES OF INTEREST FOR COMMUNITY PHARMACY PRACTICE

www.fda.gov/cder/drug/shortages/default.htm
    FDA site for information on drug shortages
http://www.fda.gov/cder/ob/
    Information from the FDA *Orange Book* regarding drug bioequivalence
    Approved Drug Products with Therapeutic Equivalence Evaluations
http://www.fda.gov/medwatch
    FDA *Medwatch* documentation via the Internet
http://www.needymeds.com/
    Program for information on indigent programs for prescription medications

http://www.usp.org/
   United States Pharmacopoeial Convention, Inc.
http://www.pharmacytimes.com/links.html
   Site established by *Pharmacy Times* with links to many other pharmacy organizations, associations, manufacturers, other agencies
http://www.ncpanet.org/
   National Community Pharmacists Association home page
http://www.ccspublishing.com/index.htm
   Library of the National Medical Society, journals, Medical Books, and Online Medical Diagnosis
http://www-sci.lib.uci.edu/~martindale/Pharmacy.html
   Martindale's Health Science Guide, Pharmacy Center
http://pharmacotherapy.medscape.com
   Medscape, site for medical information
http://altmed.od.nih.gov/
   Government's site for information on natural products/alternative remedies
http://igm.nlm.nih.gov/index.html
   Web site for MEDLINE searching; Internet Grateful Med
http://www.nih.gov/health/
   NIH site for health and medical information
http://www.intellihealth.com/
   Web site for medical information, health news
http://www.fda.gov/
   FDA home page
http://www.fda.gov/cder/drug/default.htm
   FDA Center for Drug Evaluation and Research home page
http://clinic.isu.edu/amcare/billing.html
   Site sponsored by ACCP that has a list of responses to question regarding payment for pharmacy services in ambulatory care setting
http://www.docguide.com/dgc.nsf/ge/Unregistered.User.545434
   Doctor's Guide home page, another site that allows potential users to register for a free site for health and medical information
http://www.mayohealth.org/mayo/
   Mayo Clinic Health information portal
http://www.pharmacist.com
   American Pharmaceutical Association (APhA), site for professional resources

CHAPTER 12: CASE EXAMPLE

The following history is a practice case for you to use when working on the development of your own interviewing and writing techniques. The written case is organized in the style that is expected of medical practitioners, and much of the same information will be expected from you in your presentations and writing.

You go with the new medical student on your team to interview Mr. Smith, and this is the information you two get from the patient:

> I fell the other day and hit the back of my head and have been having trouble with my balance and vision ever since. I came to the hospital last Saturday after falling and hitting my head. I was squatting down to pick up a steel rod. When I went to stand-up, I fell backwards and hit the back of my head on the corner of a bench. It didn't bother me none; I just got a big goose egg. I got some double vision, although it ain't really nothing. My wife says I came in with bad speech after. I have a headache that just won't go away no matter what I do, and I am dizzy from it. I reckon these have been going on for at least a month, but I didn't want to worry Edna. I thought the headaches were just sinus. I took some of that ibuprofen for colds from the druggist. If I had to tell you how much these headaches hurt, they are probably about medium. Maybe a 5 or 6 out of 10. I haven't thrown up at all, so I guess it ain't the flu, but it sure has been mighty bad this last week. I am afraid to drive Edna to the store. Edna here says my temper is short, and that's not usual for me. I can put up with an awful lot of aggravation, after all I have been married to her for 25 years.

How will you write this in a medical chart? What kind of information is this, subjective or objective? How should it be organized? The medical student has dictated the chart note below, based on Mr. Smith's interview and other information obtained. Read the note; then, before reading her impression and plan, consider your own and write it down, check to see how well you do. Then move on to the ambulatory and hospital practice cases in Chapters 15 and 16.

MEDICAL STUDENT'S NOTE

Saturday, 10-6-01. 1400

Subjective

Chief Complaint (CC)

"I fell the other day and hit the back of my head, and have been having trouble with my balance and vision ever since."

History of Present Illness (HPI)

A 71-year-old right-handed male fell on Wednesday 10-3-01, while squatting down to pick-up a heavy steel rod used in his printing business. He describes grasping the steel rod in his hands from a squatting position, and, while attempting to stand up, fell backwards, hitting the back of his head on the corner of a metal workbench. He does not know if he lost consciousness. Per patient report, the skin on his head was not lacerated in the fall—"just a big goose egg." Patient complains of diplopia, slurred speech, headache, and ataxia, which have been problematic since the fall. On further questioning the patient admitted that, although he has not fallen previously, he has been having problems with his balance, occasional slurred speech, double vision, driving, and word finding for over a month. Patient reports that at approximately the same time these symptoms developed he began having headaches that were transient in nature. The headaches were mild and responsive to ibuprofen initially. However, they have become worse over the past 2 weeks and described as continuous and intense. Pain is nonresponsive to analgesics and is rated 5–6/10. Occasional nausea occurs, but patient denies vomiting. All symptoms have worsened over the last week according to patient. Significant other, reports an increase in irritability with a short temper that is unusual. Patient has not exercised in over a week because of ataxia.

Past Medical History (PMH)

Patient had a lower back injury 15 years ago that resolved with physical therapy, controlled hypertension (HTN); patient states he is slightly hard of hearing (HOH) but has no other significant medical problems and no prior history of headache or neurologic problems.

Family History

Father died at age 80 from a sudden myocardial infarction (MI); mother died at 85 from cancer, type unknown. Family history of cardiovascular disease, arthritis, cancer, and stroke in several of the patient's 10 siblings. Patient has two sons and one daughter, one son with HTN; otherwise children are alive and well, as are six grandchildren.

Psychosocial History (Psych/Soc Hx)

Married for 50 years. He, his wife, and son run a printing business. The patient smoked for several years in his 20s. ETOH = average of 1 drink a month. Physical activity: walking several miles 3–4 times a week. Diet: 3 meals a day–mostly freshly prepared with few preservatives.

Review of Symptoms (ROS)

Denies shortness of breath (SOB), difficulty swallowing, choking after swallowing liquids or solids, numbness or tingling, weakness, gastrointestinal (GI), genital, urinary (GU) difficulties, skin rashes, or sexual dysfunction.

Objective

Allergies

No known drug allergies (NKDA).

Medications

Hydrochlorothiazide 25 mg QD, ibuprofen 400 mg PRN for headaches, and a multivitamin QD.

Physical Exam

Vital Signs

BP: supine 132/76, P 80; sitting 132/74, P 82; standing 130/74, P 82. Height 74 inches, weight 178 lbs.

Constitutional

A 71-year-old right-handed, well nourished, well-developed male, neatly dressed with some aphasia noted.

Cardiovascular

Carotid arteries, $\varnothing$ bruits upon auscultation. $\varnothing$ jugular venous distention (JVD) or edema.

Musculoskeletal

Neck supple without lymphadenopathy or thyromegaly.

Mental Status

Alert to time, person, and place (A & O $\times$ 3).

Recent and Remote Memory

Can name the presidents back to Nixon and can also detail who the Broncos played last week and the score.

Abstraction

"The grass is always greener on the other side of the fence." Is able to explain the meaning.

Attention Span and Concentration Span

Intact as evidenced by serial 7s to 86.

Language

Some word-finding problems noted as well as some slurring of speech; could not find the name for the collar of a shirt or the cap for a pen.

Response Time

Somewhat slow to answer questions.

Cranial Nerves

CN #1 not tested, CN #2 pupils approximately 2 cm and sluggish to react to light, CN #3, 4, 6 coarse nystagmus on lateral gaze with hypometric saccades and bilateral internuclear ophthalmoplegia—the adducting eye will lag behind the abducting one (INOs), CN #5 & 7 intact as evidenced by intact facial sensation in the trigeminal area and symmetrical smile, CN #8 unable to hear finger rub bilaterally, CN #9 & 10 midline uvula and ability to swallow intact, some slurred speech (? damage to CN #10 or 12), CN #11 intact—head rotation complete, shoulder shrug unable to break, CN #12 slurred speech noted, tongue without fasciculations or deviations.

Funduscopic Exam

Diminishment of red reflex L>R, disc edges were blurred, slight papilledema bilaterally, no hemorrhages or exudate.

Sensory

Position (great toe) intact bilaterally. Vibratory diminished bilaterally R>L.

Pinprick patchy right lower extremity (RLE) up to knee level, intact on left lower extremity (LLE). Temperature 80% RLE 100% LLE. Romberg + with retropulsion.

Motor

Strength 5/5 all, Tone ∅ ⇑,   Bulk ∅ atrophy

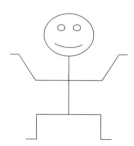

Abnormal Movements

Tremor: + right & left on extension   Unable to complete task R>L
Fasciculations ∅   Finger-to-Nose dysmetria noted R>L
Clonus ∅   Heel–Shin dysmetria noted bilaterally
Rapid Alternating Movements: □

Gait: Wide-based ataxic, catches right toe when walking.

Tandem unable to perform because of ataxia. Heel Walk retropulsion. Toe Walk unable to perform because of ataxia.

Reflexes: Grade 0–4 2/2 all muscle groups, upper and lower extremities.

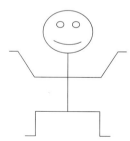

Jaw jerk 1, Snout −, Glabellar −, Babinski −

Assessment

Impression

Recent onset of headaches, ataxia, falls, slurred speech, diplopia, & anomia.

Rule Out (R/O)

Transient ischemic attacks (TIAs), stroke, tumor, syncope, medications, alcohol, intracranial bleed, skull fracture, and toxic exposure.

Plan (Include Laboratory Studies, Diagnostic Tests, Consults, Patient Education, etc)

CT Scan

Rationale

This will rule out a fracture and intracranial bleed or embolic event. It potentially will rule out a tumor if the tumor is large.

Patient Education

Tell the patient what test is being done and why. Patient hit his head, and this is reason enough to perform a scan. Explain how the test is done and how long it will take.

If the CT is negative:

Obtain an MRI with Contrast

Rationale

Tumors or lesions will enhance with an MRI scan.

Patient Education

Same as with CT scan.

Toxicology: Screen for Heavy Metals

Rationale

Patient has been in the printing industry for a number of years and has been exposed to lead and toxins in ink.

Patient Education

Explain the reason for the blood draw and what a positive result will mean.

Toxicology: Screen for Illegal Drugs

Rationale

Is there a rationale for doing this? Must you inform a patient who is alert and aware of what you are doing?

Complete Metabolic Panel

Rationale

To evaluate for hypokalemia and hyponatremia from diuretic use. Evaluate abnormal levels to see if there is a possible correlation with symptoms. BUN, creatinine, and liver function test results are important to evaluate because of patient age and possible encephalopathy, uremia, and liver failure.

Patient Education

Explain venipuncture to patient for this and following procedure. Inform the patient why the results may be useful.

Complete Blood Count (CBC)

Rationale

Investigate possible occult bleed.

Patient Education

Same as above for venipuncture and why test results may be useful.

Electrocardiogram (ECG)

Rationale

If ECG is abnormal, this could provide an explanation for the fall.

Patient Education

Explain patch placement, safety of test, and what abnormal outcomes may mean.

A P P E N D I X   L

MANAGED CARE SUGGESTED RESOURCES

RECOMMENDED READING

Baldor RA. Managed care made simple. Cambridge: Blackwell Science, 1996.
Ito S, Blackburn S, eds. A pharmacist's guide to principles and practices of managed care pharmacy. Alexandria, VA: Foundation for Managed Care Pharmacy, 1995.
Wertheimer AI, Navarro RP. Managed care pharmacy: principles and practice. New York: Pharmaceutical Products Press, 1999.

WEBSITES

Academy of Managed Care Pharmacy
www.amcp.org
American Pharmaceutical Association
www.apha.org
American Society of Health-System Pharmacists
www.ashp.org
Managed Care Digest (Aventis)
www.managedcaredigest.com

This Website accesses the nationally renowned Managed Care Digest Series. The material is presented to help develop strategies, control costs and assess value by providing real-world applications for information management coupled with the latest health economic data.

ON-LINE GLOSSARIES

Pam Pohly's Net Guide: Glossary of Terms in Managed Health
www.pohly.com/terms.html
DHHS Glossary of Managed Care Terms
http://aspe.os.dhhs.gov/Progsys/Forum/mcobib.htm
Managed Care Resources Inc. Managed Care Terms and Definitions
www2.mcres.com/MCR/mcrdef.htm
CareWorks Managed Care Dictionary
www.careworks.com/dict.htm

RESIDENCIES

If you wish to pursue a career in managed-care pharmacy, many postgraduate training (residency or fellowship) programs are available. These 1- or 2-year programs provide extensive experience in managed-care environments. The following is a partial list of organizations offering managed-care residencies.

- Advanced Paradigm Clinical Services
  Hunt Valley, MD
- Blue Cross Blue Shield of Alabama
  Birmingham, AL
- Blue Shield of California
  San Francisco, CA
- Blue Cross and Blue Shield of Kansas City and Pharmacia Corporation
  Kansas City, MO
- Express Scripts
  Bloomington, MN
- Harvard Vanguard Medical Associates
  Boston, MA
- Health Partners of the Midwest/St. Louis College of Pharmacy
  St. Lois, MO
- Henry Ford Health System
  Bingham Farms, MI
- Humana Inc.
  Louisville, KY
- Kaiser Permanente of Colorado
  Littleton, CO
- Kaiser Permanente of Georgia
  Duluth, GA
- Merck-Medco Managed Care, L.L.C.
  Franklin Lakes, NJ
- Prescription Solutions
  Costa Mesa, CA
- Rutgers State University/Horizon Blue Cross Blue Shield of New Jersey
  Newark, NJ
- Rx Care
  Nashville, TN
- University of Maryland College of Pharmacy
  Ellicott City, MD
- University of Oklahoma College of Pharmacy
  Oklahoma City, OK
- University of the Sciences in Philadelphia
  Philadelphia, PA
- Walgreens Health Initiatives
  Deerfield, IL

A P P E N D I X   M

HOSPITAL PATIENT-MONITORING FORM

Pt. Name:	ID#:	Rm#:

Ht:	Wt:	Age:	Race:	Gender:

Admit:	MD:	Allergies:

CC:

HPI:

PMH:	PSH:
FH:	SH:
Home Meds:	Problem List:

Hospital Meds:

Date	Dose/Route/Sig	D/C

ROS/PE:

GEN:
HEENT:
NECK:
CV:
LUNGS:
ABD:
GU:
EXT:
NEURO:

Vitals/Labs:

Date									
BP									
HR									
RR									
Temp									
Wt									
Ins/Outs									
Na									
K									
Cl									
CO_2									
BUN									
SCr									
Calc CrCl									
Glu									
$HgbA_{1c}$									
Ca									
Phos									
Mg									
T Prot									
Alb									
AST									
ALT									
Alk Phos									
LDH									
GGT									
Bili Tot									
Amylase									
Lipase									

WBC									
RBC									
Hgb									
Hct									
MCV									
MCH									
MCHC									
PLT									
Neut									
Lymph									
Mono									
Eos									
Baso									
Sed rate									
PT									
INR									
PTT									
Retic									
CK									
CKMB									
Trop									

UA, C&S, Drug levels, etc.

Progress Notes:

PERSISTENT VEGETATIVE STATE

A MultiSociety Task Force was set up in 1991 to achieve an authoritative consensus on the medical aspects of the diagnosis and prognosis of persistent vegetative state (PVS); it resulted in the publication of the most current and authoritative medical facts on PVS in the *New England Journal of Medicine* in 1994.[1]

Several societies, including the American Academy of Neurology (AAN) and the American Medical Association, have published their consensus statements on the ethical appropriateness of withdrawal of hydration and nutrition in these patients. In 1988, "A General Consensus Statement on Guidelines on the Vegetative State" by the AAN[2] was ultimately approved as the official policy of the AAN. Part I was a discussion of the basic medical facts of PVS, including the most prominent clinical features of the syndrome. It asserts that the diagnosis can be made with a high degree of medical certainty and that these patients are incapable of experiencing pain or suffering because of the loss of cerebral cortical functioning. The AAN believed it was important, as only a neurological organization can state with sufficient expertise and credibility that PVS patients cannot experience (consciously perceive) pain and suffering. Part II was the explanation of why artificial hydration and nutrition are forms of medical treatment and why the same factors that govern the withdrawal or withholding of other forms of medical treatment should also apply to artificial nutrition and hydration. These guidelines are consistent with the AMA positions on Witholding or Withdrawing Life-Prolonging Medical Treatment,[3] the President's Commission for the Study of Ethical Problems in Medicine and Biomedical and Behavioral Research,[4] and the report of the Hastings Center.[5] They stated that the artificial provision of nutrition and hydration is a form of medical treatment and may be discontinued in accordance with the principles and practices governing the withholding and withdrawal of other forms of medical treatment.. The Academy stated that it recognized that the decision to discontinue the artificial provision of fluid and nutrition may have special symbolic and emotional significance for the parties involved and for society. Nevertheless, the decision to discontinue this type of treatment should be made in the same manner as other medical decisions, i.e., based on a careful evaluation of the patient's diagnosis and prognosis, the prospective benefits and burdens of the treatment, and the stated preferences of the patient and the family. In caring for hopelessly ill and dying patients, physicians must often assess the level of medical treatment appropriate to the specific circumstances of each case. This includes (1) the recognition that a patient's right to self-determination is central to the medical, ethical, and legal principles relevant to medical treatment decisions. (2) In conjunction with respecting a patient's right to self-determination, a physician must also attempt to promote the patient's well-being, either by relieving suffering or addressing or reversing a pathologic process. Where medical treatment fails to promote a patient's well-being, there is no longer an ethical obligation to provide it. (3) Treatments that provide no benefit to the patient or the family may be discontinued. Medical treatment that offers some hope for recovery should be distinguished from treatment that merely prolongs or suspends the dying process without providing any possible cure. Medical treatment, including the medical provision of artificial nutrition and hydration, provides no benefit to patients in a PVS, once the diagnosis has been established with a high degree of medical certainty.

Part III of the AAN Consensus Statement[1] was the ethical position that supports the fundamental right of patients to make their own decisions concerning treatment and attempts to reconcile the potential conflicts between the wishes and rights of patients and their families and the views and responsibilities of those healthcare providers who feel that withholding artificial hydration and nutrition may be contrary to their own ethical integrity and professionalism. The statement strongly encourages the use of institutional ethics committees as one means of resolving possible conflicts in order to obviate need for court action.

Part IV was the explanation that there are no significant medical or moral distinctions between withholding and withdrawing treatment. The reluctance to withdraw life-sustaining treatment once started has been a major issue for neurologists caring for individual patients and for the courts. The statement takes a strong position: that any important medical/ethical distinction between the withholding and withdrawing treatment belies common sense and is inconsistent with good medical practice. Given the importance of an adequate trial period of observation and therapy for unconscious patients, a family member must retain the ability to withdraw consent for continued artificial feedings well after initial consent has been provided. Otherwise, consent will have been sought for a permanent course of treatment before the hopelessness of the patient's condition had been determined by the attending physician and become fully appreciated by the family.

Further management guidelines were published by the American Academy of Neurology in 1995. This included the statement that physicians and family must determine appropriate levels of treatment relative to the administration or withdrawal of medications and other commonly ordered treatments, supplemental oxygen and use of antibiotics, complex organ-sustaining treatments such as dialysis, administration of blood products, and artificial hydration and nutrition. Once PVS is considered to be permanent, a DNR order is appropriate. A DNR order includes no ventilatory or cardiopulmonary resuscitation. The decision to implement a DNR order, however, may be made earlier in the course of the patient's illness if there is an advance directive or agreement by the appropriate surrogate of the patient and the physician (or physicians) responsible for the care of the patient.

Further management guidelines were published by the American Neurological Association Committee on Ethical Affairs Persistent Vegetative State in 1993. They stated that PVS patients are nonautonomous because they lack the capacity for decision making. Thus, it is incumbent on physicians and family to make some very difficult decisions for the patient. These decisions include (in order):

1. Most importantly, what the patient's preferences were
2. Therapeutic effectiveness—should medical management utilize therapies that at best maintain the status quo
3. Quality of life ("personhood"): Is this a life worth living
4. Economics—what resources should be spent on a PVS patient considering the health needs of others

Guidance in making some of those decisions may come from several sources, including:

1. Advanced Directives—written documents, signed by the patients, indicating their wishes regarding life support or designating who can make treatment choices if they cannot. These documents may or may not deal specifically with PVS. They can be in the form of:
   A. Living Will—written legal document, singed by the patient, indicating his or her wishes re: life support
   B. Durable Power of Attorney for Health Care, or health care proxy—person appointed to act and decide for the patient in issues limited to health care
   C. Durable Power of Attorney—formally granting another person authority to act and decide for the patient
2. Health Care Surrogate—some jurisdictions have provisions for appointing a health care surrogate. When the patient has not provided an advance directive, the healthcare provider, usually the attending physician, will seek a "health care surrogate" who will decide on behalf of the patient. The health-care provider should seek a surrogate who is the highest priority person according to the following list:
   • The patient's guardian
   • Spouse
   • Adult son or daughter of patient
   • Either parent of the patient
   • Adult brother or sister of patient
   • Adult grandchild of patient
   • Close friend of patient
   • Guardian of patient's estate

3. Who decides?
  A. The patient, via advance directives. An advance directive is an expression of the patient's wishes. It may also be coupled with the naming of a health care proxy or issuing of a durable power of attorney for health care. Providing directives and naming an agent are conceptually distinct actions.
  B. The family. Some advance directives clearly designate a family member or another person as the decision maker.
  C. The physician. In some instances families turn to the physician as the decision maker because they genuinely believe that the physician will make the best care decision after weighing all the medical facts. Ultimately, the physician may be asked to make the decision for discontinuation of nutrition and hydration.
  D. The state. The applicable law of the jurisdiction relating to all the issues will influence any course of action.
  E. The hospital. It has happened that the view of physicians and families differ from those of hospital administrators (although this is less and less common). Disputes over differing views require judicial resolution.
  F. Religion. Religious opinions may impact on decision making concerning PVS.

The conclusions of the ANA were that physicians are often called on to assist in difficult ethical and moral decisions for their patients at a time when scientific knowledge to validate these decisions is incomplete. We cannot make early, precise, and unerring outcome predictions about an individual PVS in all instances, but we can make accurate ones most of the time. They urged physicians to urge their patients to consider their own values and to clarify, as much as possible, their preferred viewpoints in advance directives.

REFERENCES

1. MultiSociety Task Force on PVS. Medical aspects of the persistent vegetative state, parts I and II. N Engl J Med 1994;330:1499–1508,1572–1579.
2. American Academy of Neurology. A general consensus statement on guidelines on the vegetative state.
3. AMA Council on Ethical and Judicial Affairs. Witholding or withdrawing life-prolonging medical treatment. Chicago: AMA, 1986.
4. President's Commission for the Study of Ethical Problems in Medicine and Biomedical and Behavioral Research. Deciding to forego life-sustaining treatment. Washington, DC: US Government Printing Office, 1983.
5. The Hastings Center. Guidelines for the termination of life-sustaining treatment and the care of the dying. Garrison, NY: Hastings Center, 1987.

INDEX

Page numbers followed by *f* indicate figures; page numbers followed by *t* indicate tables.

ss or s̄s̄ (abbreviation), definition of, 164*t*
S₁, 241
S₂, 241
S₃, 241
S₄, 241
Saline, normal, 171, 173
Sample selection, in research study,
        internal validity and, 195*t*
Sample size, in research study, literature
        evaluation and, 188*t*, 190*t*
Schedule I drugs, 68
Schedule II drugs, 68
    filling prescriptions for
        partial filling and, 77–78
        presentation to pharmacy and, 72–74
Schedule III drugs, 68
    filling prescriptions for
        presentation to pharmacy and, 72
        refills and, 77
Schedule IV drugs, 68
    filling prescriptions for
        presentation to pharmacy and, 72
        refills and, 77
Schedule V drugs, 68
    filling prescriptions for
        presentation to pharmacy and, 72
        refills and, 77
Schisto~, as prefix/root word, 141*t*
Sclero~, as prefix/root word, 141*t*
Scoli~, as prefix/root word, 141*t*
Scope of practice, legal requirements for
        filling prescription and, 72
Screening, definition of, 157
Scruples, in apothecary system, 165, 165*t*
Search strategy, for drug information
        requests, 182–183, 184–185*t*
Secondary literature, responding to drug
        information requests and,
        182–183, 186, 187*t*
Sedimentation rate (ESR), 122
Segs (neutrophils), 86–87
Selection bias, resource allocation and,
        18–19, 25–26
Self-examination
    breast, 244
    testicular, 245–246
Self-insured, definition of, 157
Semi~, as prefix/root word, 135*t*
Sender, in communication model, 38

Sept~, as prefix/root word, 137*t*
Serum concentrations, for drug therapy
        monitoring, 259–260, 260*t*
Serum glutamic oxaloacetic transaminase
        (SGOT). *See* Aspartate
        aminotransferase
Serum glutamic pyruvic transaminase
        (SGPT). *See* Alanine amino-
        transferase
Serum osmolality, 101
Service-learning rotation, goals of, 10, 11*t*
Setup area (prescription), in community
        pharmacy, 354
Sex~, as prefix/root word, 137*t*
Sexual history, 246
SGOT (serum glutamic oxaloacetic
        transaminase). *See* Aspartate
        aminotransferase
SGPT (serum glutamic pyruvic
        transaminase). *See* Alanine
        aminotransferase
Shannon-Weaver model of
        communication, 37–38
Sharps, handling/disposing of, 235
"Shift to the left," 87
Siegler method of "four boxes," for
        ethical decision making, 21–23,
        22*f*
Significance, of research study, literature
        evaluation and, 189*t*, 195*t*
Significant figures, 162–163
Single-blinding, in research study,
        literature evaluation and, 188*t*,
        191*t*
Sinistro~, as prefix/root word, 138*f*
Skilled nursing facility (SNF), definition
        of, 157
Skin, assessment of, 237
SMCR model of communication, 38
Snellen test, 238, 238*f*
SNF. *See* Skilled nursing facility
SOAP notes, 322–323
    ambulatory care example of, 410–412
Social bias, resource allocation and, 26
Social history
    drug therapy monitoring and, 257–258,
        258*t*, 446
    patient education in ambulatory care
        and, 407